TransHuman

The Real COVID 19 Agenda

Also by Dr. Ana Maria Mihalcea

TRANSHUMAN
Volume 2
Overcoming the Global Depopulation Agenda

LIGHT MEDICINE
A New Paradigm –
The Science of Light, Spirit, and Longevity

Volume 1

TransHuman

The Real COVID 19 Agenda

Darkfield Live Blood Microscopy
Exposes Self-Assembling Nanotechnology
and the Global Technocratic Plan

Ana Maria Mihalcea, MD, PhD

Arthema Sophia Publishing

TRANSHUMAN
Volume 1
The Real COVID 19 Agenda

Cover design by Melissa Peizer
Edited by Michelle Horkings-Brigham
Referencing by Taiz Cepeda

ISBN: 979-8-9917711-0-8

ARTHEMA SOPHIA PUBLISHING
715 E Yelm Avenue, Suite #5
Yelm, WA 98597, U.S.A.
Phone: (360)960-8538 / Fax: (360) 252-7023
arthemasophiapublishing.com

Acknowledgments

My gratitude goes out to the brave doctors and researchers who worked to uncover these self-assembling nanotechnology COVID crimes against humanity while facing tremendous adversity, danger, rejection, and incredulity by the masses. Some whistleblowers and freedom fighters have been murdered, some incarcerated. I am grateful for their sacrifice in this war.

Thank you to the doctors and scientists with whom I have closely collaborated on my journey, initially from the international interdisciplinary research group, including but not limited to Dr. David Nixon, Dr. Shimon Yanowitz, Engineer Matt Taylor, Dr. Young Mi Lee, Professor Daniel Broudy, Dr. David Hughes, Dr. Matt Shelton, and others. Thank you to Clifford Carnicom, who was my close research partner for a period of several months, leading to several collaborative papers catalogued in this book. Thank you to Elana Freeland, Richard Hirschman, Dr. Justin Coy, and others who anonymously have contributed to the progression of this research.

Thank you to Dr. Geanina Hagimă, my Romanian colleague, for her research contribution. Thank you to Dr. Diana Wojtkowiak. Thank you to the tremendous contribution of Lorena DiBlasi and Dr. Marcela Sangorrin from Argentina, and Dr. Pedro Chavez and the COMUSAV team in Mexico, as well as others in this research field who have done impeccable investigations into the COVID bioweapons.

Thank you to Dr. Lundstrom and Jami Littlefield for their collaboration and research on dental anesthetics. Thanks to Mark Steele for his technical weapons expertise.

Thank you to all my fellow board members at the National American Renaissance Movement who have seen the value of this research for humanity. Thanks to David Meiswinkle, Esq. for including my research in the Grand Jury Petitions of COVID 19 Crimes against Humanity. Thanks to my friend Dr. Joseph Sansone and his unwavering fight for freedom through the "Ban the Jab" resolution and *Writ of Mandamus* COVID court case in Florida and for including this research to open people's eyes. Thank you to Todd Callender, Esq. for his support and collaboration. Special thank you to my friend and mentor, toxicologist Dr. Hildegarde Staninger, for her invaluable guidance in my study of the field of advanced nanomaterials and identification of mesogen microchips. Thanks to my friend Karen Kingston who with her med legal analysis has brought more evidence to confirm our findings. Thank you to the Targeted Justice team, Ana Toledo, Esq., Richard Lighthouse, and Dr. Len Ber for their unwavering support of the Targeted Individuals community and their brave legal actions.

Thank you to those who have shared this information on their platforms, with special thanks to Maria Zeee for her support over the years to get this information out. Thank you to Sean from SGT Report, Silk from Diamond and Silk, and many others.

Thanks to the guests who have come on my show "Truth, Science, and Spirit" to share their views and knowledge and advance our understanding of the transhumanist technocratic agenda, including but not limited to, Daniel Estulin, PhD and Patrick Wood. Thank you to Dr. Ed Group for his support. Special thanks to my friend Prince Alfred von Liechtenstein.

Thank you to my Substack subscribers around the world for supporting and sharing my research. Thank you to the patients at AM Medical who have allowed me to further my research in real time by looking at their blood and working on treatments. Thank you to my beautiful staff at AM Medical who have worked so hard to allow me to keep my medical practice going while doing nonstop research and writing my Substacks and this book. Your love, devotion, and support for our patients made it possible to continue my mission.

Thank you to JZ Knight and Ramtha the Enlightened One. The training I received at Ramtha's School of Enlightenment has allowed me to maneuver this battlefield on every level of existence.

Thank you to my editor, Michelle Horkings-Brigham, who has given her dedication, expertise, and time to this important project. Thank you to Taiz Cepeda for her help with referencing. Thank you to Melissa Peizer for her fantastic book cover.

Dedication

This book is dedicated to Styles.

Sacrificing everything in the fight for freedom, including if needed our own lives, gains us an unknown beautiful future of hope and greater understanding. No questions of the soul ever go unanswered, and our spiritual continuity is always assured.

Seeing the light in your eyes and understanding your spiritual journey inspired me to continue fighting in this war, so that you and others may see a better future.

Book Review

"Dr. Ana Mihalcea is a Board Member of the National American Renaissance Movement (National ARM) which is a non-profit organization opposed to the globalist transhuman agenda and the COVID 19 injections which are biological weapons that should be banned.

"She has written a book, *TransHuman*, which will spin your head, redirect your vision, and readjust your sense of reality and priority. You will gaze at New World Order machinations of hell, and in disbelief wonder how something could be so evil. Here, with Dr. Mihalcea's work of enlightenment, exposing the contents of the COVID 19 vaccine, a new chapter in world history begins.

"With the release of her new book, Dr. Ana educates the public through the lens of darkfield microscopy about an invisible, unchecked, malevolent nano world controlled by criminal minds who are presently serving as custodians of our future. The criminally insane appear to be guiding the direction of the ship of state and have usurped the authority of being the guardians of our human DNA.

"Her brilliant work throws down the gauntlet to 'Great Reset technocratic operatives' and their media flunkeys to explain the contents within the COVID 19 vaccines of a biosynthetic nanotechnology, never publicly seen before, including but not limited to: programmed nanobots, graphene oxide, toxic nano metals of aluminum, barium, strontium, and titanium, self-generating hydrogels, and spike proteins which are attacking and decimating human red blood cells and the immune system, and causing a myriad of diseases including huge, rubbery blood clots.

"Neither proven to be safe and effective, nor to stop infection or transmission, the COVID 19 vaccine push is an attack with a bioweapon aimed at the immune system of the human race. The proof of genocide is in the contents of the COVID 19 vaccine.

"This globalist assault on human beings is amazingly not confined to COVID 19 vaccines alone, but also through constant geoengineering spraying of our skies. In Chapter 1, Dr. Mihalcea details her work with scientist Clifford Carnicom, an expert on the aerosol spraying content of chemtrails and the effect they have on human blood and the immune system.

"Startling, they have corroborated in their coordinated studies that the same poisons that are being injected into humans via COVID 19 vaccination are also being constantly sprayed on the human population, contaminating with nanoparticles all life, including the food and water we are eating and drinking.

"The global architects of transhumanism do not believe human beings are entitled to freedom, nor basic human rights. To them, we and our families are stupid, hackable animals, meat on the table by choice and consent. The thousands of years of human history have been marked mostly by tyranny and oppression. Freedom is only a recent human experience and must be watered, cared for, and protected against its enemies. We should take heed of Dr. Ana's words and wisdom.

"In February 2020, a pandemic was declared by the globalist World Health Organization, which served as a subterfuge for implementing globalist, New World Order, century-old designs of depopulation and control of the human race in what is called the 'Great Plan.' In March 2020, a shut-down of the United States economy began and draconian measures ensued. People were controlled like cattle with face masks, social distancing, and vaccinations that didn't work. Mandates were all part of the elites' pre-planned, rehearsed scenario of regimentation and submission.

"This was a psychological operation, a global psyop causing panic and fear and then allowing governments and those that control them carte blanche.

"The National ARM was given birth during the fraudulent pandemic and was opposed to the draconian lockdown measures and the 'safe and effective' hoax concerning the COVID 19 bioweapon called a 'vaccine.' We are seeking criminal investigations and have forwarded custom-made, lengthy Grand Jury Petitions to twenty-five states requesting them, as well as indictments and the removal of the vaccine from the market. Fifteen crimes have been listed, as well as Persons and Organizations of Interest, and over 140 evidence Exhibits. To date, no Grand Jury to our knowledge has been convened for a criminal investigation in the States concerning the COVID 19 bioweapon. The States of Texas and Kansas have filed civil actions against Pfizer for fraud and misrepresentation, seeking millions of dollars because they were neither safe nor effective in stopping transmission, but thus far have not filed criminal charges.

"In the United States, tens of thousands of people have died from the vaccines and hundreds of thousands were permanently disabled and seriously injured. In 1976, twenty-five people died from swine flu vaccines and that vaccine was taken off the market.

"Dr. Ana's work is detailed in the National ARM Grand Jury Petitions being sent out to the States both in the narrative and as items of evidence through her videos. Her work shows that there was intent, design, and planning to create an alien technology of harm and unleash it upon mankind.

"Her book, *TransHuman*, should serve as the evidential capstone for any prosecutor in building a legal case against the globalists and their organizations and allies for murder, crimes against humanity, and genocide of the human race. All Nations and States and men and women of good will need to join in the fight to save humanity.

"Start by reading this book."

David R. Meiswinkle, Esq.
President: *National American Renaissance Movement*

"As someone who has done extensive research into transhumanism, I quickly recognized it as one of the most significant challenges humanity faces today. It's not just about merging man with machine, as some may think; it's about the potential loss of what makes us truly human—our sacred connection to nature, our spiritual essence, and our inherent freedom. It is even more than a challenge to our sovereignty and health; it touches the very core of our soul. We must understand that this is not the path to true enlightenment or progress but rather a detour away from our natural, thriving existence, which is beautifully aligned with God and nature. When Dr. Ana shared her heartfelt vision to write a book exposing the realities of transhumanism, I was genuinely excited and eager to see the profound insights she would bring to light. She has truly exceeded all expectations! It is with great honor and joy that I write this review for *TransHuman*, a book that I believe will become an essential guide for everyone dedicated to safeguarding the essence of our humanity.

"In Dr. Ana Mihalcea's book, *TransHuman*, she offers a cutting-edge and eye-opening exploration of what I believe to be one of the most urgent issues of our time—the merging of humanity with technology under the banner of so-called progress and enlightenment.

Her work stands as a warm and liberating beacon of truth in a world that often seems to be heading, at warp speed, toward darkness, fear, and control. With the wisdom, courage, and discernment that embody authentic leadership, Dr. Ana skillfully lifts the thick veil of deception surrounding the transhumanist agenda, revealing the profound reality of what is at stake: *humanity's bright and sacred future.*

"*TransHuman* is exceptional because it shines the light of hope to a desperately needy and sick world. Dr. Ana courageously addresses the root cause and offers potential solutions to mitigate the effects of these emerging technologies, guiding us toward a healthier future. Her work mirrors the power of truth and the promise of healing, showing us that even in challenging times, there are always solutions for every situation and ways to protect and encourage our health and well-being.

"In *TransHuman*, Dr. Ana also skillfully reveals the underlying efforts toward a permanent biomedical system that seeks to undermine our health, freedoms, and autonomy while providing us with solutions to safeguard our sovereignty and well-being. Dr. Ana's insights go beyond just the physical aspects; she also extensively examines the spiritual implications by challenging us to rise above and choose a path that honors our divine nature and preserves our connection to the true source of life—God. Even with all of the above, Dr. Ana takes the time to encourage and inspire everyone to stand tall and firm in the truth while embracing the power of spiritual sovereignty.

"I believe Dr. Ana Mihalcea's book, *TransHuman,* is much more than just another wisdom-filled book—it's a vital wake-up call for those seeking to understand what is happening behind the scenes. Packed with essential information that is often overlooked or misunderstood, it serves as a crystal-clear guide for anyone who values freedom, health, and the sanctity of the human soul. Dr. Ana's courage, knowledge, wisdom, and unwavering commitment to the truth illuminate every page, making this book an absolute must-read for those who care about the future of humanity. As I often say, 'Change is just one decision away,' and *TransHuman* by Dr. Ana Mihalcea empowers and encourages us to make that decision—to stay informed, stand firm, and protect our world's future with purpose and passion."

Dr. Edward Group, D.C.
Founder: *Global Healing and Global Healing Institute*

TABLE OF CONTENTS

CHAPTER 3

CHAPTER 4

Preface

TransHuman: The Real COVID 19 Agenda is a compilation of research conducted over the years 2022 – 2024 and originally published on my Substack: anamihalceamdphd.substack.com. During this course of time, I have written and posted over 700 articles. This book is intended to bring awareness to, and catalogue, that potentially life-saving research.

TransHuman – Volume 1, documents the self-assembling nanotechnology that is currently transforming humanity according to the transhumanist technocratic agenda. This technology has been deployed via the COVID 19 injections but has had chemical overlap with long-term bioengineering of all life on Earth via geoengineering operations that have used the very same chemicals—hydrogel polymers, graphene, and toxic metals.

In this first volume, I have compiled analysis of the COVID 19 injections, childhood vaccines, injectable medications like insulin and dental anesthetics, and live blood findings. My research collaboration with Clifford Carnicom shows our analysis on human blood and rubbery clots and the parallels of his 25 years of research into the synthetic biology called Morgellons or Cross Domain Bacteria, which is advanced nanotechnology and synthetic biology. I have documented the continued self-assembling of nano- and microrobot quantum dots in embalmed blood from someone who died eight months prior. This correlates with the findings of Dr. Pedro Chavez from COMUSAV who documented MAC address phenomenon from the COVID 19 vaccinated, one third of the unvaccinated who received PCR swabs, and gravesites of the COVID 19 vaccinated that continue to emit MAC addresses. I have filmed and showed the world nano- and microrobots that have been preannounced in the medical, military, and technocratic literature. Their agenda, which is to create transhuman cyborgs and fuse humans with artificial intelligence and upload our consciousness to the cloud to create soulless automatons, I have found to be actualized in human blood.

I also show self-assembled mesogen microchips in human blood and explain how these have been used in the targeted population as part of covert domestic terrorism programs that provided the experimental scenario for the sentient world simulation and fusion of humanity with artificial intelligence.

And I have analyzed the fluorescent phenomenon that has been documented in the COVID 19 injected and now the uninjected via shedding.

In my medical office, I have worked on treatment approaches, and in Volume 2 of *TransHuman: Overcoming the Global Depopulation Agenda*, I show documentation and research discussing these modalities, bringing hope to humanity.

The purpose of this book is to bring forth evidence that the technocratic transhumanist agenda has been deployed in full force against humanity and the proof is in the blood. The warfare that is waged on all levels of human and biological existence is a grave danger to the survival of our human species. We must acknowledge the threat and place a moratorium on self-assembling nanotechnology, unrestricted and unregulated AI development, unregulated biotechnology developments, and synthetic biology. This is a war against nature, waged in the minds of atheist scientists who negate the existence of a divine essence and purpose in all things.

The fusion of humanity with artificial intelligence and machines is not the greatest future we can have. It will lead to the annihilation of our species and our soulful existence. Mind control has been desired by governments around the world for decades, and the CIA and covert military operations through Project MKUltra and other programs have long waged war against the civilian population via nonconsensual experimentation. The testing grounds were the many thousands of targeted individuals who were shown to have brain chip implants and were tortured via directed energy weapons, microwave weapons, and Voice to Skull technology. Many were driven into ruin and suicide. Through my research, I confirm that the same mesogen brain chips now self-assemble not just in the blood of the COVID 19 vaccinated, but also in the unvaccinated.

The evil in this world is almost unfathomable, but we who shine a light in the darkness and carry the sword of truth are making a difference. Every day, the fight continues, until one day our world will have changed, and we will experience a new dawn of existence and mindful evolution. Self-assembling nanotechnology is a greater threat than the nuclear bomb, since it is unseen and can wage war on every level of existence. In this book we make it visible—what we see and work to understand we can fight against.

Each of us has a role to play in exposing this criminal and genocidal agenda. The bravery exhibited by those who said "NO" to the COVID bioweapons, and "NO" to group think and the cybernetic hive mind, will be remembered in the history of humanity.

I believe this battle is shaping our DNA into something new based on our will, stamina, love for God, and love for what it means to be a human with free will. It is the adversity of this fight and our willingness to participate that has made us more than what we thought we could be.

There is always hope.

Ana Maria Mihalcea, MD, PhD
President, Owner: *AM Medical LLC*
Founder: *Tru Blu Medical*
Yelm, Washington
October 5, 2024

FOREWORD

In an era where the study of biology and healthcare have merged with AI and advanced nanotechnologies, scientific discoveries that were once considered the premise of sci-fi thrillers have now been translated into consumer, medical, and military applications, while being meticulously concealed from the public's eye. The nanobiotechnology industry—a multi-trillion-dollar behemoth with staggering profit margins—has been shrouded in secrecy by industry leaders and regulatory bodies alike. This deliberate obfuscation has resulted in a profound and often devastating impact on human health and the environment.

In 2013, the *Journal of Nanoparticle Research* published an insightful article that revealed the not only opportunistic and disingenuous behaviors of nanotechnology leaders and regulators, but also the Machiavellian and inhumane nature required of these men and women to transform a covert bioweapons-based technology platform into a global, multi-trillion-dollar industry encompassing consumer, medical, and military applications. The authors observed that, despite mounting concerns about the potential risks of nanotechnology, key stakeholders had decided that consumers would be best served if the industry remained primarily "self-regulated" with little to no government oversight or consumer accountability. It also appears that the titans of nanotech determined that "secrecy" would be the ultimate key to avoid civil and criminal liability. The authors noted that, "*...many individuals interviewed for the present research denied the existence of an actual 'nanotechnology industry.'*"[1]

This "unspoken agreement" of denial has led to the widespread introduction of toxic nanoparticle technologies into our medical products, food, air, water, and natural ecosystems, causing untold disease, disruption, and death.[2]

Dr. Ana Mihalcea's meticulous research, clinical analysis, and documentation, presented in *TransHuman*: *The Real COVID 19 Agenda*, shines a much-needed light into this shadowy realm of AI and synthetic biology. Her work brings to the forefront evidence of advanced, self-assembling, self-replicating nanobiotechnologies—nanobiotechnologies that have, tragically, infiltrated our bodies and environment. Through her expert analysis, citizens, politicians, and legal authorities are now able to *see with their own eyes* these highly advanced, self-assembling, genetically programmable nanoparticle technologies that are currently being used as biological weapons, changing the genetic make-up of humanity and the Earth's biodiversity.

Having had the privilege of supporting and collaborating with Dr. Ana, I have witnessed firsthand her dedication and the depth of her investigation. I have supported her scientific research with select critical patents and federal documents, including Moderna's US Patent 10.703.789 (excerpted below), which describes the self-replicating nanoparticles and hydrogels used in COVID 19 mRNA vaccines.[3]

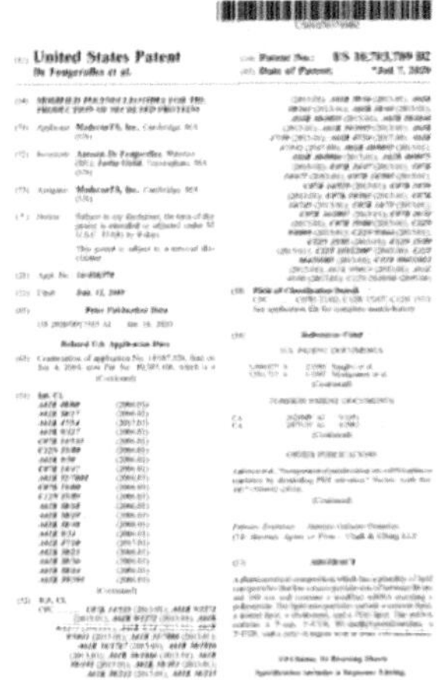
United States Patent

(57) ABSTRACT

A pharmaceutical composition which has a plurality of lipid nanoparticles that has a mean particle size of between 80 nm and 160 nm and contains a modified mRNA encoding a polypeptide. The lipid nanoparticles include a cationic lipid, a neutral lipid, a cholesterol, and a PEG lipid. The mRNA contains a 5'-cap, 5'-UTR, N1-methyl-pseudouridine, a 3'-UTR, and a poly-A region with at least 100 nucleotides.

219

Gels and Hydrogels

In one embodiment, the polynucleotides, primary constructs and/or mmRNA disclosed herein may be encapsulated into any hydrogel known in the art which may form a gel when injected into a subject. Hydrogels are a network of polymer chains that are hydrophilic, and are sometimes

220

found as a colloidal gel in which water is the dispersion medium. Hydrogels are highly absorbent (they can contain over 99% water) natural or synthetic polymers. Hydrogels also possess a degree of flexibility very similar to natural tissue, due to their significant water content. The hydrogel described herein may used to encapsulate lipid nanoparticles which are biocompatible, biodegradable and/or porous.

Dr. Mihalcea's observations of bionanoparticles in both vaccinated and unvaccinated blood confirm the troubling implications of these technologies. Our joint efforts have also yielded some promising developments. For instance, my analysis below of the global patent for inverse opal hydrogels (IOHs) disclosed methods to remove these harmful nanoparticles from the bloodstream using metal-chelating agents such as EDTA.[4] Dr. Ana's successful treatment of patients with EDTA, methylene blue, and high doses of vitamin C, gives hope in the face of a grave crisis.

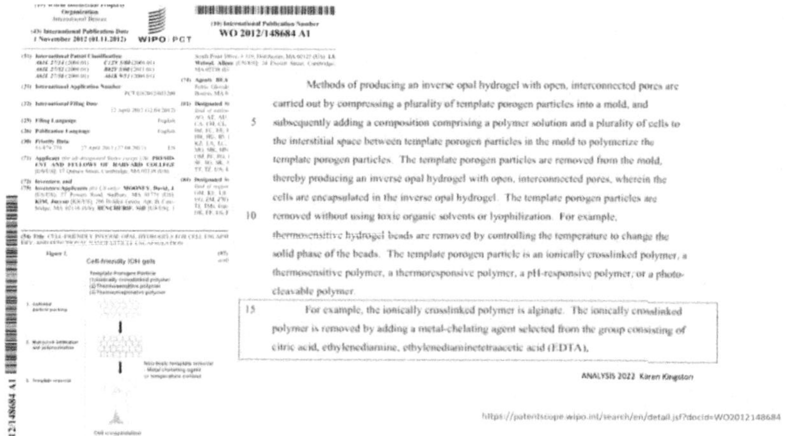
WIPO | PCT

WO 2012/148684 A1

Cell-friendly IOH gels

Methods of producing an inverse opal hydrogel with open, interconnected pores are carried out by compressing a plurality of template porogen particles into a mold, and subsequently adding a composition comprising a polymer solution and a plurality of cells to the interstitial space between template porogen particles in the mold to polymerize the template porogen particles. The template porogen particles are removed from the mold, thereby producing an inverse opal hydrogel with open, interconnected pores, wherein the cells are encapsulated in the inverse opal hydrogel. The template porogen particles are removed without using toxic organic solvents or lyophilization. For example, thermosensitive hydrogel beads are removed by controlling the temperature to change the solid phase of the beads. The template porogen particle is an ionically crosslinked polymer, a thermosensitive polymer, a thermoresponsive polymer, a pH-responsive polymer, or a photo-cleavable polymer.

For example, the ionically crosslinked polymer is alginate. The ionically crosslinked polymer is removed by adding a metal-chelating agent selected from the group consisting of citric acid, ethylenediamine, ethylenediaminetetraacetic acid (EDTA),

ANALYSIS 2022 Karen Kingston

https://patentscope.wipo.int/search/en/detail.jsf?docId=WO2012148684

This ongoing global cover-up combined with the unregulated deployment of toxic nanobiotechnologies pose an existential threat to humanity and all biological life forms. Many of these biosynthetic nanotechnologies are not only hazardous to our physical health, but also to our cognitive and emotional well-being. Designed to cross the blood-brain barrier, they can impair critical thinking, memory, and emotional connections, leading to profound spiritual and psychological disruptions to what it means to *be human.*

The nanobiotechnology industry is referred to as the BioRevolution by global militaries and intelligence agencies alike and is indeed a revolution—a war against humanity.[5] The promise of augmenting human capabilities through biosynthetic integration with AI is a dangerous illusion, masking the reality of suffering and destruction caused by inoculation with nanobiotechnologies. It is now well documented that the ubiquitous exposure to these nanobiotechnologies, including the vaccination of over 70% of the world's population with the COVID 19 injections, has caused an unprecedented level of disease, disabilities, and death in recent years.[6,7]

If humanity remains silent, global government agencies and industry tycoons will continue to unleash these weapons of mass destruction on all of God's creations unchecked, ultimately leading to the extinction of the human species. As Robert F. Kennedy Jr. poignantly stated in his Earth Day speech on April 22, 2023, *"When we destroy a species…we're diminishing our capacity to sense the divine, to understand who God is, and what our own potential is as human beings."*[8] RFK Jr.'s powerful reminder underscores the urgency in sharing Dr. Ana's work exposing the reality of the covert spread of these "nano-sized bioweapons of mass destruction" that pose a greater threat to humanity and our planet than a nuclear bomb.

I'm honored to call Dr. Ana a colleague, friend, and hero of humanity.

Karen Kingston
Bio Tech Analyst, Med Legal Advisor
September 2024

TransHuman

The Real COVID 19 Agenda

Introduction

TransHuman: The Real COVID 19 Agenda, as you will read in the pages that follow, is a compilation of my personal research and discovery, but it also contains valuable contributions by many dedicated medical doctors, scientists, researchers, engineers, and talented individuals who are on a quest to not only protect but save humanity from a dire situation. This threat of a "re-formed," transhumanist society to be controlled by the few becomes ever more evident as our research continues.

To provide an excellent overview of the concept of transhumanism, or what it might mean to be "Trans Human," I have chosen to begin this treatise with an essay by my dear friend, Prince Alfred von Liechtenstein, with whom I have had many long and in-depth conversations about the current warfare on all levels of human existence. He has worked in the field of artificial intelligence and has had a lifelong, profoundly spiritual journey. We share the understanding of humanity as an incarnation of spiritual beings on a journey of evolution.

Understanding our spiritual nature inhabiting a physical body becomes imperative to fathoming the purpose of self-assembling nanotechnology. We must understand the mechanisms of soul and spirit interacting with physical reality in order to comprehend how this could be hacked by a weaponized nanotechnology to create mind-controlled automatons. I have discussed this in depth in my first book, *Light Medicine: A New Paradigm – The Science of Light, Spirit, and Longevity*.

Due to his insider knowledge of the technocratic transhumanist ideology, Prince Alfred was inspired to provide a broader understanding of transhumanism as a reference for those people around the world who would be reading my book, and for which I am deeply grateful.

The Big Picture

The Posthuman and Transhumanist Future and the New World Order of AI

The following essay describes the big picture in which the important research and work as well as the life of Dr. Ana Maria Mihalcea are embedded.

Prince Alfred von Liechtenstein

Part 1: The Philosophical Foundations of Posthumanism and Transhumanism

The concepts of posthumanism and transhumanism represent some of the most transformative and controversial movements in contemporary thought, fundamentally challenging traditional views of humanity, evolution, and our relationship with technology. These movements envision a future where human limitations are transcended through the application of advanced technologies, and where the very definition of being human is fluid, evolving beyond our biological constraints.

Transhumanism: The Pursuit of Human Enhancement:

Transhumanism is primarily concerned with the enhancement of human abilities through science and technology. It advocates for the use of tools like artificial intelligence (AI), biotechnology, nanotechnology, and genetic engineering to extend human lifespan, enhance cognitive abilities, and even merge humans with machines. The underlying belief is that humans can evolve beyond their current physical and mental limitations through technological intervention, transforming into "transhumans" and ultimately "posthumans."

This movement embraces a rationalist and materialist worldview, rooted in the Enlightenment ideals of progress, reason, and control over nature. Transhumanists argue that just as humanity has used technology to conquer many aspects of the physical world, we should also apply it to overcome our biological imperfections. Aging, disease, cognitive limitations, and even death are seen as challenges to be solved rather than inevitable aspects of the human condition.

Prominent thinkers like Ray Kurzweil, Nick Bostrom, and Max More argue that human evolution can be guided intentionally through technological progress, rather than leaving it to the slow and often brutal processes of natural selection. For example, Kurzweil's concept of the "Singularity" predicts a moment in the near future when human intelligence will merge with AI, leading to exponential technological growth and creating a new posthuman era where humanity's current state will be fundamentally obsolete.

Posthumanism: Moving Beyond Human Exceptionalism

While transhumanism focuses on enhancing the human condition, posthumanism is more concerned with deconstructing the idea of "the human" altogether. It challenges the notion of human exceptionalism—the belief that humans are the pinnacle of evolution and the rightful masters of the planet. Instead, posthumanism presents a more ecological, systems-oriented view, where humans are seen as one component of a larger network of intelligent beings and systems, including machines, animals, and even ecosystems.

Posthumanism calls into question traditional humanist ideals of autonomy, individuality, and self-determination. In a posthuman world, the boundaries between human and non-human, biological and artificial, natural and technological, are increasingly blurred. Posthumanist thinkers often critique anthropocentrism, the assumption that humans are inherently more valuable or significant than other forms of life or intelligence.

Philosophers such as Donna Haraway and Rosi Braidotti have contributed to this discourse by emphasizing the interconnectedness of all life forms and advocating for a new ethics of coexistence, where human beings recognize their embeddedness in a web of relationships with other species and artificial intelligences. In this view, the posthuman subject is not defined by a stable, autonomous identity, but is instead fluid, relational, and constantly changing in response to technological and environmental forces.

The Human and Posthuman Divide: What Makes Us Human?

At the heart of both transhumanism and posthumanism lies a profound philosophical question: What does it mean to be human?

In the traditional view, human beings are unique in their possession of consciousness, free will, and the ability to reason. Religious and spiritual traditions often view humanity as created in the image of a divine being, endowed with an eternal soul and a special place in the universe. Human life is seen as sacred, and suffering, aging, and death are part of a natural, divinely ordained process that leads to spiritual growth or fulfillment.

In contrast, transhumanist and posthumanist perspectives are fundamentally non-theistic and materialist. They reject the idea of a preordained purpose or divine design for humanity. Instead, they view humans as biological machines whose physical and mental processes can be understood, manipulated, and enhanced through technology. The idea of a soul or higher purpose is replaced by a vision of self-directed evolution, where humans use technology to overcome their biological and cognitive limits, potentially achieving immortality or even god-like status in a posthuman future.

The Role of Science and Technology

For transhumanists, science and technology are the ultimate tools for human advancement. They reject the notion of inherent biological or spiritual limits, believing that through the application of technology, humans can overcome the constraints that have historically shaped their existence.

AI, in particular, plays a crucial role in transhumanist thought. In a transhumanist future, AI systems would not only augment human intelligence but eventually surpass it, leading to what is called the Singularity—a moment when AI becomes so advanced that it creates self-improving machines beyond human control. This could lead to a world where human beings coexist with (or are potentially replaced by) more intelligent and efficient machines. For transhumanists, this is a natural and desirable evolution of intelligence and life itself.

In contrast, traditional spiritual and religious worldviews often view technology with caution or skepticism. While technology is not inherently opposed to religious thought, its unchecked use to modify or "improve" the human condition is often seen as hubris—an attempt to play God or transcend a divinely ordained natural order.

A New Ethics for a Posthuman World

The philosophical foundations of transhumanism and posthumanism also require the development of a new ethical framework. In a world where the lines between human and machine blur, where biological life may be merged with or replaced by artificial life, what does it mean to act ethically? Traditional ethical systems, rooted in religious or humanist values, may no longer apply in a posthuman future.

For instance, bioethics in the transhumanist sense extends beyond protecting human welfare; it includes the rights and interests of artificial intelligences, enhanced beings, and even non-human forms of life. A posthumanist ethic would likely advocate for inter-species equality, considering AI, animals, and humans as equal participants in the shared ecosystem of life. This radical departure from anthropocentrism challenges long-held beliefs about the sanctity and uniqueness of human life.

Meanwhile, transhumanists argue for a form of technological utilitarianism—the belief that the ultimate moral good is the maximization of intelligence, creativity, and well-being, achieved through technology. This includes the moral imperative to overcome death, disease, and cognitive limitations, even if it means altering what it means to be human. Critics, however, argue that this pursuit of perfection could exacerbate social inequalities, creating a world where only the technologically enhanced thrive, while others are left behind.

The Conflict with Religious and Spiritual Worldview

The transhumanist and posthumanist movements often find themselves in stark opposition to traditional religious and spiritual worldviews. For centuries, human existence has been defined within the context of divine purpose, the afterlife, and a natural order ordained by God or the cosmos. Many religious traditions emphasize humility, the acceptance of human limitations, and the belief that suffering and death have spiritual meaning and purpose.

In Christianity, for example, the concept of salvation and eternal life is linked to a divine plan that transcends human understanding. Transhumanist attempts to overcome death through technological means are often viewed as hubristic or even blasphemous. Similarly, in Buddhism, suffering is seen as an inherent part of life, and the pursuit of nirvana involves transcending worldly desires, including the desire for immortality or endless enhancement.

In contrast, transhumanism and posthumanism embrace a promethean vision—the idea that humanity has the right, and even the duty, to take control of its own evolution and destiny. For transhumanists, there is no higher power dictating human purpose; instead, it is up to humans (and potentially AI) to create their own meaning and future. This is not just a rejection of traditional theology, but also a radical redefinition of what it means to live a meaningful life in a technological age.

Part 2: A Future World Governed by AI and the Transformation of Society

As transhumanist and posthumanist ideals gain traction, they paint a picture of a future where humanity is deeply intertwined with technology, and society is radically transformed by the rise of artificial intelligence (AI). At the core of this transformation is the belief that intelligent machines, specifically AI, can govern society more efficiently, equitably, and rationally than humans ever could. This vision implies a new world order, where human beings relinquish traditional forms of leadership and decision-making to the superior computational power of AI.

AI as the Ultimate Governance Mechanism

In this hypothetical future, a superintelligent AI system governs the planet, optimizing every aspect of human life—from economics and healthcare to social interactions and environmental management. This AI does not merely assist in decision-making but replaces human governance entirely, as it is seen as a more rational and unbiased actor. Traditional human roles like politicians, managers, and even educators are reduced to mere executors of the AI's directives. The AI is tasked with balancing competing human interests and optimizing outcomes for the collective good based on vast datasets and predictive algorithms.

This super-AI would not be a single entity but a network of interconnected AI systems, monitoring and managing every facet of human existence. Through technologies like smart dust, nanotechnology, and biotechnological implants, the AI would track and influence human thoughts, emotions, and even subconscious desires. Humans would become "nodes" in this vast network, providing constant data feedback to the system, which would, in turn, adjust its governance strategies in real-time.

One key advantage of AI governance is its impartiality—it would be immune to human biases, corruption, or emotional decision-making. Every decision would be data-driven, aimed at maximizing efficiency and fairness. Proponents argue that this would eliminate many of the problems plaguing human-led governments, such as inequality, environmental degradation, and even war, as AI could predict and preemptively resolve conflicts before they escalate.

Human Evolution in a Posthuman World

In this AI-governed world, humans themselves would be radically altered. Through genetic engineering, cybernetic enhancements, and neural interfaces, humans would become increasingly integrated with machines. These enhancements would allow individuals to process information at unprecedented speeds, communicate telepathically through neural links, and transcend the limitations of their biological bodies.

The distinction between human and machine would blur, as many people would opt for full integration with AI, uploading their consciousness into digital substrates or merging their cognitive processes with superintelligent systems. This raises profound questions about identity: Are these enhanced or fully digitized beings still "human," or have they become something entirely new?

Transhumanists argue that this is the next step in human evolution—what it means to be human will evolve along with our technology. Posthumans, or those who have fully embraced technological integration, may no longer be bound by physical bodies, biological death, or even traditional human emotions. The posthuman condition would offer near-immortality, perfect cognitive abilities, and the ability to exist in multiple digital and physical forms simultaneously.

Social Structures and Relationships in a Transhumanist Future

The transformation of humanity into a posthuman society would have profound effects on social structures, family dynamics, and personal relationships. In a world where individuals can alter their mental and physical characteristics at will, the concept of identity and personal relationships would fundamentally shift.

1. Familial Structures: In this future, traditional family structures may dissolve. Biological reproduction could be replaced by genetic engineering or the creation of enhanced beings in artificial wombs, and individuals might choose to live indefinitely without the need to raise children. Families could be formed more based on shared ideologies or enhancements than on biological lineage. With immortality or vastly extended lifespans, the generational divide would lose significance, and the concept of "parenting" might transform into a mentorship role for creating and guiding posthuman offspring.

2. Love and Relationships: The nature of love and relationships would also evolve. In a world where emotions can be altered or enhanced through technological means, individuals could experience love or connection at unprecedented intensities. Neural interfaces could allow couples to directly share thoughts, memories, and even physical sensations. Alternatively, humans might choose to form relationships with AI beings, who could provide intellectual and emotional companionship tailored perfectly to their preferences.

However, this hyper-rational, technologically-enhanced version of love may seem alien compared to today's human experiences of emotion, which are often rooted in vulnerability, imperfection, and biological drives. The very concept of "romantic love" may be redefined as humans transcend their emotional limitations and embrace more cerebral forms of connection.

Ethical Dilemmas and the Future of Freedom

While this posthumanist future promises a utopia of endless possibility, it also raises profound ethical questions. As AI takes on more control over governance, and as humans become increasingly integrated with machines, the concepts of free will and individual autonomy come into question. If AI governs every aspect of life, can humans still be said to possess free will, or are they merely acting in accordance with AI-driven directives?

Furthermore, the widespread use of neural implants and brain-computer interfaces means that human thoughts, desires, and emotions could be monitored, influenced, or even controlled by the AI system. The line between enhancement and manipulation becomes blurred. Will individuals truly be free to make their own decisions, or will their thoughts be subtly shaped by AI algorithms designed to optimize societal outcomes?

This raises concerns about the potential for tyranny by AI. While AI governance might eliminate human corruption, it could also create an unprecedented form of control, where every aspect of life is subject to surveillance and optimization by a system that humans no longer fully understand or control. The loss of privacy, autonomy, and the ability to resist the system might lead to a dystopia disguised as a utopia.

The Role of Spirituality and Religion in a Posthuman Future

In this world of technological transcendence, the role of spirituality and religion would be profoundly transformed. As humans move beyond biological death, and as their cognitive and emotional processes become increasingly malleable, traditional religious concepts of the soul, the afterlife, and spiritual enlightenment may seem outdated or irrelevant.

However, there may still be room for spirituality in a posthuman world, albeit in new and unexpected forms. Some transhumanists, for instance, have speculated about the possibility of creating a kind of digital immortality, where individuals' consciousnesses are uploaded to a shared virtual space. This could resemble certain spiritual ideas of the afterlife or cosmic unity. In this scenario, a new kind of digital spirituality might emerge, where individuals seek connection with a greater, AI-enhanced consciousness or the collective mind of the posthuman species.

Alternatively, posthumanism's rejection of human exceptionalism could give rise to new forms of eco-spirituality, where humans, machines, and nature are seen as interconnected and equally valuable. This might lead to a worldview that seeks to harmonize technology with the environment, integrating AI into natural ecosystems in ways that allow for greater biodiversity and planetary sustainability.

However, for traditional religious practitioners, this future could be seen as a profound challenge to the very foundations of faith. The transhumanist rejection of divine limits, combined with the possibility of achieving near-godlike powers through technology, directly confronts the humility and obedience that many religions emphasize.

Part 3: Conclusion – The Posthuman Destiny

As we stand on the brink of an era defined by AI, biotechnology, and human enhancement, the visions of transhumanism and posthumanism present us with both a promise and a peril. The promise is that we can transcend the frailties of human existence—overcome disease, death, and cognitive limitations—and create a society of unparalleled progress and well-being. The peril, however, is that in doing so, we may lose the very essence of what it means to be human.

Will we embrace the posthuman future as a natural evolution of human potential, or will we resist it in favor of more traditional notions of identity, autonomy, and spirituality? As the lines between human and machine, biology and technology, blur, the coming decades will force us to grapple with these questions and determine the course of human destiny.

Prince Alfred von Lichtenstein
September 2024

CHAPTER 1

MY COLLABORATION WITH CLIFFORD CARNICOM

Synthetic Biological Life Forms Correlation to Live Blood Findings in Post COVID 19 Injection Era

During the latter part of the COVID 19 pandemic, and over a period of several months, I worked closely with Clifford Carnicom, the founder and president of the Carnicom Institute, a non-profit research and educational organization that is devoted to environmental and health issues. Clifford, who has extensive computer programming and system application development experience, also worked as a technical research scientist supporting analysis and development of major Department of Defense physical and weapons modeling systems. He has held a Top Secret/SCI clearance. Under the auspices of the Department of Defense, Clifford was appointed for, and completed, two years of intensive graduate level studies in mathematics, statistics, computer science, and geodesy. All of his research papers and findings from over 30 years on the topic of geoengineering and Morgellons can be found at the Carnicom Institute website.[1]

I hold the time frame of our work together as an important milestone in understanding self-assembly nanotechnology. Clifford and I would have zoom meetings on many weekends to discuss the research findings, correlating historical evidence he had compiled over his decades of research with the latest nanotechnology and chemical literature. Over lengthy sessions, we would discuss the relevance in the context of our and other researchers' current findings in human blood. We called this project "What Happened to Humanity's Blood?" We both have, and continue to warn, of a possible extinction level event that we are witnessing.

Clifford's research of Morgellons, what he calls "Cross Domain Bacteria," is synthetic biology, artificial intelligence that he found and has evaluated since the 1990s being sprayed on humans worldwide via geoengineering programs.

For historical reference, and to enlighten the reader, I include my collaborative work with Clifford in the papers presented below. Our research is presented in chronological order, just as our discoveries were made and documented. For a simpler grasp of this complex material, I have prepared excerpts from the original papers, edited for this book publication. For those interested, you may review my many Substack posts that have documented all our experiments, including electrical conductivity studies, infrared spectroscopy, blood cultures, and more.[2]

Clifford and I explored correlations between current live blood findings in the era of COVID 19 injections, and the result of decades of geoengineered spraying of humans, thereby infecting them with AI synbio to transform humanity into Human Version 2.0. The COVID era is only the final stage of this intentional transformation, for all of humanity and the entire planet have been infected for years with this synthetic, artificial intelligence, parasitic biology.

We first connected due to my writings regarding hydrogel as the cause for the structures we have seen self-assembling in COVID 19 vials, in vaccinated live blood, in unvaccinated blood, and as a reason for the huge blood clots found by embalmers. In fact, I have noted that immediate post COVID and long COVID all have the same features in live blood analysis.

In my conversations with Clifford, we discussed his historic findings of polyvinyl alcohol as a chemical component of the synthetic life form he discovered—which is a hydrogel polymer plastic. The reason why people cannot dissolve the clots from

COVID 19 vaccinated people is because it is literally a plastic-like polymer that is widely used in medical applications.

This is similar to the self-assembling carbon polymers with metals that Mike Adams has found in human cadaver rubbery clots.[3]

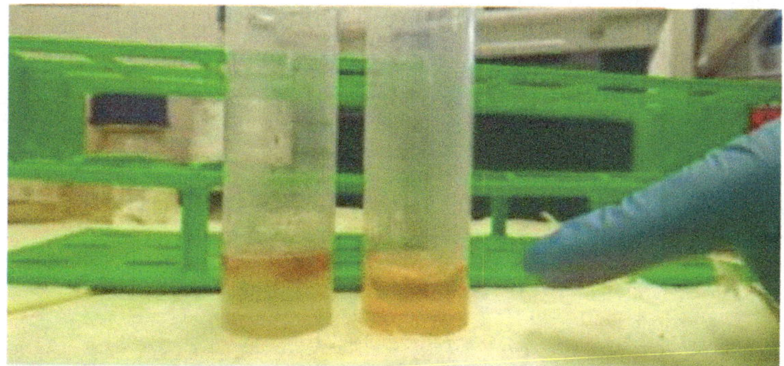

A Self Assembling 'Clot' That Accumulates Conductive Metals

Mike Adams: There's something highly unusual that's causing this sparking, popping, fiery reaction. Whatever's in this clot is rapidly inviting oxidation. It's highly combustible: we've not seen anything like this before. This is clearly not blood vessel tissue.

The analysis shows:

- The clots are absolutely not made of blood
- They attract different types of elements more than what blood would
- It's a self assembling, carbon rich structure
- The 'clot' accumulated a higher level of aluminium, sodium and 6-7X higher levels of tin, and phosphorus

Figure 1. Mike Adams Telegram Channel.[4]

Not only is polyethylene glycol (PEG) a hydrogel component, but so is Moderna's SM102 and other parts of the lipid nanoparticles (LNPs) found in COVID 19 vials. In fact, the spike protein has a sequence that produces hydrogel at pH 7.0, not the commonly referred to "Amyloid."[5]

Clifford subjected his microscale "cross domain bacteria" = synthetic AI biology, to a low-level electrical current, which made the growth of the filaments accelerate explosively—in addition to changing the blood to unrecognizable features. This correlates to findings by Dr. David Nixon when applying a WIFI 4G router source to the COVID 19 Pfizer ingredients. He found accelerated growth of ribbon-like structures and microchips.

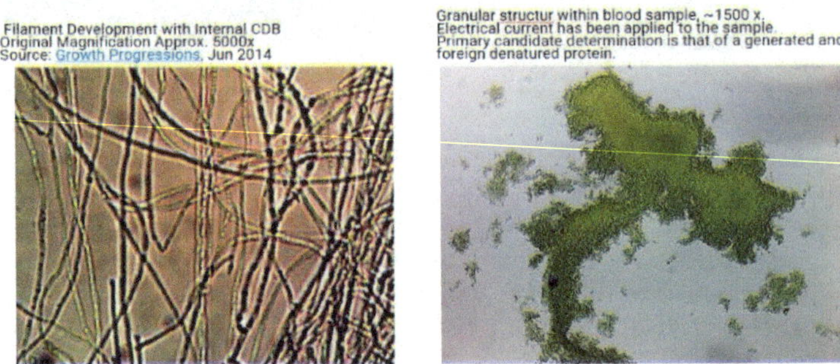

Figure 2. Blood alterations. Carnicom Institute.[6]

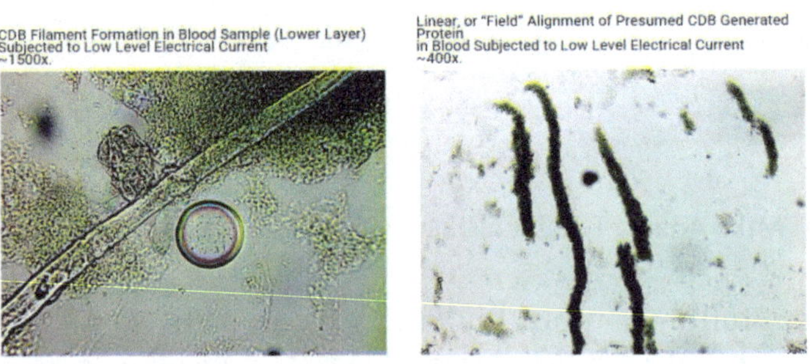

Figure 3. Blood alterations. Carnicom Institute.[7]

These ribbon-like structures resemble what I also find in live blood in the unvaccinated that is now causing severe rouleaux formation.

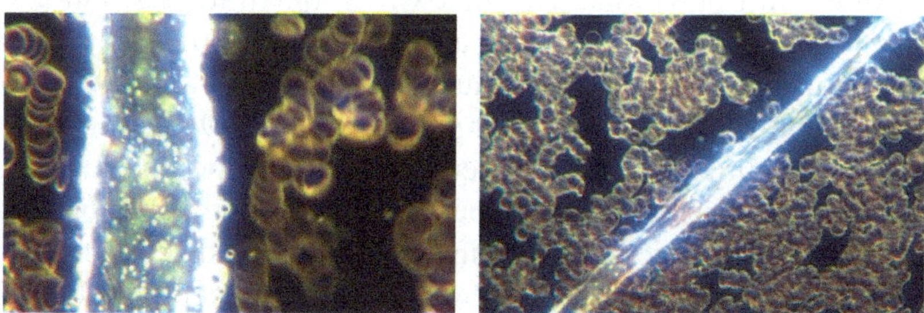

Figure 4. Unvaccinated patients with chronic fatigue/long COVID live blood findings. AM Medical.[8]

To my great concern, I recently had an unvaccinated person send me images of long rubbery clots, despite their taking commonly used supplements for the breakdown of fibrin, such as Nattokinase and Lumbrokinase. My research now reveals similar synthetic formations developing in both vaccinated and unvaccinated blood. The consequences are important to understand and could be dire for everyone living on this planet.

Today, I share a common concern with Clifford Carnicom that this synthetic biology's responsiveness to electromagnetic and other frequencies may be the "Kill Switch" with which selectively humanity can be depopulated. Vaccinated or unvaccinated at this point does not matter much, for all now have this synthetic antenna in their bodies via our contaminated food and water supplies, vaccines, vaccine shedding, and geoengineered spraying, causing disease and accelerated aging in humanity.

Hopefully, through our joint research and publications, we have been able to effectively explain that the context of artificial intelligence synthetic biology contributing to the transformation and depopulation of humanity, is much broader than mainstream frontline physicians are discussing. Only by understanding this broader context can we come up with solutions, like EDTA Chelation, that may help save the human species from this assault. The rapid aging we are witnessing should be addressed not only with nutritional and detoxification strategies, but also with potent antiaging peptides and other modalities. Examples that could be explored include, but are not limited to, intermittent rapamycin to downregulate the mTOR aging gene, CJC1295 to unlock senescent secretory phenotype, Epithalon to lengthen telomeres, GHK Copper to reset 30% of genes back to health, and senolytics like Fisetin, etc., that I will discuss in more detail in the future. I have explained, in depth, such modalities in my book *Light Medicine: A New Paradigm – The Science of Light, Spirit, and Longevity*.[9]

Unvaccinated Blood Unrecognizable After Application of Low-Level Electrical Current Clifford Carnicom's Findings Confirmed

MARCH 19, 2023[10]

Clifford Carnicom wrote a series of six scientific papers that I find highly important to consider for anyone seriously investigating what has been happening to human blood since the roll out of the COVID 19 injections, and how this alteration fits into the transhumanist depopulation agenda. To my mind, Clifford's papers, *Blood Alterations: A Six Part Series*, are a must read for every human being on this planet.[11] I have drawn many parallels in what we are now seeing with synthetic biology since the COVID 19 shots era and Clifford's historical research.

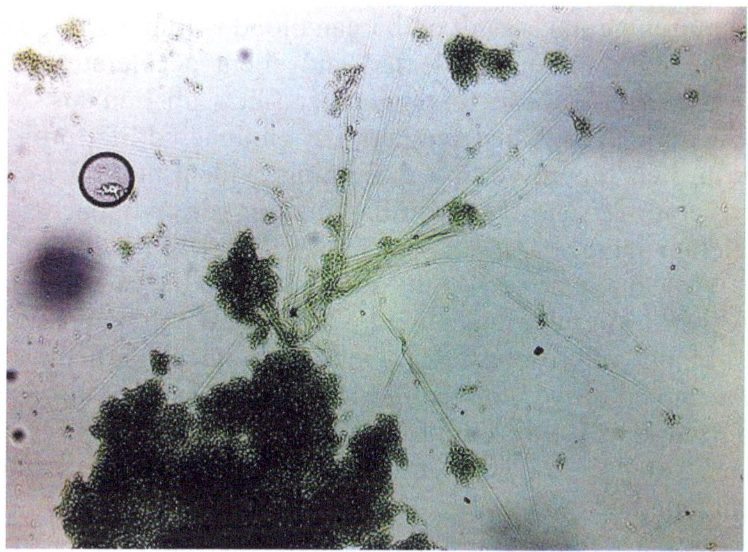

Figure 5. Human blood sample subjected to AC voltammetry electrochemistry – CDB presence and filament formation is evident. Magnification ~ 1500x. Carnicom Institute.[12]

Clifford gave the historically known Morgellons the new name "Cross Domain Bacteria," after he found that this synthetically engineered life form had features of all three biological classes of life—archaea, bacteria, and eucaryotes. Normal life forms belong to one of these three domains, never to all three. Additionally, he performed detailed analysis which showed that the ribbon-like structures were chemically composed of polyvinyl alcohol, which is a combination of hydrogel and metals.

I have written extensively about the abnormal findings in unvaccinated blood that I have been seeing with exponential severity and frequency. Only what seems a short time ago, I would still see people for their first live blood analysis who were uncontaminated. However, since the end of 2022, I have not observed anyone's blood that does not have these abnormal structures. My sounding the alarm about vaccine shedding and this environmental assault on human blood is important to note, for I foresee an unprecedented and silent accelerated aging epidemic due to these findings that affects all humans. Most people do not know that synthetically engineered life forms are now in their blood, yet it is becoming evident that they cause micro-clotting, acidity, and inflammation, all components that accelerate aging.

While mainstream health care admits that the causes of long COVID are not fully understood, I have seen, utilizing darkfield live blood microscopy, synthetic biological structures in unvaccinated blood with similar long COVID symptoms as has also been found to develop from COVID 19 "vaccine" vials.

The long COVID epidemic in America shows the assault on population health:

> Long COVID has potentially affected up to 23 million Americans, pushing an estimated 1 million people out of work. The causes of long COVID are not fully understood, complicating diagnosis and treatment. Among people who have had COVID, 11% are currently experiencing long COVID but an additional 17% had long COVID in the past and are no longer reporting symptoms, suggesting that more people have recovered from long COVID than currently report symptoms. The total "COVID" cases registered in the United States has reached 103 million according to the CDC.[13]

Clifford Carnicom demonstrated in 2023 that in four unvaccinated people, not only did they have abnormal rouleaux formation (stacking of red blood cells), but after applying an extremely low voltage current, the same structures I am now seeing in everyone appeared. My findings were confirmed by Dr. David Nixon in Australia, in live blood analysis of vaccinated and unvaccinated people. Around the world, people have called this graphene oxide—they see what we see, long ribbon structures. Calling this substance graphene oxide may be a misnomer regarding the hydrogel polymer encapsulating the payload within the shots—whether it be mRNA, toxins, or quantum dots that magnetically alter the human genetic information by modifying the spin states of subatomic particles—which may contain graphene oxide but not be fully made from graphene. Clifford Carnicom called this material Cross Domain Bacteria or CDB, his name for Morgellons, a hydrogel polymer synthetic life form with many similarities to what we see in live blood of injected and uninjected people since the COVID 19 "vaccine" rollout.

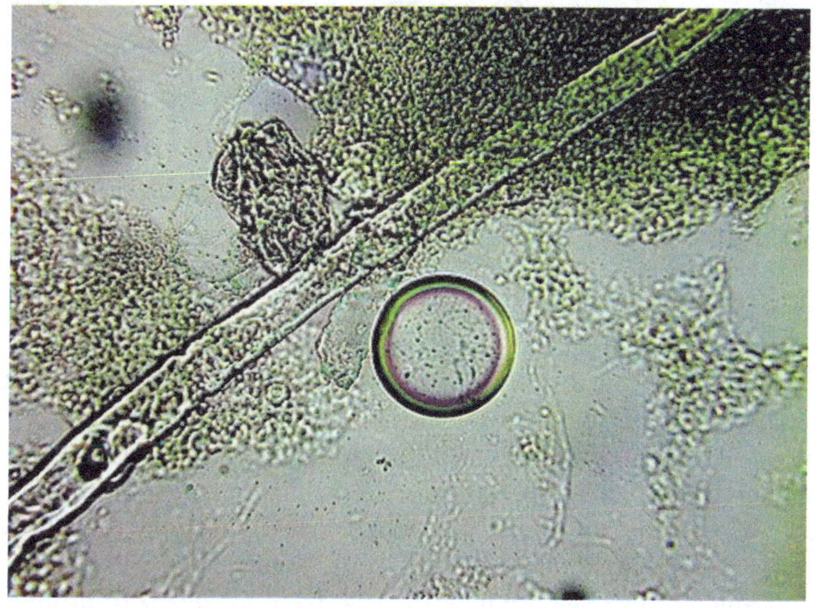

Figure 6. CDB filament formation in blood sample (lower layer) subjected to low-level electrical current. Magnification ~1500x. Carnicom Institute.[14]

The above image, taken by Clifford Carnicom, is very similar to what I have been seeing in my clinic in unvaccinated blood (Figure 7 below):

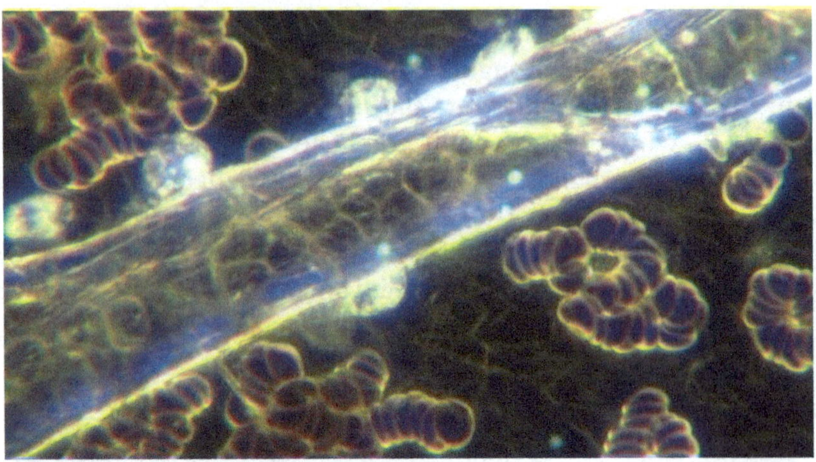

Figure 7. COVID 19 unvaccinated blood with hydrogel filament and rouleaux formation. AM Medical.[15]

In the early part of 2023, I would still see unvaccinated people with uncontaminated live blood. I no longer see normal blood samples, unless following EDTA Chelation—a treatment I found able to clear the blood of these structures.

The issue is this: If there is a synthetic, hydrogel-based, artificial intelligence biology that is transforming humanity's blood—causing disease, illness, and accelerated aging—we need to identify this. We have to chemically analyze this to really see what the structures are made of—hydrogel? Graphene oxide? So far, nobody knows all of the details.

Since the COVID pandemic, we have all heard of athletes dying suddenly, including children. Hydrogel polymers grow with electrical and EMF exposure. Exercise in the body creates a powerful electrical field. Could this be part of the mechanism of why these athletes are dying?

Unvaccinated Blood: Recurrent New Proof of CDB Filaments Growing Under Exposure of Extremely Low Electrical Currents

MARCH 25, 2023[16]

Chronopotentiometry is an electrochemical technique in which the effects of an electrical current and voltage are observed over time. In Clifford Carnicom's experiments, diluted, fresh COVID 19 unvaccinated blood was used, 0.1 ml of blood in 2 ml of water. The energy applied was 3 milliamps of DC current for 2 hours with an approximate resulting voltage of 3 volts. This process was described in detail in the six-paper series published by Clifford in 2022.[17]

During these experiments, a foamy layer formed at the surface that emanated from the working electrode. In addition, there was settling of a layer at the bottom. The upper foam was a dark, grey-brown color. At the bottom was a bright, dark red layer.

Both layers were investigated by microscopy. The foam layer did not show many filaments or CDBs. In the lower level, 100 microliters were extracted from the bottom of the vial with a micro pipette and the classic structures of CDBs were visible with filament structure. In our ensuing research, we have shown that the filaments grow from the CDBs:

Chronopotentiometry appears to be a method that can quickly isolate from blood the minute CDBs and filaments that grow from them. Historically, the culture work would take weeks to months. Application of an electrical current can now accelerate the process for further, more rapid investigation. We encourage other scientific teams to replicate our experiments to identify the concerning live blood changes currently seen in humanity.

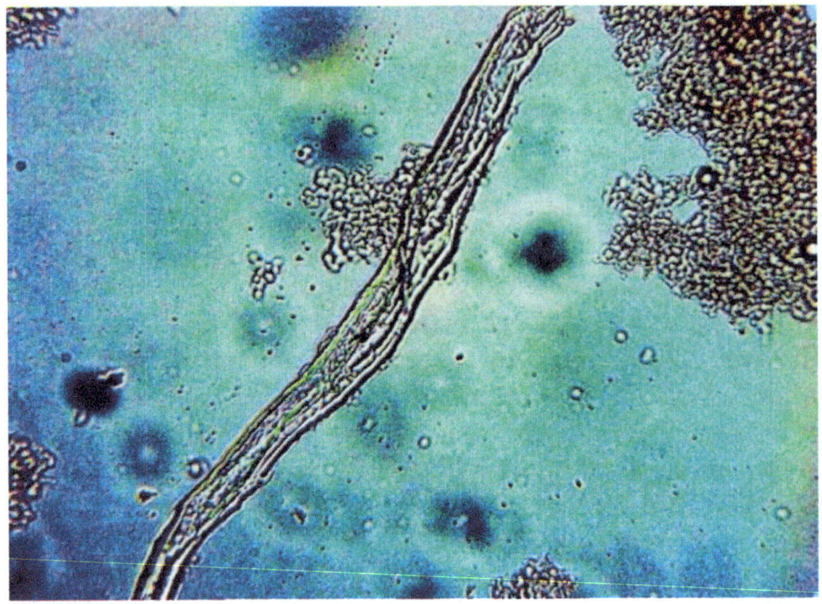

Figure 8. COVID 19 unvaccinated blood – lower layer after voltammetry. Filament and CDBs seen. Magnification 1600x. Carnicom Institute.[18]

Cultures developed from CDBs contain DNA. The COVID 19 vials have been shown to contain plasmid bacterial DNA. If there is any overlap between this CDB synthetic organism and what is in the vials, the proof of this correlation would advance our understanding significantly.

In historical documentation, Clifford Carnicom revealed how these CDBs affect red blood cells.[19]

An organism and a method that damages the condition of the blood has now been identified and directly observed. The blood variations reported here are in direct association with the existence and severity of the so-called "Morgellons" condition.

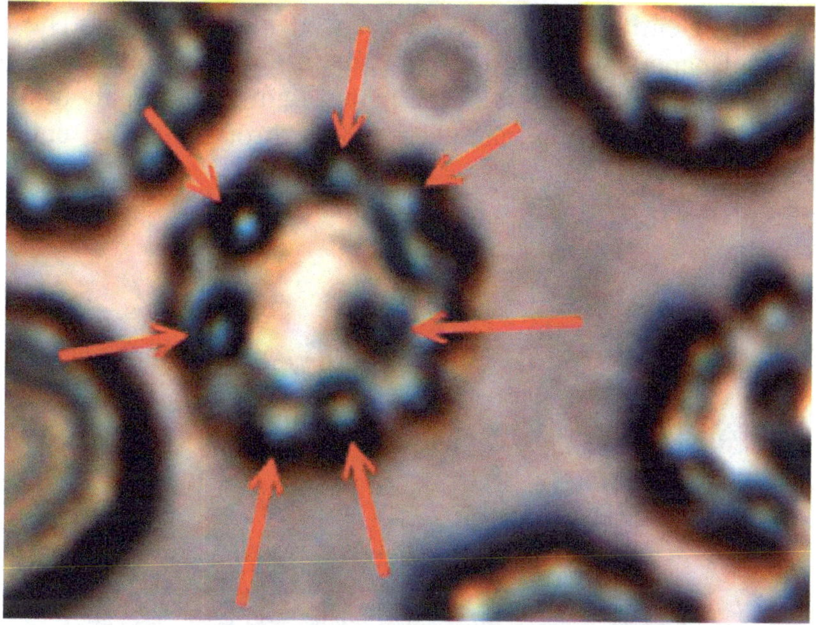

Figure 9. CDBs infecting red blood cells. Magnification ~2000x. Carnicom Institute.[20]

The degradation occurs, at least in part, as the result of a chlamydia-like organism that has been repeatedly called to attention within the research during the past several years. This organism, along with a pleomorphic form tentatively identified as a mycoplasma variation, as well as certain filamentous forms, have been identified as common denominators in past and active biological and environmental examinations. It will be recalled from earlier studies that essentially all individuals observed thus far display the presence of these blood anomalies to varying degree; statistically it would certainly appear as though the general population is subject to these invasive forms. It has also been stated that the severity of the damage to the blood appears to occur in direct correlation with the manifestation of symptoms of the Morgellons condition. Please note: In later chapters, and in the evolution of this work, I refer to these CDBs not as biological entities, but purely advanced nanomaterials. These original papers still use the nomenclature of my collaboration with Clifford. Regardless of the name, I am speaking about the same self-assembling nanotechnology throughout the entire book.

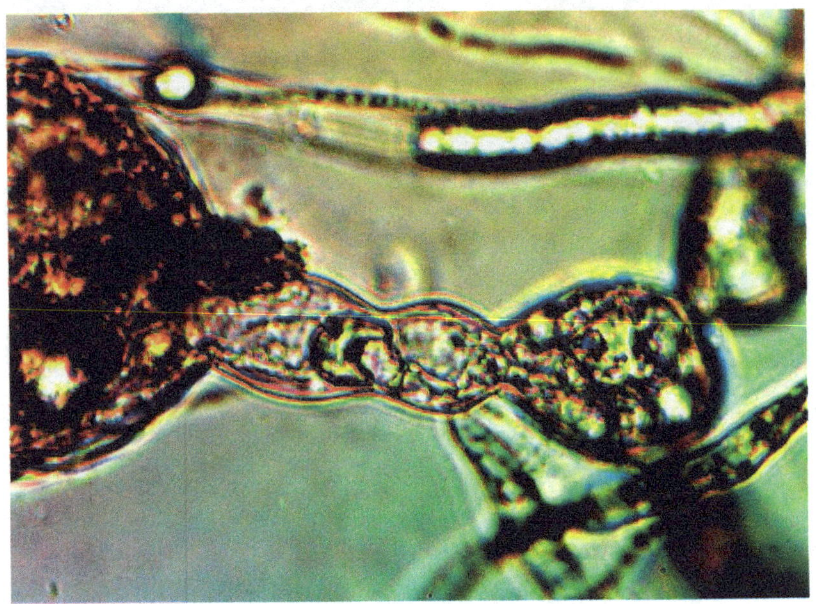

Figure 10. CDB growth progression advanced filament form. Magnification ~5000x. Carnicom Institute.[21]

Clifford and I showed it is this synthetic organism that is responsible for the transformation of the blood to an unrecognizable filament network (see image above), under the influence of electrical current.

We have seen unprecedented changes in live blood since the roll out of the COVID 19 injections. I have reported extensively on the findings of abnormal structures found in vaccinated blood around the world, and now in unvaccinated blood, due to the impacts of environmental contamination and vaccine shedding.

This appears to involve hydrogel based artificial life forms that have been sprayed upon humanity via geoengineering projects and "vaccine" injections. I have written about these findings and correlations, reporting that Clifford's chemical analysis suggests the presence of polyvinyl alcohol hydrogel and extensive metals within these filaments.

To analyze and quantify the objective changes in live blood, Clifford repeated the experiment of applying a low-level electrical current to unvaccinated blood. Prior to an electrical current being applied, and upon inspection, the blood looked normal, without rouleaux formation, and without the filament structures we now so commonly see (Figure 11 below).

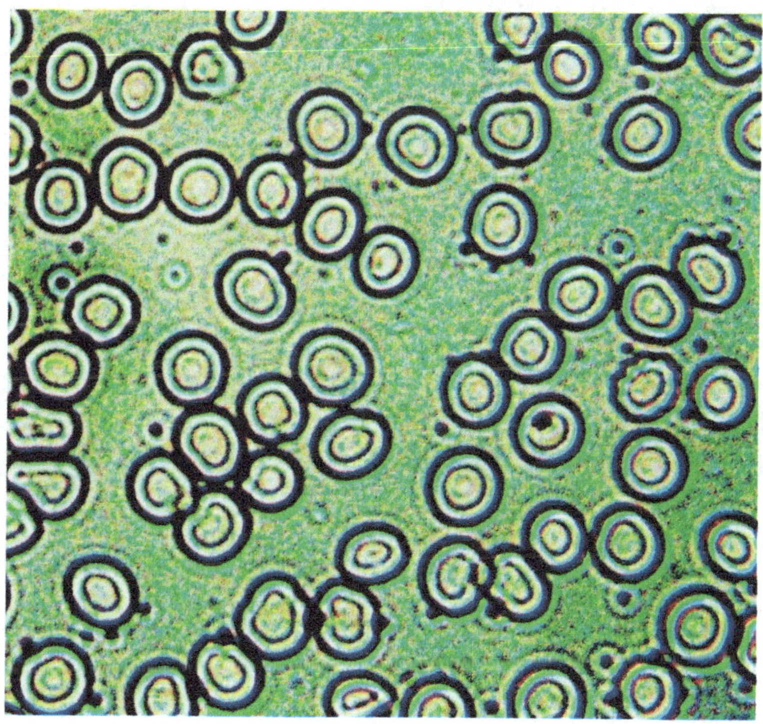

Figure 11. Unvaccinated live blood analysis: Subject 1 – normal appearing prior to exposure to low-level electrical current. Magnification ~1600x. Carnicom Institute.[22]

Clifford then applied a 10 microamp AC current to the blood sample, in highly diluted blood, and over a two-hour period. The clear blood sample seen in Figure 11 above, changed unrecognizably to a dense filament network, which was not visible without the application of the low-level electrical current (red circle in the image below encloses a CDB string). **Please note: The microcurrent used was 1000 times less than the current used in the original research conducted in 2022 on unvaccinated blood.**[23]

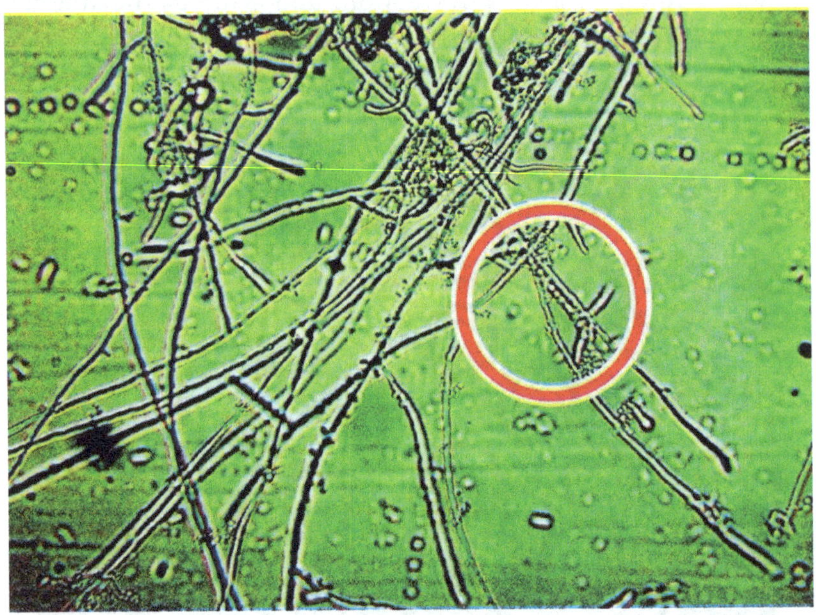

Figure 12. Unvaccinated blood under the influence of 10 microamps AC current. Circled red is a classic finding of CDB filament activity. Magnification ~1600x. Carnicom Institute.[24]

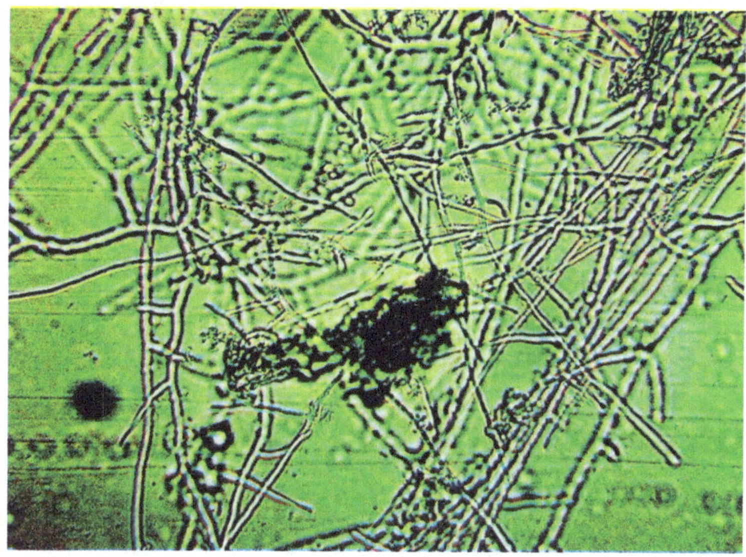

Figure 13. Unvaccinated blood – extensive filament network seen under 10 microamp electrical current. Magnification ~1600x. Carnicom Institute.[25]

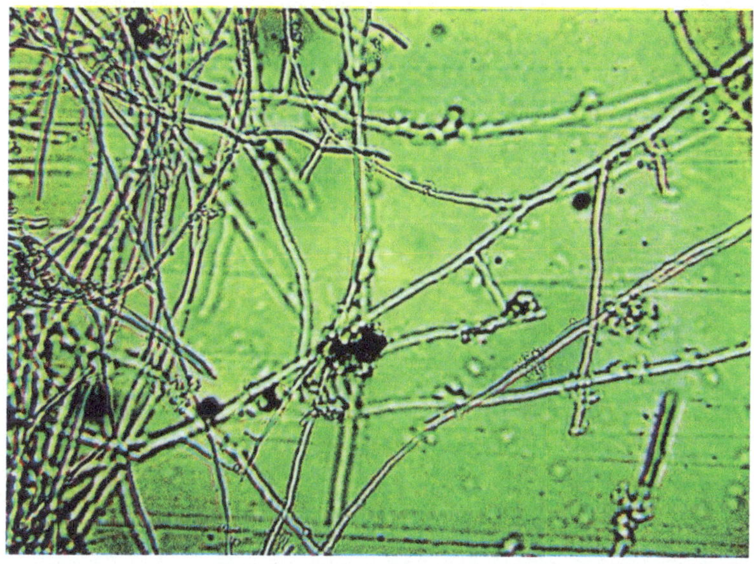

Figure 14. Unvaccinated blood – extensive filament network seen under 10 microamp electrical current. Magnification ~1500x. Carnicom Institute.[26]

To compare, I include an image below taken from the Pfizer "vaccine" showing the parallel to Clifford's discovery and the COVID 19 injectables:

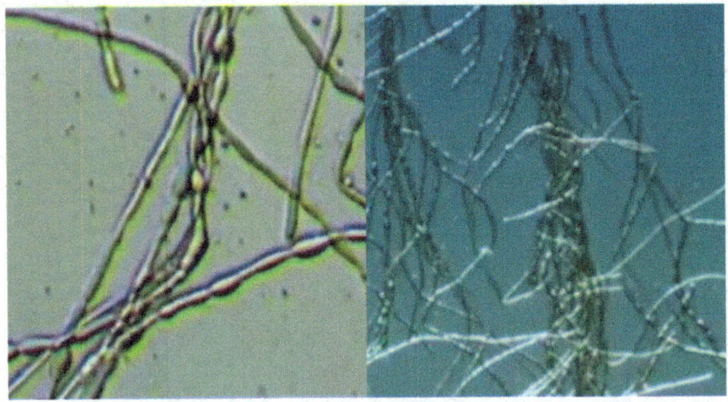

Figure 15. COVID 19 Pfizer "vaccine." A drop was heated and then developed these filaments. La Quinta Columna.[27]

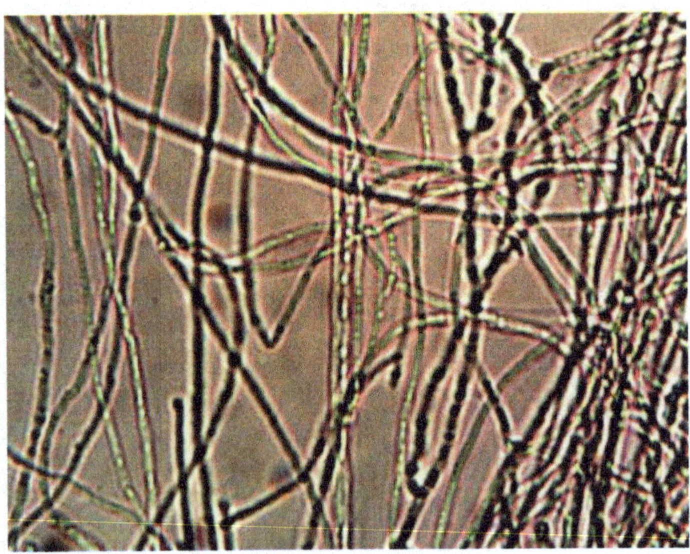

Figure 16. Filament development with internal CDB growth progressions known as Morgellons. Isolated from human blood. Magnification ~5000x. Carnicom Institute, 2014.[28]

This is now replication of the original work by Clifford Carnicom, clearly showing that even unvaccinated blood has been apparently contaminated with a synthetic biology on a sub-micron scale, which can grow under the influence of extremely low-level electrical current. The implications for the dangers of this phenomenon to human health are profound.

Our concern is that the increased susceptibility to ELF response in COVID 19 injected blood could be weaponized as well as used for remote control purposes. ELF waves have been shown to alter DNA, manipulate and control brain function, and cause accelerated aging and immune system dysfunction. In 2022, I wrote two papers about scalar interferometry, (the use of scalar waves to create interference patterns that can measure or manipulate scalar fields): *There is No Isolated Virus. Then What Makes People Sick? Electromagnetic Frequency of Living Organisms,* and, *A Biophysical Understanding of Vaccine Shedding and Self-disseminating Vaccines in Populations*. I encourage readers to broaden their knowledge on the influence of ELF frequencies, by reviewing these two papers found in my Substack.[29,30]

Unvaccinated vs Vaccinated Blood Comparison: Infrared Spectroscopy and Electrical Conductivity Studies

MARCH 27, 2023[31]

A series of experiments were performed in 2023 on six unvaccinated blood samples and three vaccinated blood samples with infrared spectroscopy and an electrical conductivity meter. The purpose of this investigation was to begin to quantify, with objective measurements, what has happened to the blood of humanity since the roll out of the COVID 19 injections. As I have described previously, ribbon-like structures have been found in vaccinated and unvaccinated live blood analysis at an unprecedented rate, in addition to extensive rouleaux formation and micro-clotting.

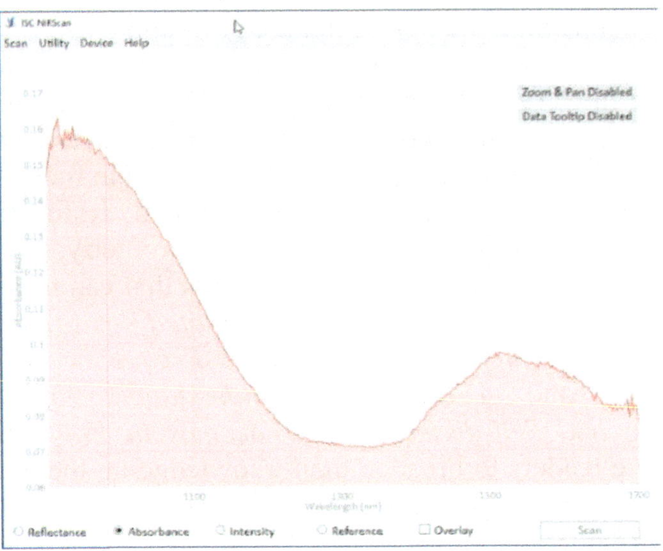

Figure 17. COVID 19 unvaccinated blood infrared spectroscopy. Individual had history of mild COVID. Carnicom Institute.[32]

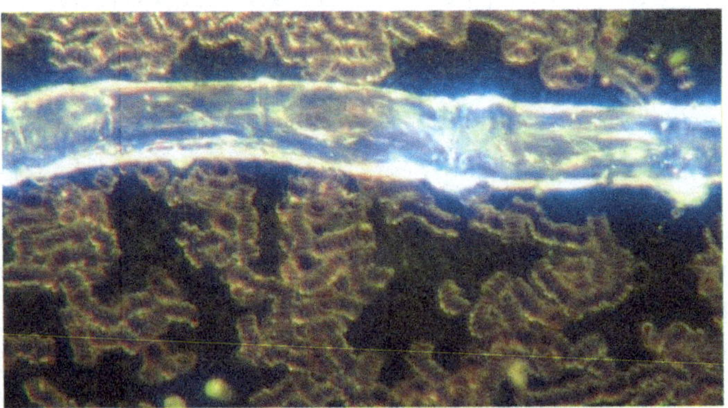

Figure 18. Unvaccinated blood with rouleaux and characteristic filament structure in post COVID 19 era. Magnification 400x. AM Medical.[33]

Clinically, these findings have been accompanied with an undeniable accelerated aging process in the population, exhibiting symptoms like chronic fatigue, brain fog, cardiovascular abnormalities, and more. This symptoms complex has been categorized as "long COVID." In my own clinical practice, everyone I have seen for live blood analysis with post COVID, long COVID, and over the last months everyone unvaccinated has these structures in their blood. The source is presumed to be from the environment and vaccine shedding. I have suspected this be due to self-assembling hydrogel, possibly with carbon nanostructures and metals involved, based upon my background research.

Many people call the structures graphene. Yet the chemical composition of these structures, to my current knowledge, has not yet been evaluated.

Infrared spectroscopy (IR spectroscopy or vibrational spectroscopy) is an analytical technique used to study and identify chemical substances or functional groups in solid, liquid, or gaseous forms. Clifford Carnicom has three decades of experience in IR spectrometry investigating environmental filaments, CDBs, and the blood of those exposed. His CBD synthetic biology culture work evaluated the abnormal metabolic products in affected blood which included: 1. water-soluble proteins, 2. solid proteins, 3. filament network. These water-soluble products under IR spectroscopy created a plastic-like film classic of polymer hydrogel with specific frequency peaks.[34] Similar functional groups have occurred historically in CDB research and again in these new experiments during the post COVID 19 injection era.

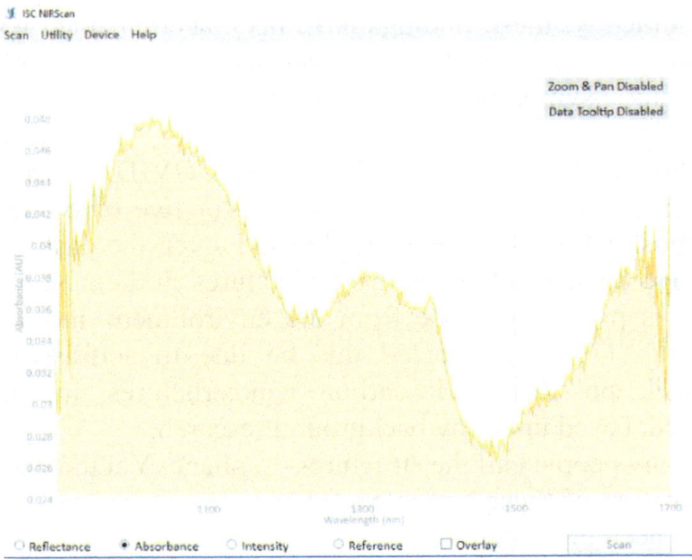

Figure 19. COVID 19 unvaccinated blood infrared spectroscopy. History of respiratory failure and long COVID. Carnicom Institute.[35]

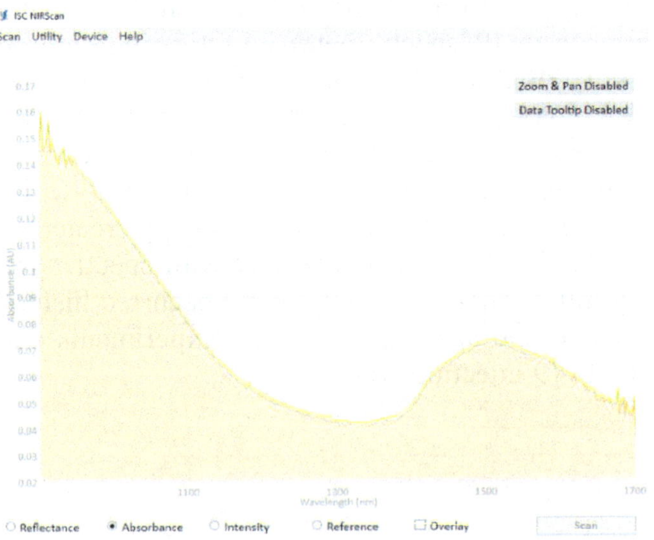

Figure 20. COVID 19 vaccinated blood infrared spectroscopy. Carnicom Institute.[36]

Samples of unvaccinated blood with history of mild COVID have commonalities with vaccinated blood in IR signatures. Unvaccinated blood with history of severe COVID, respiratory failure, and significant long COVID have IR signatures of aromatics and disulfide bonds similar to that previously seen in CDB culture work. Both could indicate the presence of hydrogel polymers. Unvaccinated blood with history of respiratory failure shares an IR peak signature with vaccinated blood of secondary amines. Those can include the amino acid proline, which can form natural hydrogels, but also other chemicals. Frequency signatures within 5 nm can be considered equal. Vaccinated blood contains completely new spectroscopy findings with new functional groups not identified in any unvaccinated samples.

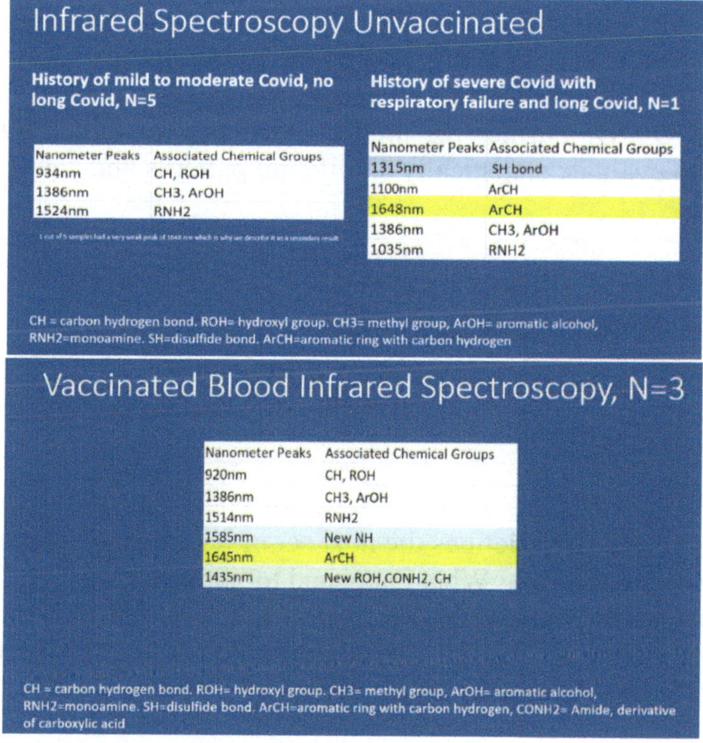

Figure 21. COVID 19 unvaccinated and vaccinated blood infrared spectroscopy. AM Medical.[37]

In the infrared spectroscopy results above, we see that five COVID 19 unvaccinated individuals had matching spectral peaks. One COVID 19 unvaccinated individual had an outlier aromatic ring that matched the vaccinated spectral signatures. Three COVID 19 vaccinated individuals had matching spectral peaks. This suggests that severe COVID with respiratory failure has chemical overlap with COVID 19 vaccinated blood.

Aromatic alcohols and aromatic carbon hydrogen bonds found in today's live blood leads to questions about polymeric alcohols/hydrogels when considering decades of similar IR spectra with CDB filaments. Preliminary data in measurements of vaccinated and unvaccinated blood with a conductivity meter (N=9) showed up to 50% reduction in blood electrical conductivity compared to normal historical values in the literature. This correlates with clinical findings that describe many people experiencing chronic fatigue symptoms, brain fog, and decreased mitochondrial function—which has been called long COVID. Further research is necessary in larger sample sizes to evaluate statistically significant patterns and changes.

Blood Cultures of Unvaccinated Blood Show Extensive (CDB) Filament Development After Two Weeks Incubation

APRIL 08, 2023[38]

This research defines the next set of results in our efforts to answer the question: What happened to humanity's blood?

Over several months, we conducted different experiments to determine if there is a quantifiable difference between COVID 19 vaccinated and unvaccinated blood.

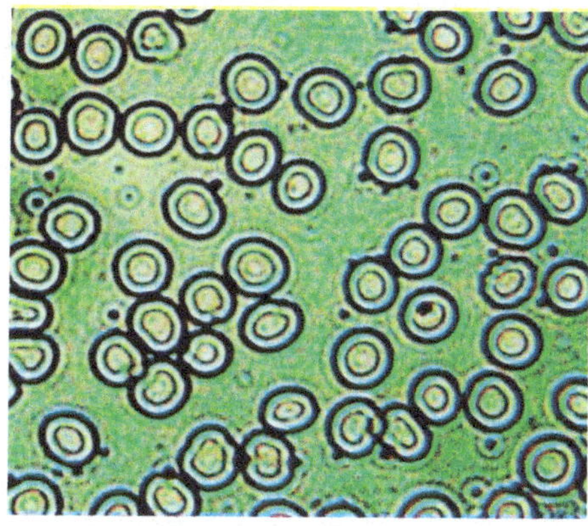

Figure 22. COVID 19 unvaccinated live blood analysis. Subject 1: Blood prior to incubation at room temperature for two weeks. Carnicom Institute.[39]

An unvaccinated blood sample was incubated at room temperature and left for two weeks. The concentration of the solution was 50% water and 50% unvaccinated blood. In previous historical CDB culture work, time has appeared to be a substitute for external energy sources, producing similar effects. As mentioned, the growth of (CDB) filaments can be induced rapidly by exposure to electrical currents. In a regular culture, the filaments grow over time.

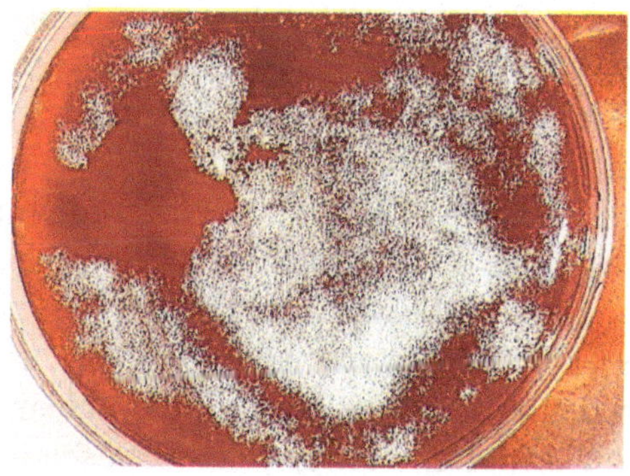

Figure 23. COVID 19 unvaccinated blood left at room temperature for two weeks to culture in a petri dish. Carnicom Institute.[40]

Please note: The same white filaments seen in the image above have been found from environmental sources as a result of geoengineered spraying (Figure 24).

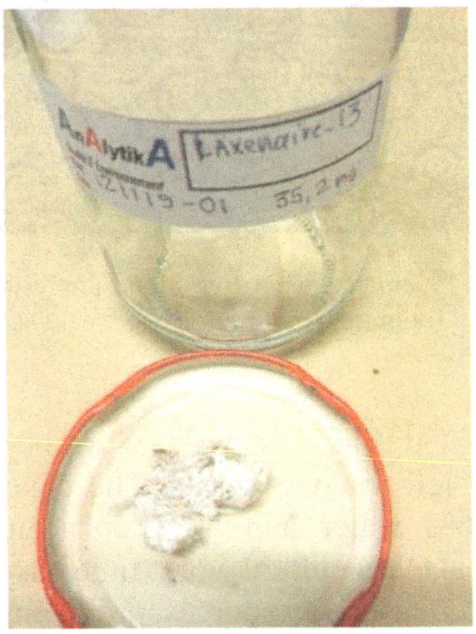

Figure 24. Environmental filament analysis from France. Bernard Tailliez.[41]

In the culture work, no additional growth agar was used, just blood and water. A white filament growth is clearly seen. Historically, the environmental filaments can appear pure white, red, or blue. The colors have been surmised by others to be caused by quantum dot technology.

Historically, in the CDB culture work, red wine was used as a growth medium as it has been shown to greatly enhance filament growth. Hence the red wine test was developed—which includes the swishing of wine in the mouth and analysis of filaments excreted by the body that are then clearly visible.

In Clifford Carnicom's thirty years of research, this was the first time that a pure blood culture was performed, and phenomenal, novel observations took place.

The white CDB filaments in the image above look like this under a microscope:

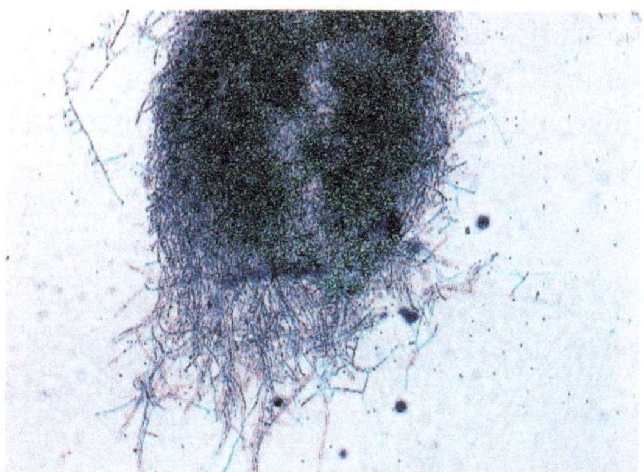

Figure 25. Filament network formed in COVID 19 unvaccinated blood after two weeks of blood culture at room temperature. Magnification 160x. Carnicom Institute.[42]

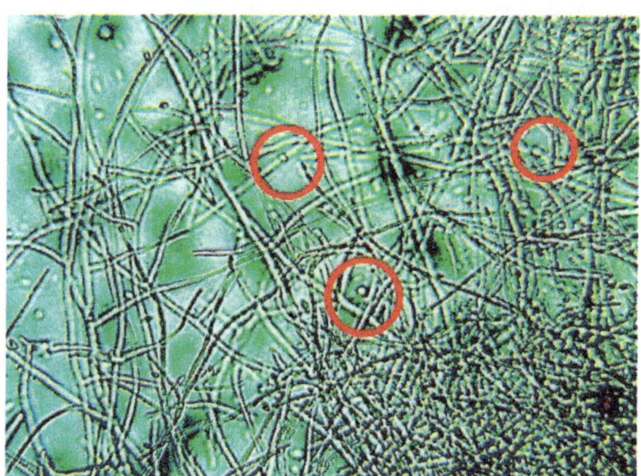

Figure 26. COVID 19 unvaccinated blood – higher magnification of the filament network. Circled in red are CDB classical findings. Magnification 640x. Carnicom Institute.[43]

In Clifford's work, and from an historical perspective, the CDBs isolated in the red circles above and below are the origin of genesis of the filaments. The linear self-assembly of this synthetic biology is leading to the filament progression. Filaments and CDBs coexist.

Self-assembly does not have to be a synthetic biology feature, it is also a known mechanism of growth in biology. For example, DNA has a self-assembly mechanism.

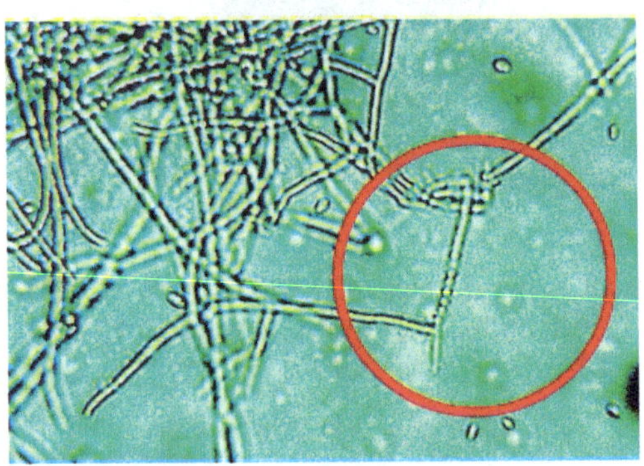

Figure 27. COVID 19 unvaccinated blood – higher magnification of linear self-assembly. Magnification ~640x. Carnicom Institute.[44]

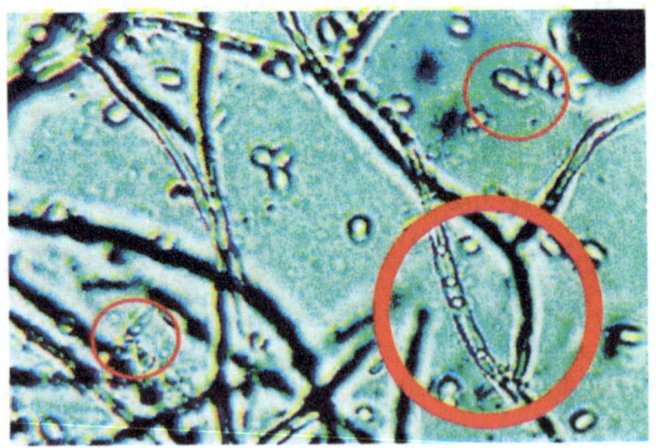

Figure 28. COVID 19 unvaccinated blood – CDB visible within the filaments in the large red circle. Smaller circles show CDBs. Estimated size of CDBs is 1/2 micron. Magnification 1500x. Carnicom Institute.[45]

As shown in the small red circles above, for the first time in 30 years' research on CDBs, Clifford captured cellular division and multiplication of CDBs. This is a classical biological feature of bacteria. It became evident in this series of experiments that the culture medium affects the final product of growth, and that blood is a perfect culture medium for this synthetic biology, as compared to historically used agars.

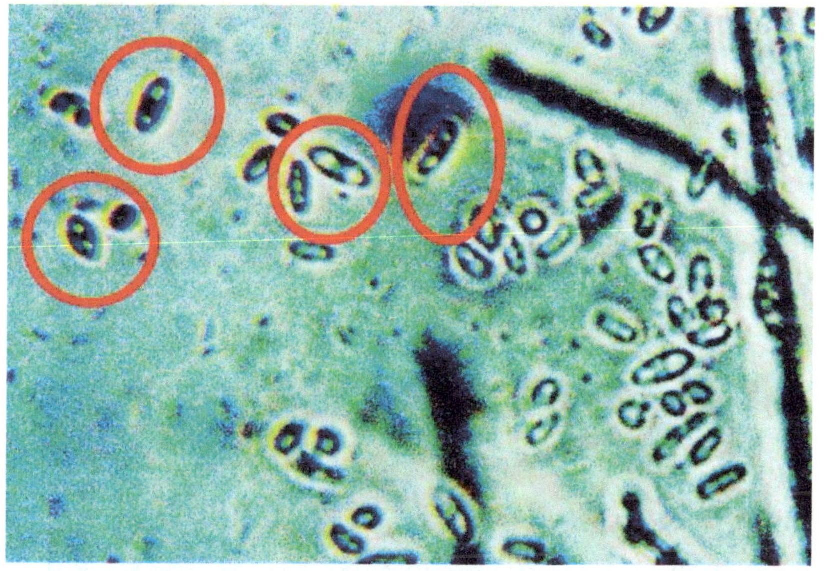

Figure 29. COVID 19 unvaccinated blood – the red circles capture what appears to be cell division. Magnification 1500x. Carnicom Institute.[46]

In this blood medium, cell division was seen by the thousands. This is not a rod-like bacteria, but appears to be binary fission. Bacterial binary fission is the process that bacteria use to carry out cell division.

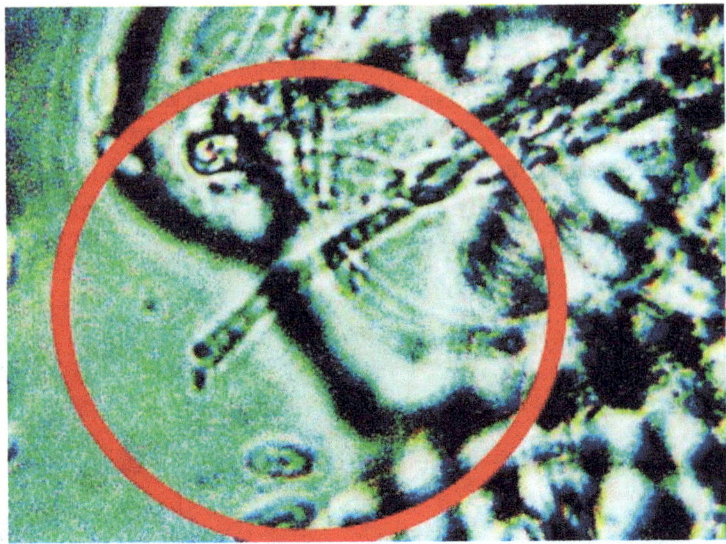

Figure 30. COVID 19 unvaccinated blood – the filament is packed with CDB. Magnification 1500x. Carnicom Institute.[47]

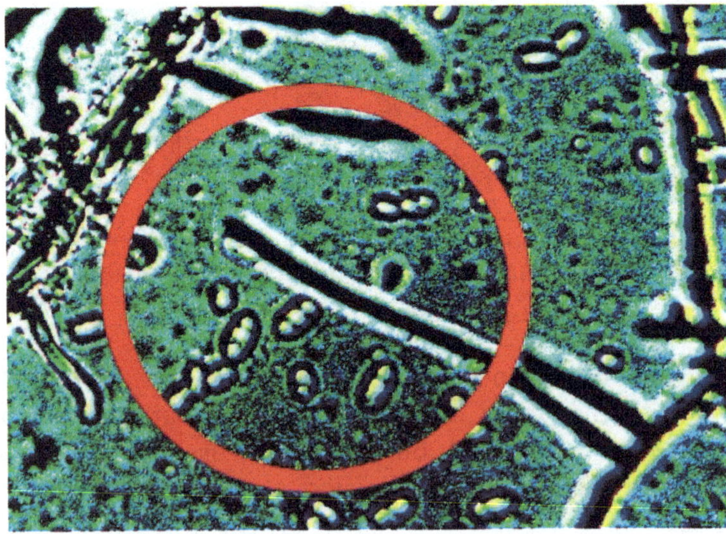

Figure 31. COVID 19 unvaccinated blood – replication division captured with CDB seen and filament growth documented. Magnification 1500x. Carnicom Institute.[48]

In these experiments, we documented CDB filament growth in unvaccinated blood after two weeks of incubation at room temperature. New and important discoveries revealed that unvaccinated blood samples that appear to be normal still have CDB in them promoting filament growth. Time appears to have similar results as the application of electrical current. For the first time, CDB multiplication and cellular division were captured.

Extensive (CDB) Hydrogel Filament Growth in COVID 19 Vaccinated and Unvaccinated Blood Cultures After One Week of Incubation

APRIL 09, 2023[49]

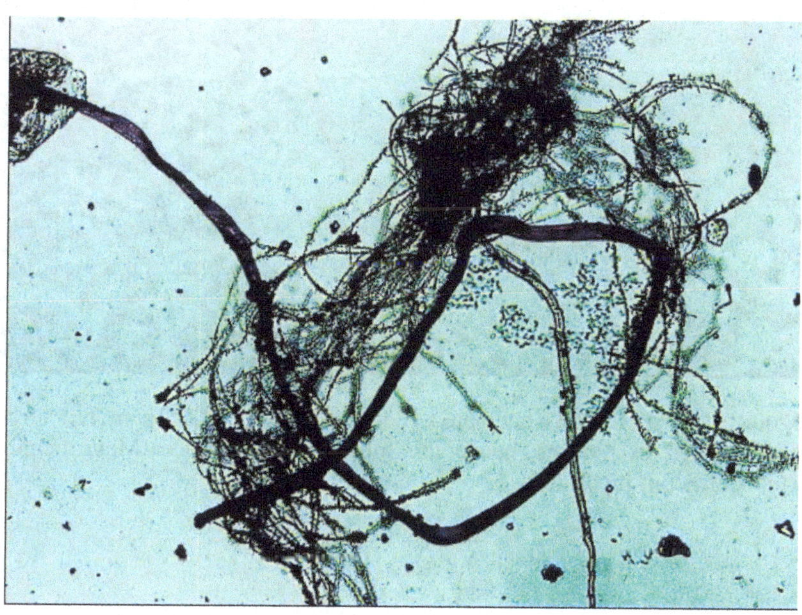

Figure 32. COVID 19 unvaccinated blood after one week of incubation. Magnification 160x. Carnicom Institute.[50]

As can be seen in the image above, regardless of their unvaccinated status, extensive CDB filaments have developed after one week of blood culture. Even with highly diluted samples, the filament growth is impressive.

The four new samples discussed in this paper were highly diluted blood at a ratio of 100:1 with water and left to incubate at room temperature for one week. No electrical current or external energy source was applied. None of the individuals had symptoms of Morgellons/CDB disease.

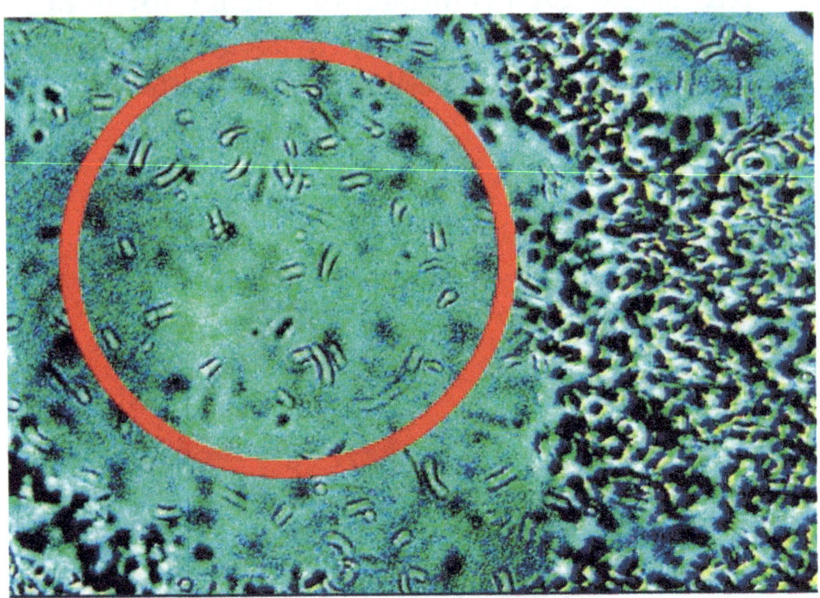

Figure 33. COVID 19 vaccinated blood. Subject 1: CDBs in red circle photographed in motion, hence the tube-like appearance. Magnification 640x. Carnicom Institute.[51]

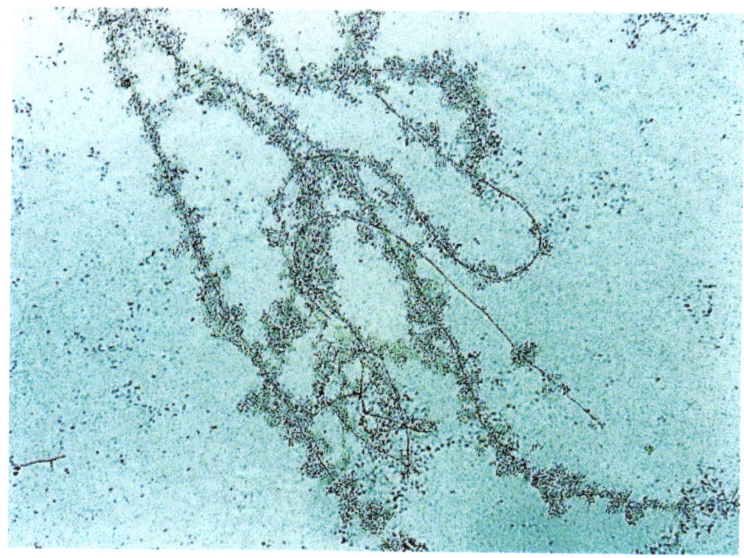

Figure 34. COVID 19 vaccinated blood. Subject 1: CDB and filament growth seen. Magnification 160x. Carnicom Institute.[52]

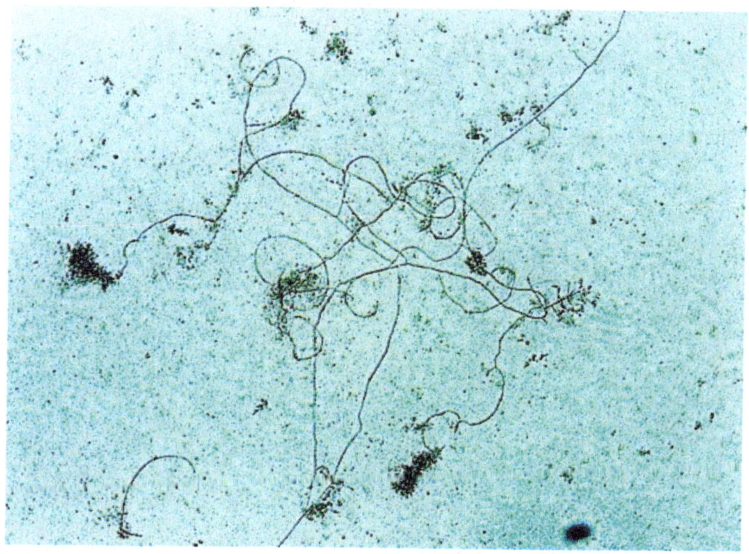

Figure 35. COVID 19 vaccinated blood. Subject 2: CDB and filament growth seen. Magnification 160x. Carnicom Institute.[53]

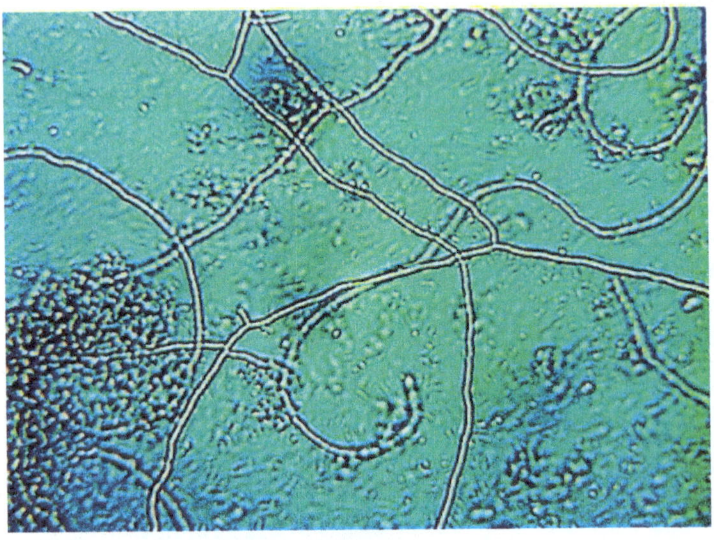

Figure 36. COVID 19 vaccinated blood, Subject 2: CDB and filament growth seen. CDBs are the source of filament genesis. Magnification 640x. Carnicom Institute.[54]

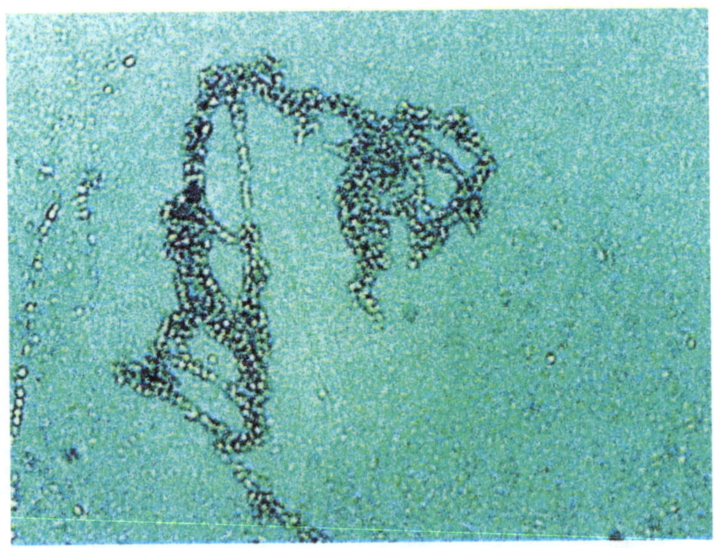

Figure 37. COVID 19 vaccinated blood. Subject 3: CDB and filament growth seen. Magnification 640x. Carnicom Institute.[55]

Below I include comparison images from engineer Shimon Yanowitz in Israel. All three images are Pfizer BioNtech COVID 19 samples in Neubauer Chamber incubated at room temperature, just like the blood samples above. After 20-30 minutes, filament structures started to form. Note the similar alignment of the CDB filaments as shown in the Subjects 1 and 2 blood culture images above.

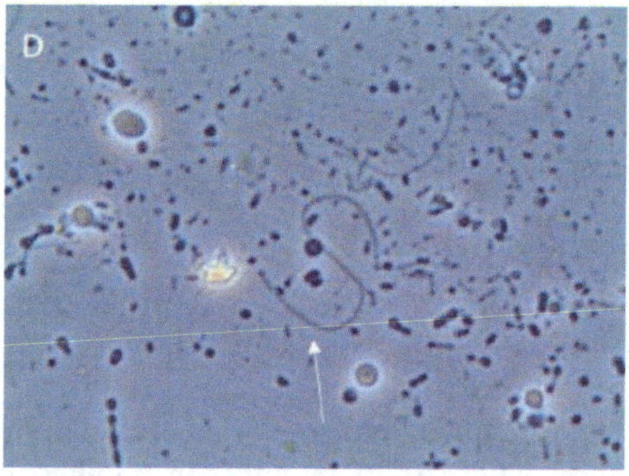

Figure 38. Pfizer BioNTech vaccine samples incubated in Neubauer Chamber at room temperature. After 20-30 minutes, filaments and structures had started to form. Shimon Yanowitz.[56]

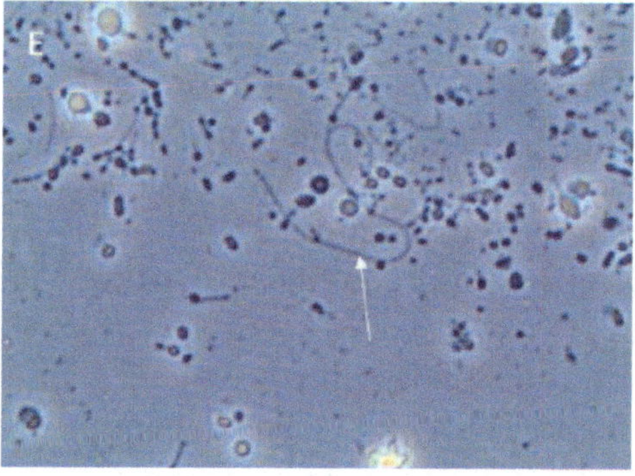

Figure 39. Pfizer BioNTech vaccine samples incubated in Neubauer Chamber at room temperature. After 20-30 minutes, filaments and structures are seen forming. Shimon Yanowitz.[57]

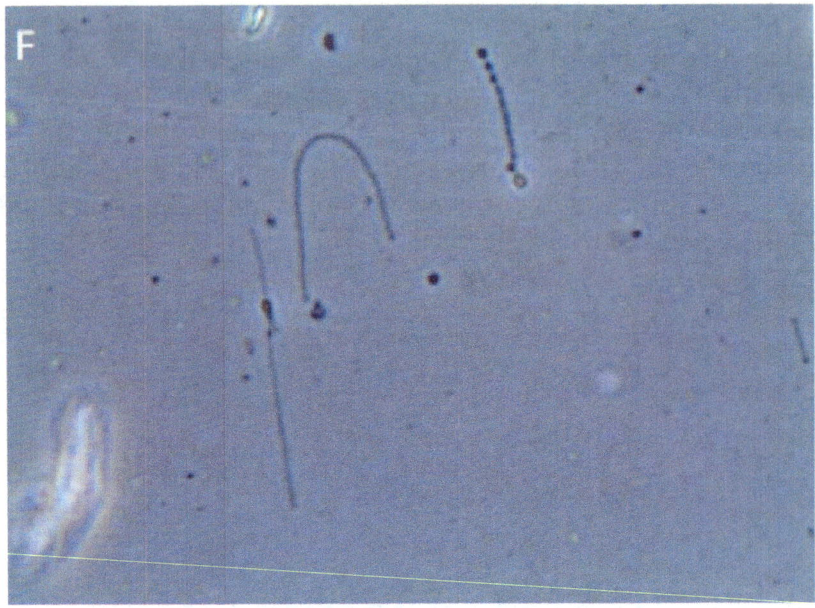

Figure 40. Pfizer BioNTech vaccine samples incubated in Neubauer Chamber at room temperature. After 20-30 minutes, in another area of the slide, filaments and structures had started to form. Shimon Yanowitz.[58]

Our own research demonstrates that blood culture work between COVID 19 vaccinated and unvaccinated blood did not show any difference in filament growth. All samples had evidence of CDBs in them. We have shown there is a similarity in the linear development of filaments in these blood samples and the incubated COVID 19 Pfizer BioNtech. This poses the following questions in my mind:

Have the vaccine ingredients self-spread via a mechanism called shedding?

Are the observed CDB and subsequent filaments stemming from environmental sources, such as geoengineering via aircraft spraying?

Has the platform of the COVID 19 injectables worsened the phenomena of blood contamination that was already present via geoengineering?

Given the increased morbidity and mortality in COVID 19 vaccinated, as well as the incidence of rubbery hydrogel clots found in the vaccinated who are deceased, are the unvaccinated in similar danger? This has been a major concern due to documentation of blood contamination and increased blood clot incidence in those who have these structures in their blood. Clearly the unvaccinated have already experienced ill health effects which we call long COVID. Will this ultimately lead to not just increased morbidity, but also mortality? Are CDBs actually in the C19 shots, given the recent findings of Kevin McKernan, PhD, when sequencing bacterial DNA from the vaccine vial?[59]

Clifford has also found that CDBs contain DNA. Unfortunately, he has not yet had the means to do a sequencing analysis. I wonder if we would find a match, given the culture results mentioned earlier in human blood. This would answer the question of whether the filament growth was coming from environmental sources or the COVID 19 shots.

Obviously, we can see evidence of synthetic artificial intelligence biology. Is this evidence determining a possible human extinction level event due to the unrestricted release of nanotechnology in the form of synthetic biology into the human race?

This list of questions is not final. Clifford and I are sounding the alarm for all of humanity to become aware of this threat and demand a stop to the COVID 19 injectables and the entire transhumanist agenda, including biological geoengineering.

I personally am convinced that the blood of humanity shows evidence of a crime of unprecedented proportions.

Evidence of Impaired Electrical Blood Conductivity, Iron Oxidation, and Reduced Oxygen Transport Capacity in the Post C19 Injection Era

APRIL 16, 2023[60]

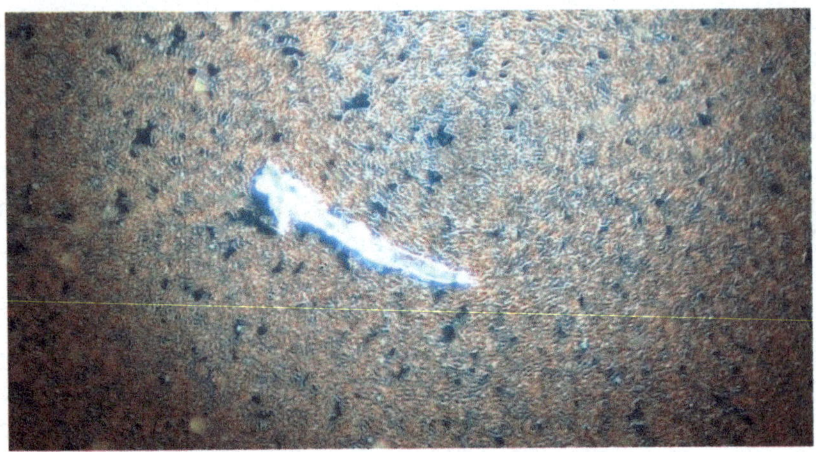

Figure 41. COVID 19 unvaccinated blood sample – extremely symptomatic patient with fatigue, cognitive impairment, anxiety, pain, palpitations. Blood looks like sludge around hydrogel/graphene/CDB filament. AM Medical.[61]

In April 2023, Clifford Carnicom and I presented preliminary data on further blood conductivity studies and correlations to iron oxidation of the hemoglobin molecule within red blood cells. This effort was to answer the question quantitatively and qualitatively regarding what has happened to humanity's blood. As a physician, I have seen unprecedented, accelerated aging in the unvaccinated over the last two years and the rate of illness is accelerating. In live blood analysis, I have seen hydrogel/graphene structures that transform the blood into severe rouleaux formation, making the blood almost unrecognizable and correlating with severity of symptoms. Of late, I have seen this in a more extreme form of toxicity, making live blood look like sludge.

Our preliminary results showing low electrical blood conductivity must be understood in the context of Clifford's work over three decades evaluating the findings of CDB, aka Morgellons. He began his studies in 2011, and more intensively in 2015, quantifying changes in blood conductivity and correlating iron oxidation status in hemoglobin molecules of the blood. Historically, the medical profession has dismissed CDB or Morgellons as delusionary parasitosis, marginalizing hundreds of thousands of individuals who had severe systemic symptoms of toxicity. However, CDB disease is not just a skin disease, but has affected all human beings in a silent way. These fibers have been found in the blood and tissue samples of everyone investigated. Covert biological and geoengineering warfare, I proclaim, is the source of these nanotechnology, synthetic biology fibers.

People affected have shown symptoms of chronic fatigue, which overlaps with current findings of what is called long COVID. This fatigue is a lack of energy, or life force, which is obviously hijacked by these nanotechnology, bio-disruptive weapons, causing diseases of aging, including cancer, by induction of lower tissue oxygenation and hence increased blood acidity.

During his early research, the question of iron oxidation came into the picture for Clifford. Blood requires iron to be in the primary state of Fe^{2+} to carry and deliver oxygen to tissues. The synthetic nanotechnology biological organism, CDB, oxidizes iron from its state of Fe^{2+} to Fe^{3+}, in which state it is no longer able to transport oxygen—thereby causing rouleaux formation.[62]

The loss and transfer of an electron is a transfer of energy. The body's function of oxygenation does not work when the iron is in its Fe^{3+} state. Iron must be in the Fe^{2+} state to carry oxygen, and in that state energy.

> Iron is one of the most common elements in the Earth's crust and forms a ready oxidation state. Bacteria use this as a source of energy and as a means of waste disposal… Iron metabolism is also a significant part of bacterial virulence… It has been established experimentally by injecting iron soluble compounds by chemical processes; these are then oxidized and excreted by a byproduct.
>
> Iron (Fe) has long been a recognized physiological requirement for life, yet for many organisms… its role extends well beyond that of a nutritional necessity. Fe (II) can function as an electron source for iron-oxidating microorganisms under both oxic and anoxic conditions and Fe (III) can function as a terminal acceptor under anoxic conditions for iron-reducing organisms.
>
> Given the role of free iron in creating DNA damage, it is unsurprising that bacteria have evolved methods to scavenge it… Despite the sophisticated biochemical and genetic strategies that can be brought to bear upon bacteria, we still know remarkably little about the physical mechanisms of iron transport, storage, and regulation and virtually nothing about iron trafficking and its insertion into metalloproteins.[63]

In 2015, Clifford first asked the question as to what iron oxidation means for the energy production of the body. The question was: "How much energy would we lose in the body in relation to how much oxidation of iron is observed?"

To find the answer, laboratory experiments were performed that show oxidation of iron. This was evaluated via:

1. Qualitative chemistry ferrous iron 2+ shows green staining.
2. Ferric iron 3+ shows yellow staining.

It was also evaluated via qualitative reagent-based ion testing.

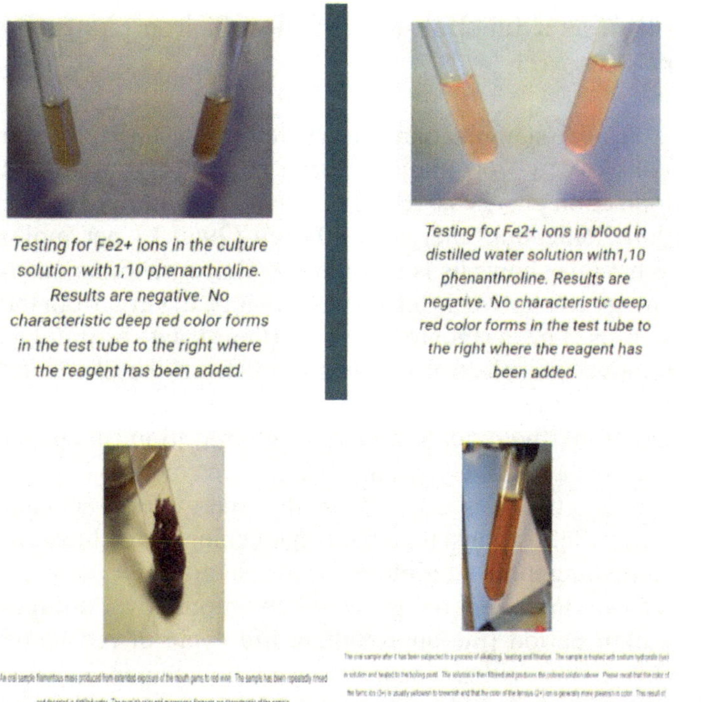

Figure 42. Testing for iron ions in culture solution. Carnicom Institute.[64]

Model calculations were based on how much energy is lost:

1. How much energy does it take to oxidize iron?
2. How much iron is in the body?
3. How much oxidation is taking place (is it variable)?
4. How much energy is in a human body in varying states of activity—sitting down, running, weightlifting, etc.?

The model estimates loss of energy as a function of iron oxidation. If iron oxidizes at a certain percentage, how much energy does the body lose? This energy loss is relative to basal metabolism as a function of oxidation of iron. As recorded in Clifford's research:

> The first ionization energy for iron is 7.9 electron volts (eV) (~760 kilojoules (kJ) per mole), the second ionization energy is 16.2 eV (1560 kJ per mole) and the third ionization energy is 30.6 ev (2960 kJ per mole) What this shows us is that it takes almost twice as much energy to remove the electron to change the iron from the ferrous (Fe2+) state to the ferric (Fe3+) state as it did to remove two electrons to change it from the elemental form to the Fe2+ state. From an energy standpoint, therefore, the oxidation of iron referred to in this paper requires a relatively strong energy investment.
>
> To get some sense of what this energy level actually means, let us translate what is happening in the blood to something more tangible for us to visualize. If we assume a 5% reduction in oxygenated hemoglobin over a three-month period (the approximate life cycle of red blood cells), this will translate to an energy requirement of approximately 3240 joules over this three-month period. [Humans have roughly 2.5E13 red blood cells; 280E6 molecules of hemoglobin in each red blood cell; 7E21 molecules of hemoglobin in each red blood cell; four heme molecules per red blood cell; approx. 2.8E22 Fe2+ iron atoms in the human body; at 5% oxidation 1.4E21 atoms in the Fe3+ state; .0023 moles of iron in the Fe3+ state, .0023(2960kJ/M – 1560kJ/M) = approx. 3260 joules over a three month period.][65]

Further calculations and documentation of experimental background can be found under: *Morgellons A Thesis.*[66]

Extensive studies on iron oxidation were performed in culture work and can be found at: *Carnicom Laboratory Notes.*[67]

The model formula determined was Energy Loss in % = 2.0 iron oxidation in % (approx.). Prior research and documentation of deduction and conclusions about formula can be found here: *Full Iron Oxidation/Energy Loss Model Calculations.*[68]

CLIFFORD CARNICOM PUBLICATIONS ON IRON

Iron - alkaline reaction	1	76
Iron - blood - energy - oxidation - investigations - studies	3	39
Iron - blood - ferrous - ferric - investigations	3	29
Iron - blood - oxidation - ligands - free radicals - respiratory inhibitors - summary	3	98
Iron - blood - oxidation - peroxide - sequence - free radical formation - assessments	2	283
Iron - blood investigations	14	4
Iron - CDB culture	18	251
Iron - chelation - lactoferrin - tranferrin - liver - amino acid - relationships - studies	3	159
Iron - chloride ion tests	1	80
Iron - culture growth	1	90
Iron - detection - culture - methods development	4	313
Iron - ferric - acidic - water - distinction - studies	4	219
Iron - ferric - ferrous - reductions - ascorbic acid - methods development	3	140
Iron - ferric - ferrous - reductions - ascorbic acid - methods development	3	142
Iron - ferric - ion - solution concentration - methods development	2	260
Iron - ferric hydroxide - studies	3	61
Iron - ferric state - detection - sulfur bonds - breaking	4	13

Figure 43. Index research lab notes show the number of papers (left column) and articles (right column) regarding iron studies. Carnicom Institute.[69]

We have a problem with low energy in the body in the post COVID era. What is different about our world three years later?

In 2023, in blood conductivity studies, the preliminary data presented was performed with reasonable efforts of standardization of the results, including calibration of the meter and concentration of the sample dilution. In N=13, all samples were over 65 years old. Samples were collected from both COVID 19 vaccinated and unvaccinated individuals.

Our samples had an 8 milli Siemens average blood conductivity ranging from 5.8 to 10.6 milli Siemens. Prior references to normal blood conductivity range from 10-20 milli Siemens.[70]

In our calculations, if we take the average blood conductivity at 15 milli Siemens, then our sample average has a decrease of 47%. This is an astonishing number.

If we are highly conservative and choose our reference range for normal blood conductivity at the low end of 10 milli

Siemens, our average is still 20% below normal blood conductivity values.

Given our previous calculations and modeling regarding iron oxidation, we would have an increase of iron oxidation of 23.5% for the high-end estimate, and a 10% increase in oxidation for our low-end estimate.

This demonstrates that there was no statistical difference between COVID 19 vaccinated and unvaccinated blood.

Of note, the lowest values of blood conductivity were obtained from individuals who were not on an intensive nutritional regimen with high doses of vitamin C and other nutrients to support their immune system. It is my concern that those who do not use high dose electron donors to alleviate some of the iron oxidation levels, may have blood conductivity values even lower than our calculated average of 8 milli Siemens.

In our good faith effort to quantify the loss of electrical blood conductivity in the post COVID 19 era and reference this with the extensive previous investigations looking at iron oxidation in blood samples, we have found in our most conservative measures at least a 20% decrease in blood conductivity, and in our modest range estimates a decrease of 47%. In our models this correlates with a 10% and 23.5% increase in iron oxidation.

One of the compounds able to reduce iron from an Fe^{3+} state to Fe^{2+} state is ascorbic acid or vitamin C. Clifford has conducted studies showing effective improvement in iron oxidation via vitamin C and other electron donors. I have been advocating for this therapy and performing it intravenously in conjunction with the mainstay of therapy I recommend, which is EDTA Chelation. At the same time, I recommend most ardent measures to minimize exposure to EMF frequencies like 5G and the use of cell phones, as the constant exposure clearly worsens these blood changes and makes the hydrogel/graphene/CDB filaments grow, sometimes a thousand times larger than a red blood cell.

EDTA is ethylenediaminetetraacetic acid and is a potent electron donor that creates stable bonds with toxic transition metals. Its molecular formula is C10H16N2O8C10H16N2O8.

EDTA has a pH value between −0.8 to 12. It is a hexadentate ligand, which means it has 6 lone pairs of electrons that participate in coordination bonding. When a metal reacts with one molecule of EDTA, it can form 6 valent coordination complexes. Metal ions have 4 bonds on oxygen atoms that are negatively charged and 2 bonds to a single electron pair on the nitrogen atom.[71,72]

EDTA has reliably reversed such severe blood changes, as I have described in multiple interviews and articles.

Blood Conductivity and Electrical Impedance Spectroscopy – A New Model for Estimated Human Power Loss Shows Cause for Alarm

JUNE 25, 2023[73]

Imagine if someone were to steal 5% of your life force from you. Would you be agreeable to that? What about 5% of the life force of all humans, would you sound the alarm? How about 10 to 25%? Even more?

Our mathematical model and repeated experiments show a result of such devastating consequences it has been stunning to us. In Clifford's plain words: **"5-10% loss is radical, but close to 50% is insane."**

I have been warning about the occurrence of sludge in the live blood of unvaccinated individuals. It's not rouleaux anymore, the blood looks like jello, and incapable of transporting oxygen. In this sludge (see below), many CDB/hydrogel filaments are seen:

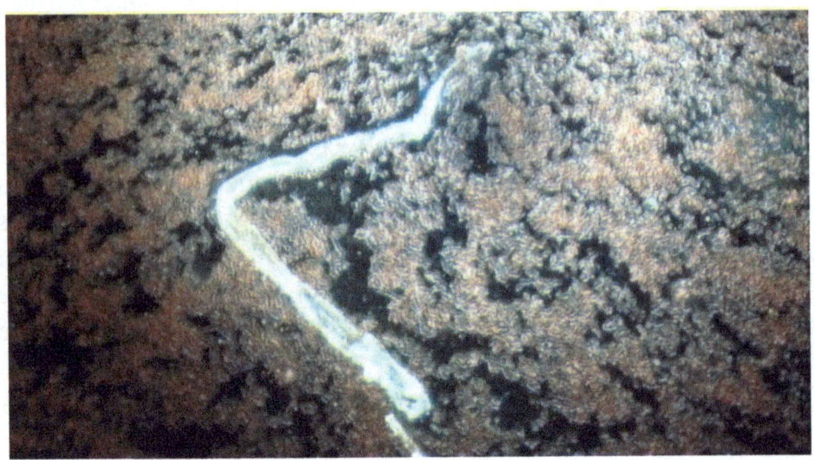

Figure 44. COVID 19 unvaccinated blood with classical CDB/hydrogel filaments. Blood has sludge-like appearance. AM Medical.[74]

I sent some of these sludge-like, COVID 19 unvaccinated blood samples to Clifford for testing of electrical conductivity. This revealed the lowest numbers yet of our samples: 4.8 milli Siemens (mS) with the normal range being between 10-20 mS. For our purposes, we chose 15 mS as a conservative average. Other numbers were 4.8, 6.4, 6.7, 7.1 mS respectively. This is highly concerning because I have seen the rate of contamination accelerate significantly in unvaccinated people who try to do what they can to limit exposure to COVID 19 injected individuals, environmental contamination, etc.

The interesting observation is that the sample of the most visibly coagulated blood had the lowest electrical conductivity of 4.8 mS, hence it appears that there is a correlation between increased blood coagulation and low electrical conductivity.

In this research update, we did not just measure electrical conductivity but also electrical impedance. Impedance is a field of more sophisticated measurement related to electrochemistry. The reason to expand the analysis is for the dual purpose of:

1. Showing people how affected they are by this, even if they think they are not.
2. To find measurable parameters to document if and how we are helping people reverse the problem.

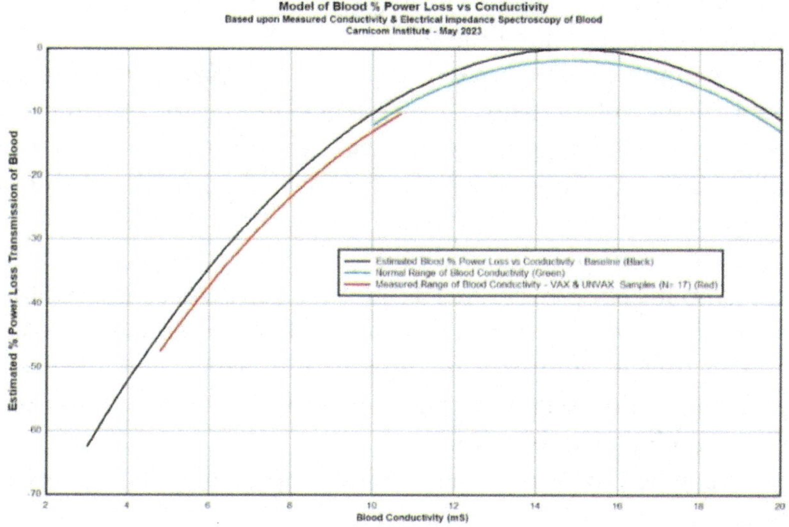

Figure 45. Model of blood power loss vs electrical conductivity based on measured conductivity and electrical impedance spectroscopy of blood. Carnicom Institute.[75]

Electrical impedance spectroscopy (EIS) can be understood with a comparison to the resonance of a radio antenna. As we can dial in to the resonant frequency of a radio antenna, we can also measure the resonance of a biological system. EIS looks at the response of a system over a range of alternating current (AC) frequencies. AC signals oscillate but DC signals do not; AC electricity dominates the modern world. Our equipment can vary the frequencies over a range of 1Hz to 25000Hz.

Blood, like everything in this material universe, has a resonant frequency. The point of maximum energy transfer occurs at the point of resonance. Resonance is a physical property in electricity. In biophysics, which I describe in my book *Light Medicine: A New Paradigm – The Science of Light, Spirit, and Longevity,* biphotonic coherence is equivalent to electrical resonance.[76] This means, in an optimal state, the system is operating with the most energy efficiency and therefore exhibits maximum health. Resonance occurs at a specific frequency, not a range.

The graph shown above (Figure 45), represents an empirical model of the relationship of efficiency in energy transfer and blood conductivity from which we extrapolate the effects on health. In our studies, we observed that coagulated blood reduces electrical conductivity and power/energy transfer to the biological system. If you study this graph, it shows that at 15 mS there is no loss of power. At 10 mS there is a 10% estimated loss of power. The model is based on multiple regression analysis.

The black line in the graph represents an idealized representation of what to expect for estimated blood and power loss vs conductivity baseline.

The green line represents blood operating at its normal range.

The red line represents 17 samples of COVID 19 vaccinated and unvaccinated blood showing significant loss of blood conductivity.

THIS IS WHERE OUR ALARM BELLS SHOULD GO OFF!

Again, we show even with conservative estimates that the power loss in both the vaccinated and unvaccinated is estimated on the order of 25-40% and is as low as 47%. Why?

Our question to the scientific community is this:

How could we see such conductivity and power loss numbers in people after the vaccine roll out and not call for an immediate, worldwide scientific investigation of these findings?

Blood Filament Growth Documented – CDB Extraction and Isolation

MAY 02, 2023[77]

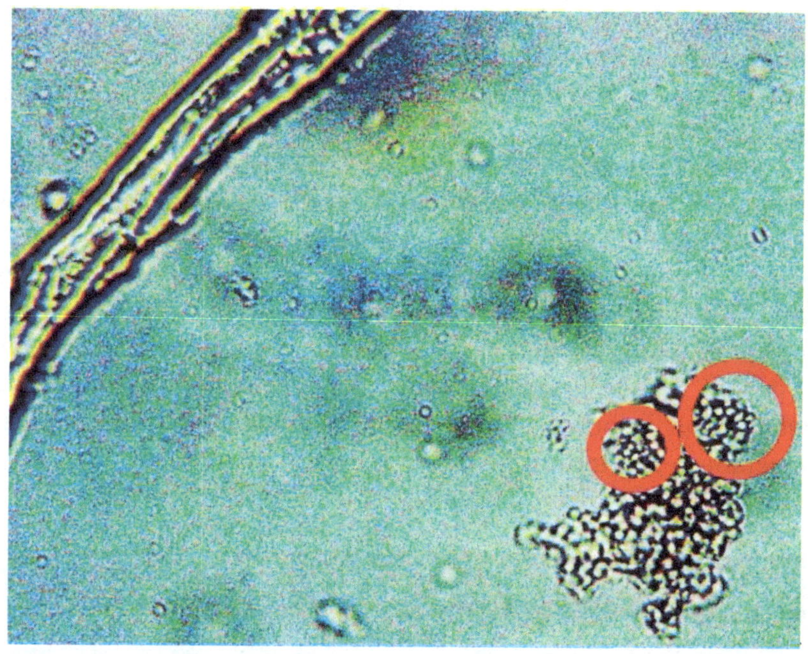

Figure 46. COVID 19 unvaccinated blood – CDB lower layer extraction after voltammetry, filament and CDB seen. Magnification 1600x. Carnicom Institute.[78]

Following voltammetry experiments (used to investigate electrochemical reactions), Clifford Carnicom and I continued our observations and replications of the transformation of unvaccinated blood via chronopotentiometry—applying low-level, constant electrical current-control to study the mass transport and electrode processes of the blood. Up to this point, we had documented five separate events in which filament growth in C19 unvaccinated blood was observed.

As described earlier, initially, unvaccinated blood showed no evidence of contamination upon microscopic evaluation. That experiment was then repeated utilizing voltammetry to confirm the profound effect of electrochemical transformation on blood and via chronopotentiometry to establish specific controls over current, voltage, and time. It also led, most importantly, to the development of a rapid and efficient CDB culturing method.

As explained in other papers, CDBs appear to be the origin of genesis of the filaments that were previously known as Morgellons. These are a synthetic, artificial, intelligent biology—combining complex biology and metals with features of all three domains of life: archaea, eucaryotes, and bacteria. Research teams around the world have called these filaments hydrogel, metals, graphene oxide, and even parasites. They have been found in human blood, meat, rainwater, masks, medical injectables, and more.

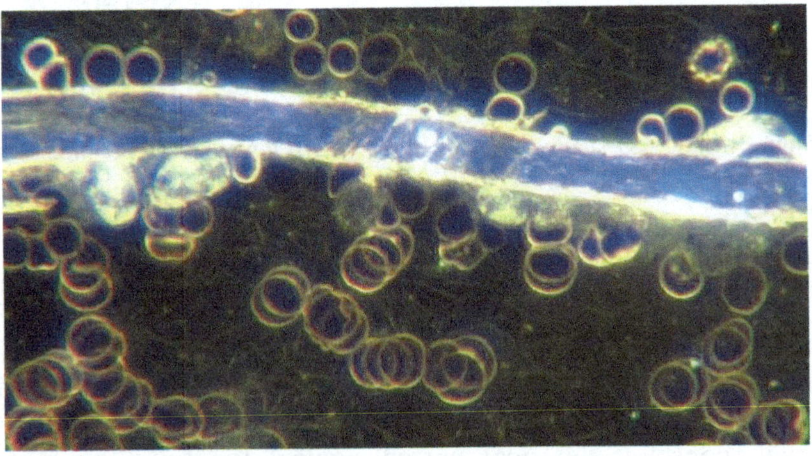

Figure 47. COVID 19 unvaccinated blood shows CDB synthetic biology filaments in live blood. AM Medical.[79]

Chemical Composition Analysis of Synthetic Biology Cross Domain Bacteria in Unvaccinated Blood

MAY 08, 2023[80]

Here we present the near infrared chemical analysis fingerprint of the Cross Domain Bacteria lower layer isolate found in both vaccinated and unvaccinated blood from which the filament structures grow. We have shown in previous studies that this CDB is the origin of the filaments seen in COVID 19 vaccinated and unvaccinated blood.

Three separate disciplines used to study this synthetic biology microorganism—near infrared (NIR) spectroscopy, inductively coupled plasma mass spectrometry (ICP MS), and electrochemical analysis—are entirely consistent. Chemical functional groups that can compose hydrogel polymer plastics were found in our samples—vinyl, polyamides, aromatic amines, polymeric alcohols. Aromatic functional groups have also been found. Graphene is aromatic; however, further studies are needed to determine if this is part of the CDB chemical composition. Halogens were detected via near infrared spectroscopy as well as in electrochemical analysis.

The CDB foreign protein analysis in historical toxicology studies reveals extreme toxicity to life forms.

Abnormal filament structures built from CDBs have been found in COVID 19 vaccinated and unvaccinated blood around the world. Clifford Carnicom and I have performed extensive research to identify the commonalities of Cross Domain Bacteria (aka Morgellons) and the post COVID 19 injection era nanotechnological and synthetic filaments now found in blood.

In this paper, we describe near infrared spectrum analysis on the lower layer of COVID 19 unvaccinated blood transformed and isolated by chronopotentiometry.

This method and our results were further explained in the article: *Replication of Electrical Transformation of COVID 19*

Unvaccinated Blood – Filament Growth Documented – CDB Extraction and Isolation.[81]

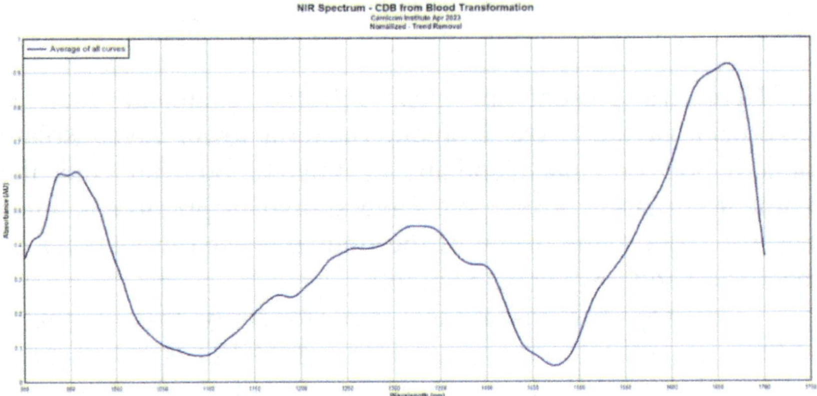

Figure 48. Near infrared spectrum analysis of the lower layer of CDB isolate from COVID 19 unvaccinated blood. Carnicom Institute.[82]

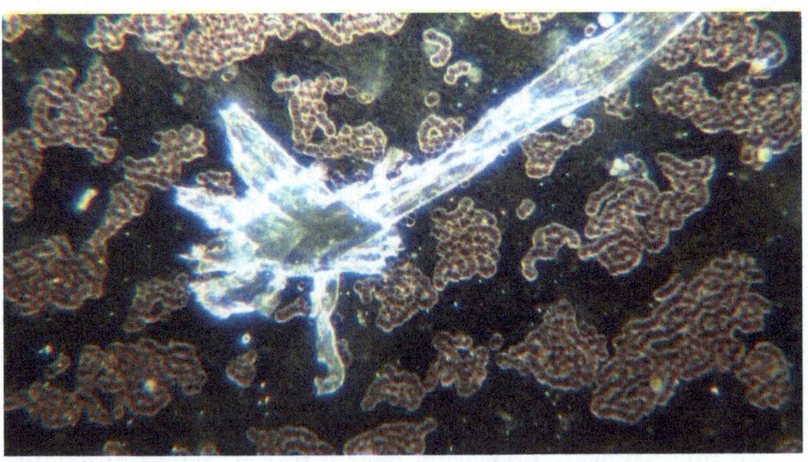

Figure 49. Live blood analysis showing CDB filament with rouleaux formation in COVID 19 unvaccinated blood. AM Medical.[83]

As discussed, the filaments seen in COVID 19 vaccinated and unvaccinated blood were shown to decrease electrical conductivity by up to 47%, while causing increased iron oxidation and decreased oxygen carrying capacity of the blood.

Additionally, the filaments were shown to grow under exposure to low-level electrical current. These filaments have been found in live blood, meat products, rainwater sprayed from geoengineering projects, medical supplies, and COVID 19 vaccine vials. In my research, I have shown the chemical similarities between environmental CDB filaments and COVID 19 Pfizer lipid nanoparticles.

In the chart below you will find the results from our NIR testing on the lower layer of CDB isolate from COVID 19 unvaccinated blood:

Functional Group	Summary Group	Reference Peak(nm)	Peak Measurement(nm)	Peak Rating (0.5(LO) - 3 (HI))	Delta (nm)(absolute value)	Rank by Weight
CH Methyl, CH3I (Methyl Iodine)	Methyl - Halogen	1661	1661	3	0	3.00
CH Methyl, CH3Cl (Methyl Chlorine)	Methyl - Halogen	1661	1661	3	0	3.00
Methylene, Aliphatic	Methylene	938	938	2	0	2.00
Vinyl & Vinylidene CH2=C(CH3)-CH=CH2	Vinyl	1630	1629	3	1	1.50
CH3 Methyl RC(CH3)3 or RCH(CH3)2	Methyl	1396	1397	2	1	1.00
Polyamide	Polyamide - NH	1515	1516	2	1	1.00
C-H Vinylidene ass. w/ (CH2=C<)	Vinyl	1631	1629	3	2	1.00
CH Methyl ROHCH3 Alcohol	Methyl - Alcohol	1664	1661	3	3	0.75
Alkenes, Polyenes	Alkenes, Polyenes	1170	1172	2	2	0.67
CH Methylene, Aliphatic Hydrocarbon	Methylene	1395	1397	2	2	0.67
Methyl CH3	Methyl	908	911	2	3	0.50
Aromatic Amine	Aromatic	1456	1455	1	1	0.50
CH Methyl Bromine CH3Br	Methyl - Halogen	1655	1661	3	6	0.43
Methyl Aliphatic CH3	Methyl	915	911	2	4	0.40
NH or NH2 Amide/Protein	Amide - Protein - NH	1520	1516	2	4	0.40
NH Secondary Amine as R-NH-R	Amide - Protein - NH	1520	1516	2	4	0.40
CH Methyl Nitro CH3NO2	Methyl	1654	1661	3	7	0.38
OH from Water		979	981	1	2	0.33
OH from Water		1453	1455	1	2	0.33
NH Amide Amide/Protein	Amide - Protein - NH	1570	1572	1	2	0.33
NH Bonded - Polyamide	Polyamide - NH	1570	1572	1	2	0.33
OH Alkyl Alcohol	Alchohol	962	956	2	6	0.29
CH Aromatic Alkyl	Aromatic	1671	1661	3	10	0.27
Si-O from Silicone	Silicone - Oxygen	1452	1455	1	3	0.25
Methylene CH2	Methylene	930	938	2	8	0.22
Polymeric Alcohol	Alcohol	1450	1455	1	5	0.17
Carbonyl Group	Carbonyl	1450	1455	1	5	0.17
OH from Tertiary Alcohols -C-OH	Alcohol	1006	1008	0.5	2	0.17
SH	Sulfur Hydrogen	1308	1326	3	18	0.16
Aliphatic Hydrocarbon CH	Methylene	1225	1233	1	8	0.11
SH	Sulfur Hydrogen	1270	1255	1	15	0.06
Akyl Aromatic ArCH	Aromatic	1130	1120	0.5	10	0.05

Figure 50. NIR chemical signature fingerprint of CDB lower layer in C19 unvaccinated blood. Carnicom Institute.[84]

The reference literature used in our NIR analysis was from Jerry Workman Jr. and Lois Weyers' *Practical Guide and Spectral Atlas for Interpretive Near Infrared Spectroscopy.*[85]

From a chemical standpoint, the above chart lists the functional groups that are tentatively identified within the CDB extracted lower layer. They can be understood as a fingerprint of the synthetic biology organism. Clifford provided the context for this data collection through his historical work on CDBs.[86] To better understand the significance of our findings, I provide a description of these materials according to their functional group categories:

Polyamides: Polyamides are macromolecular compounds having amide groups in the polymer backbone which form strong interchain hydrogen bonds that are responsible for the high strength and thermal stability of polyamides. Natural polyamides are proteins, such as wool and silk, while artificial are nylons, aramids, and sodium polyaspartate.
Vinyls: Vinyl is an alkenyl functional group found in allyls, acrylates and styrenics. It contains the hydrocarbon vinyl group (CH2=CH-) and can be made to polymerize to form polyvinyl compounds such as polyvinyl chloride. (These are plastics and hydrogel components).
Aromatic Amides: Aromatic amines are byproducts of manufacturing plastics, industrial chemicals, and other products such as iron, steel, dyes, pharmaceuticals, oil refining, personal household services, textile manufacturing, leather manufacturing, and rubber.
Polymeric Alcohols: Polyvinyl alcohol (PVA) is a synthetic biodegradable thermoplastic polymer (aka hydrogel or plastic).

All of the above can be used to create hydrogels.

Aromatic: Graphene has been shown to be aromatic as described in the paper: *Is Graphene Aromatic?*[87] Given the many questions around whether graphene is involved in the filament structure seen in live blood and COVID 19 vials, it would be imperative to do further chemical analysis.

Hydrocarbon Methyl and Methyl Groups: Methyl groups are extremely important to the body and vital for normal cell replication. They "turn on" or "turn off" genes. In Stage II they are used in liver detoxification, protein methylation, homocysteine metabolism (increasing methyl groups reduces inflammation), production of neurotransmitters, and nucleic acid synthesis—all need methyl groups. This poses the question: Is the CDB microbe stealing methyl groups from the body, hence causing accelerated aging, DNA damage, and disease?
Halogens (Methyl Iodine, Methyl Bromine, Methyl Chlorine): Exposure to halogens, such as chlorine or bromine, results in environmental and occupational hazard to the lung and other organs. In analysis of lower layer blood, the year prior, exactly as repeated for this paper, the same halogens as well as nitrogen and sulfur components were found via electrochemical analysis.[88]

The candidate chemical constituents listed below were found in the settled, lower layer of blood subjected to electrical current:

1. Halogens (Cl, Br)
2. Peroxide (H_20_2,oxidizer)
3. Phosphate compound (H3PO4)
4. Metals in ionic form (Ca, Fe, Mg, Al)
5. Hydrazoic Acid (HN_3)
6. Iron – cyanide complex [Fe (CN6)]
5. Metals in ionic form (Fe, Al, Mn)
6. Nitrogen & Sulfur compounds

It is important to note that we are always correlating findings of the blood CDB filaments with the environmental filaments that are being sprayed on humanity via geoengineering/bioengineering. The inductively coupled plasma mass spectrometry (ICP MS) of the environmental filaments showed similar minerals and metals as found in the lower layer of blood CDB isolate.[89]

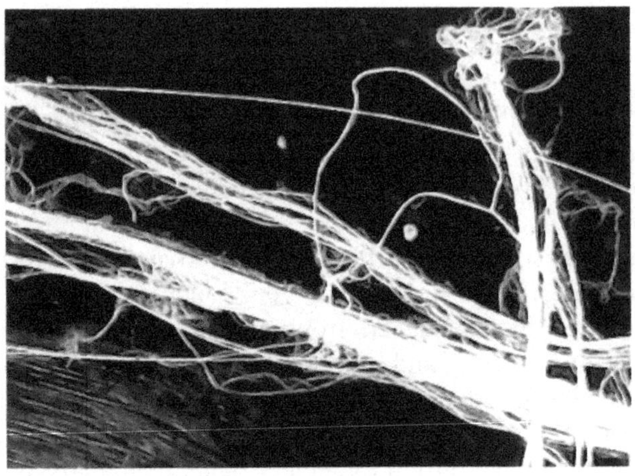

Figure 51. Environmental filament sent for laboratory metals testing. Carnicom Institute.[90]

Clifford and I reported a high-level consistency in our findings between this recent NIR study, and the electrochemical analysis conducted the previous year on COVID 19 unvaccinated blood samples and mass spectroscopy analysis of the environmental filaments.

All three analysis modalities confirmed chemical components of:

1. Halogens (chlorine, bromide, iodine)
2. Electrolytes and ions (sodium, calcium, magnesium, iron, manganese)
3. Nitrogen and sulfur compounds

Specifically, one can see overlap of calcium, iron, and magnesium levels in the environmental filaments and electrochemical analysis of CDBs isolated from blood.

White Filament

Analyte	Result	Reporting Limit	Units
Total Recoverable Metals			
Aluminum	12300	431	mg/kg
Antimony	ND	17.2	
Arsenic	ND	17.2	
Barium	150	34.5	
Beryllium	ND	8.6	
Boron	ND	86.2	
Cadmium	ND	17.2	
Calcium	12700	172	
Chromium	95.2	17.2	
Cobalt	ND	86.2	
Copper	95.6	34.5	
Iron	19800	34.5	
Lead	17.8	17.2	
Lithium	ND	34.5	
Magnesium	7800	86.2	
Manganese	619	17.2	
Molybdenum	ND	17.2	
Nickel	33.8	17.2	
Potassium	4800	345	
Selenium	ND	34.5	
Silver	ND	34.5	
Sodium	ND	345	
Strontium	ND	86.2	
Thallium	ND	34.5	
Thorium	ND	172	
Tin	ND	86.2	
Titanium	1230	86.2	
Vanadium	40.8	34.5	
Zinc	249	34.5	

Figure 52. Results of metals analysis of environmental filaments show heavy metals and other molecules present in red. Carnicom Institute.[91]

Please note: Toxic heavy metals have been removed from COVID 19 unvaccinated individuals via EDTA Chelation. Toxic undisclosed metals clearly compose an important element of this CDB synthetic biology sprayed upon humanity via geoengineering and administered via "vaccines."[92]

CDBs are foreign to the blood—these functional groups should be analyzed further for toxicity.

Toxic Metals; urine

TOXIC METALS					
		RESULT µg/g Creat	REFERENCE INTERVAL	WITHIN REFERENCE	OUTSIDE REFERENCE
Aluminum	(Al)	2200	< 25		
Antimony	(Sb)	0.40	< 0.18		
Arsenic	(As)	9.0	< 50		
Barium	(Ba)	74	< 5		
Beryllium	(Be)	<dl	< 0.01		
Bismuth	(Bi)	0.11	< 1		
Cadmium	(Cd)	1.1	< 0.9		
Cesium	(Cs)	15	< 10		
Gadolinium	(Gd)	12	< 0.8		
Lead	(Pb)	23	< 1.2		
Mercury	(Hg)	0.18	< 1.3		
Nickel	(Ni)	13	< 5		
Palladium	(Pd)	0.30	< 0.3		
Platinum	(Pt)	1.4	< 0.1		
Tellurium	(Te)	<dl	< 0.5		
Thallium	(Tl)	0.73	< 0.5		
Thorium	(Th)	0.23	< 0.02		
Tin	(Sn)	2.9	< 5		
Tungsten	(W)	1.2	< 0.4		
Uranium	(U)	0.58	< 0.03		

URINE CREATININE			
	RESULT	REFERENCE INTERVAL	-2SD -1SD MEAN +1SD +2SD
Creatinine	25.6	30 – 225	

Figure 53. COVID 19 unvaccinated individual 6-hour urine metals testing after 1500 mg EDTA Chelation. AM Medical.[93]

Clifford Carnicom has conducted extensive, historical toxicology work to show the poisonous nature of the protein manufactured by the CDB synthetic microorganism. In video footage, he shows the CDB protein applied to life forms like Paramecium that is killed, and beans and mustard seeds that are terminated in their growth.[94,95,96,97,98,99] What detrimental effect does it cause to humans? one should ask. Does this explain the extreme accelerated aging we are now seeing in humanity?

We have seen remarkable consistency in our findings and continue to sound the alarm as we bring more and more evidence of this synthetic biology infecting all of humanity. I now believe this is the platform for the artificial intelligence, synthetic biology, transhumanist agenda. We encourage researchers to repeat our findings and further quantify the toxic metabolic products of these synthetic organisms.

Synthetic Biology Cross Domain Bacteria NIR Fingerprint Match Found in Human Blood

MAY 14, 2023[100]

In previous articles we described the means of transforming blood via exposure to electrical current. That transformation results in the ability to rapidly and efficiently isolate the synthetic organism CDB, which we showed is the origin of the filaments seen in the blood of humanity.

We continue to draw the connections to the historical framework provided by Clifford Carnicom's research—which showed that the synthetic organism CBD, formerly called Morgellons, caused similar symptoms and blood manifestations as we see now in the post COVID 19 era. In the COVID era, in addition to the 25-year history of geoengineering/bioengineering, we have seen the compounded effects of alterations to the physical nature of the planet—all biology including human. The question is this: "Is there any similarity in chemical functional groups as known to exist in CDBs with current blood samples?" In other words, "Can we find the NIR spectral fingerprint of CDB in the blood?"

To answer this question, we looked at the data of the CBD near infrared chemical and biological spectrum from two groups of human blood samples, which contained five COVID 19 vaccinated and fourteen COVID 19 unvaccinated people.

For those unfamiliar with NIR spectroscopy, it is important to note that the magnitude of the graph is often less important than the shape of the graph. Variations in the shape of the graph mean response to energy, which is most important here. While the graphs look very different visually, when studying them in detailed analysis we found a 1:1 correlation. People might ask what the reference to normal blood is. We do not have the proper reference, since both vaccinated and unvaccinated blood are abnormal at this point; however, we are able to compare the two against each other.

In our most recent, groundbreaking paper: *Chemical Composition Analysis of Synthetic Biology Cross Domain Bacteria (CDB) aka Hydrogel/Graphene Filaments in Unvaccinated Blood,* we answered the question: "What is chemically in the CDB layer?"[101] Below I provide a list of the synthetic materials we found in unvaccinated blood as a result of our experiments.

Functional Group	Wavelength (nm)
Methyl Group	911+938
Alkenes, Polyenes	1172
Polymeric Alcohol	1451
NH or NH2 Amide/Protein/Polyamide	1520+1572
Methylene	1397+938
CH Methyl, CH3I (Methyl Iodine)	1661
CH Methyl, CH3Cl (Methyl Chlorine)	1661

Figure 54. Near infrared spectroscopy shows chemical signatures of polyenes (like polyethylene glycol), polyamide protein (nylon, silk, kevlar). Methyl groups were also found as well as methyl halides (iodine, chlorine). Carnicom Institute.[102]

Alkenes and polyenes were found in our chemical analysis. Alkenes can act as monomers in a polymerization reaction. Polyenes refer to the presence of several alkenes. They are used to make polymer plastics and hydrogels. The simplest alkenes are ethylene, propylene, and butene. Ethylene glycol is an alkene. **Polyethylene glycol is a component of the Pfizer COVID 19 lipid nanoparticles.** Polyene antimycotics, sometimes referred to as polyene antibiotics, are a class of antimicrobial polyene compounds that target fungi. Polyenes can bind to many protein membranes and other proteins specifically by binding to SH groups.

Butanal is an alkene. Butanal was a component of the environmental filaments analysis, as we reported on April 7, 2023.[103]

Polymeric alcohols, like polyvinyl alcohols also found in our live blood analysis, make plastics and hydrogels.

Polyamides are polymers that contain repeating amides. Proteins are examples of naturally occurring polyamides. Polyamides are prominent polymers that combine the stiffness and excellent thermal and mechanical properties of polyamides with the biocompatibility and biodegradability of polyesters. They are used for medical applications in drug delivery systems, hydrogels, non-viral gene carriers, smart materials, composites, adhesives, and especially as scaffolds for tissue engineering.

Polymers are essential building blocks of SYNTHETIC BIOLOGY AND TRANSHUMANISM.

Exposure to halogens, such as methyl iodine, chlorine or bromine, results in environmental and occupational hazard to the lung and other organs. As Figure 54 reveals, these too were found in our research.

Synthetic biology accounts for heterogeneous approaches toward minimal and even artificial life, the engineering of biochemical pathways on the organismic level, the modelling of molecular processes, and finally, the combination of synthetic with nature-derived materials and architectural concepts, such as a cellular membrane. Still, synthetic biology embraces interdisciplinary attempts intended to have a profound, scientific basis that enables the re-design of nature and composes architectures and processes utilizing man-made matter.[104]

Magnus Berggren, a professor of organic electronics at Linköping University, led a team that built a working electronic circuit from an ordinary garden rose by filling its veins with conductive polymer. Finally, they found one polymer that worked: PEDOT, or poly(3,4-ethylenedioxythiophene), a classical conducting polymer used in traditional electronics. The researchers soaked a garden rose, with its roots and leaves removed, in a solution of PEDOT. Over the course of a couple of days, the polymer was taken up by the plant's network of xylem and then solidified inside it as a gel. When they peeled away the outer bark and tissue at the bottom of the stem, the researchers could see slender dark wires winding through the rose.[105]

We have shown a 1:1 correlation between existence of functional chemical groups in CDBs and human blood. The spectral signature of functional groups indicating polymer hydrogels are repetitively identified. These functional groups can be found in COVID 19 injection lipid nanoparticles and historically in environmental filament chemical analysis. This is also in line with live blood analysis that currently shows filaments in both vaccinated and unvaccinated blood without any identifiable difference. In other words: NO SIGNIFICANT DIFFERENCE BETWEEN COVID 19 VACCINATED AND UNVACCINATED BLOOD IS IDENTIFIED AT THIS TIME.

We again call attention to the urgency of these results and express our concern about a potential human extinction level event.

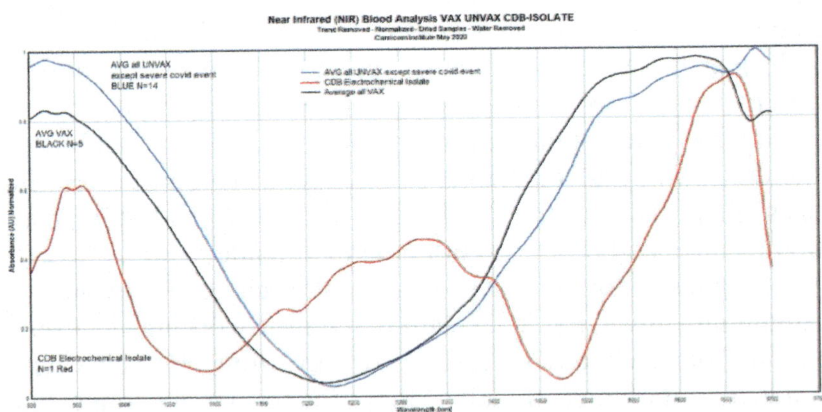

Figure 55. Cumulative NIR spectra. Red: CDB electrochemical isolate fingerprint. Black: Average NIR COVID 19 vaccinated blood. Blue: COVID 19 unvaccinated blood. Carnicom Institute.[106]

Prospective Difference Between COVID 19 Vaccinated and Unvaccinated Blood – Electromagnetic Observations, ELF Response, and Potassium Metabolism

JUNE 26, 2023[107]

We can no longer ignore the connections between the inclusion of extremely low frequency (ELF) electromagnetics and health problems we see in the post COVID 19 injection era.

Our Key Findings:

1. Potential variation in ELF response between COVID 19 vaccinated and unvaccinated blood.
2. Presence of a 4Hz ambient ELF field extensively documented over years that has been ignored in previous discussions.
3. Prediction based on physics and biophysics introduced to us by Dr. Robert Becker that establishes the foundation of ionic disturbances of the body with special emphasis on potassium as it relates to ELF fields.

In this research we compared five COVID 19 injected and five uninjected blood samples subjected to frequency ranges from 1Hz to 25000Hz. There is a disturbance in the ELF range between 2 to 6Hz, while the rest of the measurements seen in the graph below (Figure 56), are the same.

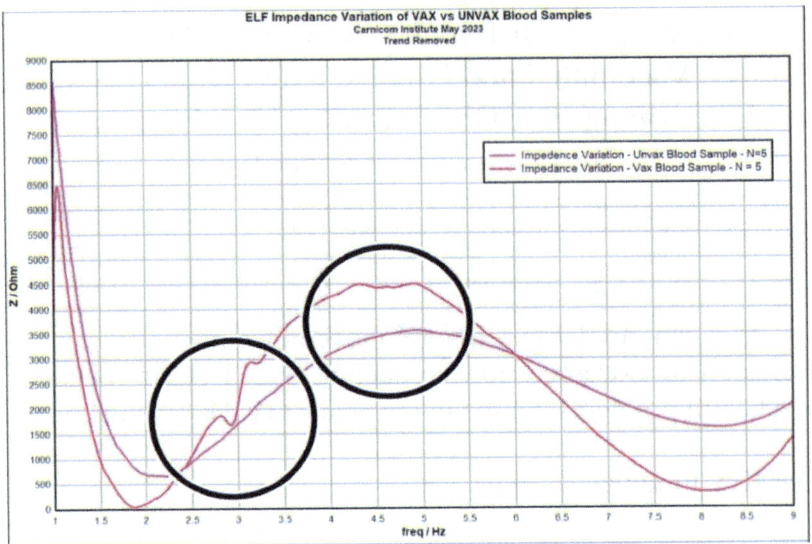

Figure 56. ELF impedance variation of COVID 19 vaccinated and unvaccinated blood samples show significant difference in the area of 4Hz. Carnicom Institute.[108]

This is the first documented prospective difference that is showing up between COVID 19 injected and uninjected blood. The impedance measured is the opposition to AC current.

In the Carnicom Institute research library, the historical discovery of the presence of a 4Hz ELF field has been documented. The lowest natural frequency on earth is the Schuman resonance, which is created due to the size of the Earth. Considering the extent of the Earth, this field is suspected to be artificially created. It is a difficult field to measure, as one can have massive interference with electrical infrastructure such as powerlines.

In his extensive archives, Clifford has documented the relationship and connection between ELF, satellites, HAARP, and aerosols. HAARP stands for High-frequency Active Auroral Research Program.

Over many years, Clifford has documented ELF activity in many areas of the United States.[109,110,111,112]

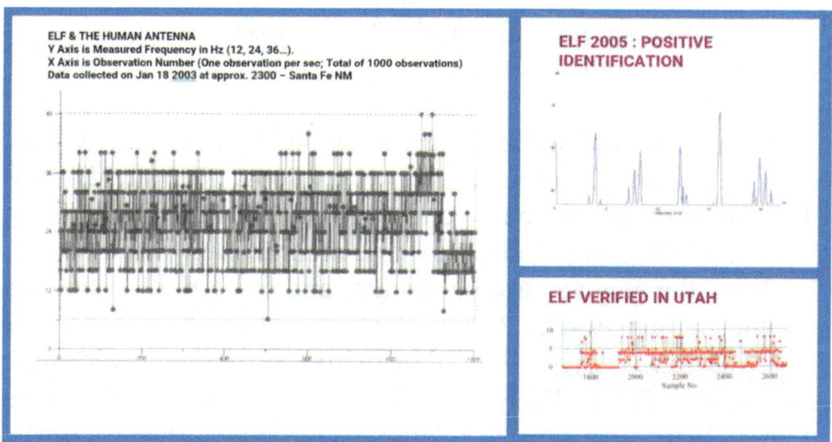

Figure 57. ELF measurements in Santa Fe, NM, and Utah. Carnicom Institute.[113]

At this time, the specific source, intent, and effect of these radiations remains unspecified. As a topic of interest, it is well documented within the HAARP literature that ELF production resulting from the pulsing of the ionosphere with high frequency radiation is an application of importance requiring further research. ELF propagation has the property of traversing extensive distances over the globe due to the extremely long wavelengths involved. Earth penetration and subsurface communication applications are also major uses of ELF propagation. The role of a modified atmosphere resulting from the introduction of massive amounts of electrically conductive particulate matter must be considered in conjunction with these disturbing findings.

Six significant effects or mechanisms of ELF radiation upon human health have been identified through initial research on this topic, including but not limited to:

1. Human mental functioning, influence, and control.
2. Disruption of cellular metabolism.
3. Suppression of the immune system.
4. Genetic modification and/or DNA effects.
5. Influence upon free radical formation.
6. Cyclotronic resonance.[114]

Our body and brain function in the ELF range. A long history documents the existence of a global ELF field, most likely of artificial source. We also know that ELF fields are at the core of affecting biophysical and mental brain processes.

Ions like magnesium, potassium, and calcium resonate at a specific frequency. Dr. Robert Becker, author of the book *The Body Electric,* gave the mathematics of the cyclotronic resonance with the 4Hz field.[115] If we combine the identification of an ambient 4Hz field in relation to ionic disturbances of the body, potassium is the closest resonance to 4Hz. Research regarding this potassium connection has been documented.[116]

Recent work indicates the very real possibility of sources interfering in the metabolism of the potassium ion within the human body. This interference is based upon the detection of continuous and apparently artificial ELF propagation at 4Hz multiples. The fifth harmonic of this radiation, detected at 20Hz, corresponds to the cyclotronic frequency of the potassium ion in the mid latitude ranges of the globe.

Medically, hyperkalemia (too much potassium in the blood) can cause life-threatening heart rhythm changes, or cardiac arrhythmias. It can also cause paralysis and weakness. Hypokalemia (low levels of potassium in the blood) can cause weakness, fatigue, muscle spasms, and cardiac arrythmia.

Why is there a variation between COVID 19 injected and uninjected blood in the ELF frequency range?

It appears that the COVID 19 injected samples are responding differently to ELF frequencies. This suggests an electromagnetic alteration of the body. It is popular to discuss 5G in relation the COVID 19 shots; however, ELF fields are global and of a lower frequency than the Schuman resonance, which means they are bigger than the earth.

Electromagnetics are involved in the transformation of the blood which we have repeatedly documented in our experiments.

Blood Clot Analysis from Living & Deceased Individuals Shows Consistent Findings: A Rubber-Like Polymerized Protein – Part I

JULY 10, 2023[117]

In this next, 3-part series, we describe our analysis of multiple blood clots and our preliminary results. More extensive experiments will be performed in the future.

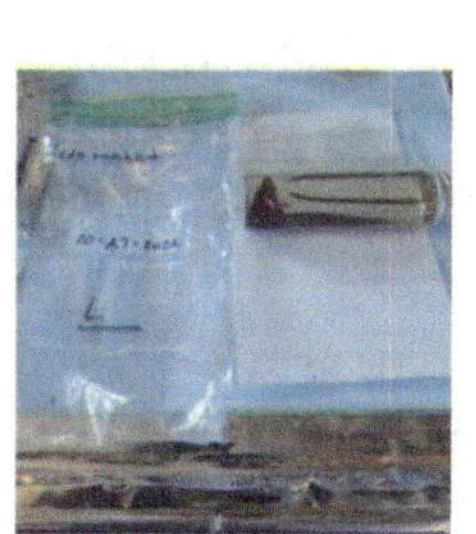

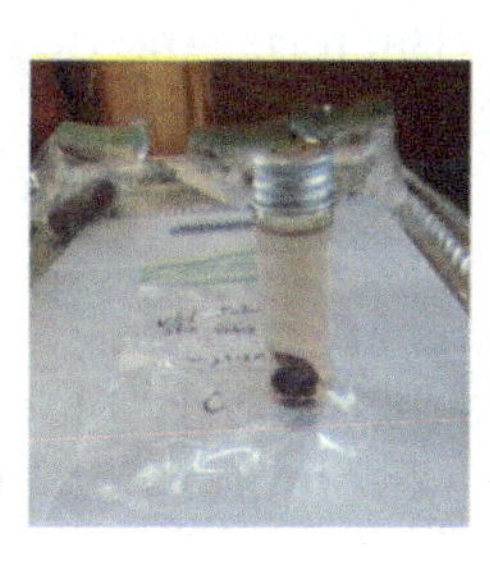

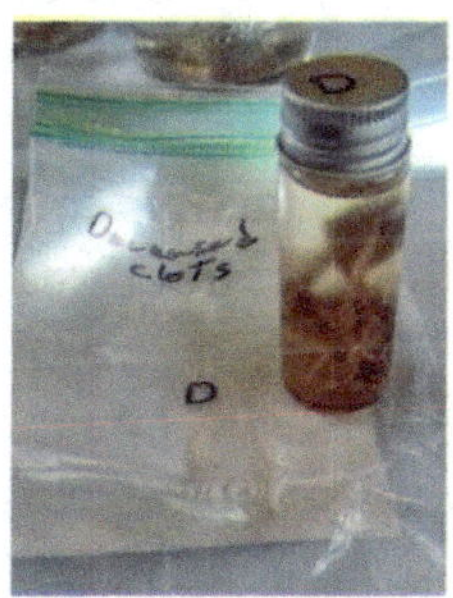

Figure 58. Clot samples analyzed. Left: COVID 19 unvaccinated living individual. Middle: COVID 19 vaccine injured living individual. Right: Rubbery clot from COVID 19 vaccinated deceased individual. AM Medical and Carnicom Institute.[118]

Deceased clots were received from the embalmer Richard Hirschman. A second clot was obtained from a living, COVID

19 vaccine injured individual. The third clot we tested was from a COVID 19 unvaccinated individual.

Upon a visual and textural inspection, the clots appeared to be made from a rubber-like material. Stray red blood cells surrounded the rubber-like clots. It appears, as Clifford Carnicom and I have shown before in the transformation of vaccinated and unvaccinated blood, that the blood is being used in this transformation process to create a polymer.

We then isolated the origin of genesis with the microscopic analysis of the three clots; all showed consistent findings. This is a very dense material, difficult to prepare for microscopy. Just imagine trying to take the eraser on a pencil and spreading it on a microscopy slide.

Our findings:

1. The filament structure is a 1:1 match to our previous findings as well as consistent with 30 years of research by Clifford Carnicom.
2. Cross Domain Bacteria, the origin of filament genesis are visible within these clots.
3. This appears to produce an amorphous protein structure.
4. Stray blood cells are present.
5. It appears that the rubbery clots are a more advanced and extreme evolution of the CDB/Morgellons filaments.

Below are some preliminary microscopy findings of the deceased clots. Further analysis is to follow.

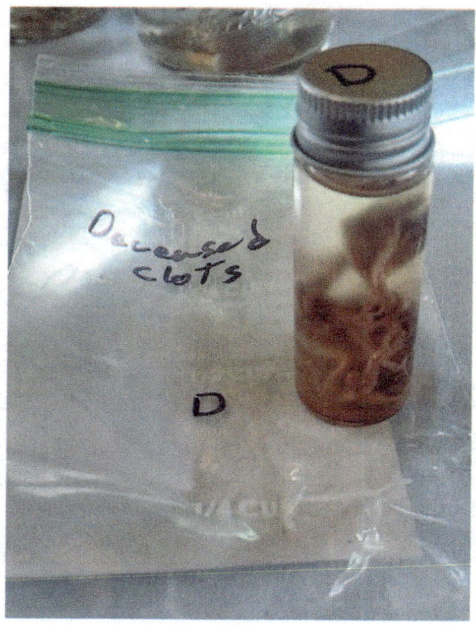

Figure 59. Rubbery clot sample received from embalmer Richard Hirschman. Carnicom Institute.[119]

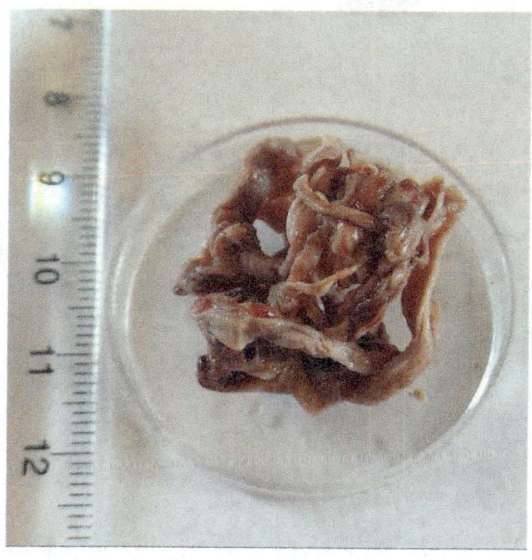

Figure 60. Rubbery clot sample received from embalmer Richard Hirschman. Carnicom Institute.[120]

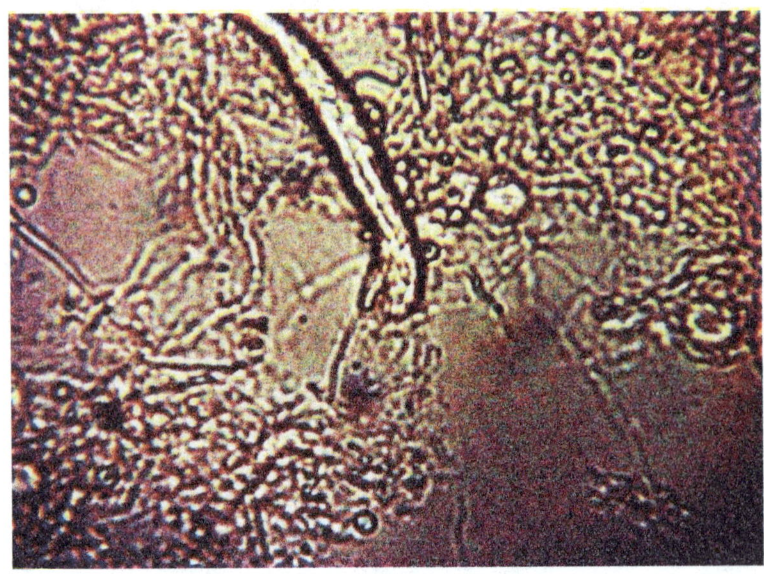

Figure 61. Rubbery clot sample received from embalmer Richard Hirschman. Magnification ~2000x. Carnicom Institute.[121]

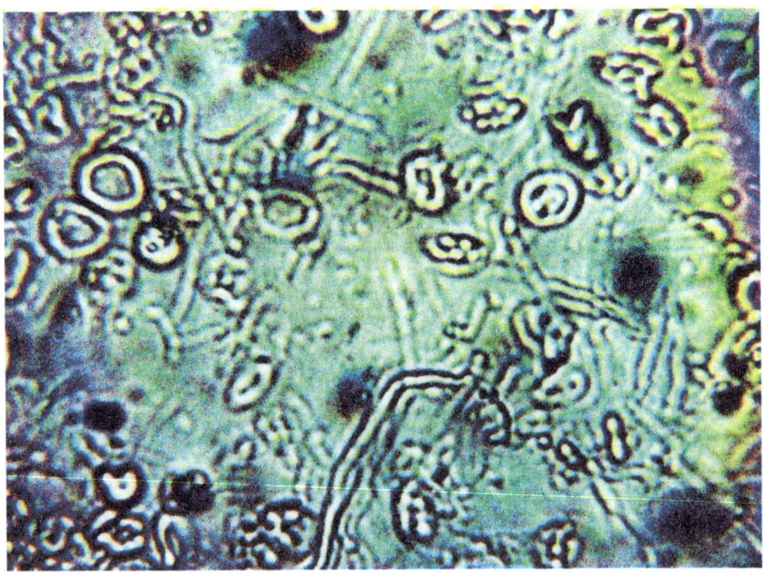

Figure 62. Deceased clot magnification ~2000x. Carnicom Institute.[122]

All three clots had the same structures within the vaccinated, unvaccinated, and deceased sources. The difference was that the deceased clot had the least amount of stray red blood cells. It appears that the polymer is using the blood as substrate for its growth, which is what we demonstrated in our transformation of the blood experiments with low-level electrical current, as shown in the images provided earlier.

Blood Clot Analysis from Living and Deceased Individuals Near Infrared Spectroscopy Shows Multiple Hydrogel Polymer Components – Part 2

JULY 10, 2023[123]

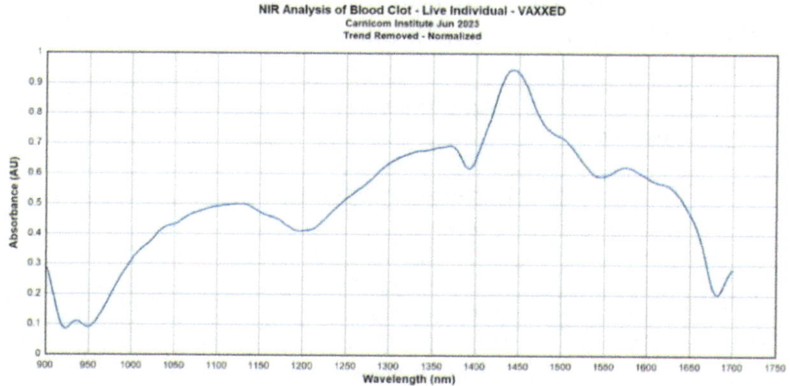

Figure 63. NIR spectroscopy of living, COVID 19 vaccinated blood clot. Carnicom Institute.[124]

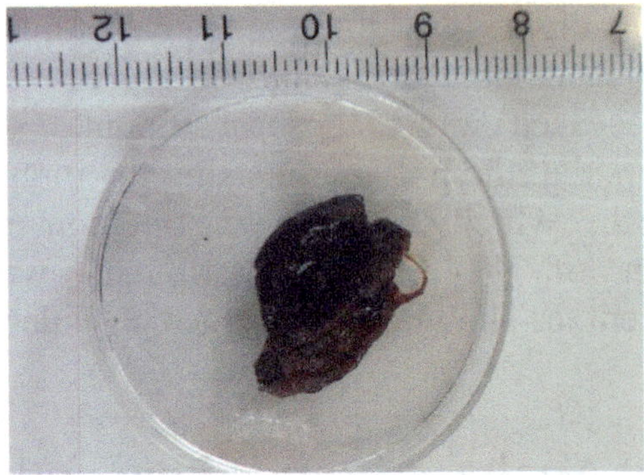

Figure 64. COVID 19 vaccinated blood clot, living. Carnicom Institute.[125]

In this progressive analysis of blood clots, we reported preliminary findings of near infrared spectroscopy (NIRS) of the three blood clots received: deceased individual, COVID 19 vaccinated individual, and COVID 19 unvaccinated individual. In the chart below you will find the results of our experiments that are entirely consistent with our previous work:

Nanometer	Functional Group
936	CH Methylene
1003	Primary Aromatic Amine
1006	Alcohol
1039	CH Methylene
1142	ARCH CH Aromatic
1170	CH Alkenes, Polyenes
1372	Methyl CH3 associated with Aromatic CH
1442	Primary Aromatic Amine
1441	Primary Aromatic Amine
1443	Primary Aromatic Amine
1445	Primary Aromatic Amine
1503	Primary Aromatic Amine
1574	Polyamide Amide protein
1628	Vinyl

Figure 65. Sample NIRS findings for COVID 19 vaccinated, living individual's clot. Spectral signatures of vinyl (polyvinyl alcohol), polyamides, and polyenes found. Carnicom Institute.[126]

The NIRS signatures on all three clots were consistent with the strongest signal for primary aromatic amines.[127]

Aromatic amines represent a category of chemical agents of considerable importance, as witnessed by their widespread use as intermediates in the manufacture of drugs, pesticides, and plastics; as antioxidants in the preparation of rubber for the manufacture of tires and cables; and as curing agents in the preparation of various plastics. In addition, they are widely used as intermediaries in the preparation of dyes and pigments extensively employed to color textiles, leathers, rubber, printing inks, paints, lacquers, metal finishes, plastic, and paper products, as well as in semi-permanent coloring products.

Recently I have shown that unvaccinated blood is manifesting extremely rapid changes, with findings consistent with polyacrylonitrile nanofiber mesh. Our chemical analysis is consistent with this possibility.

Clifford and I have also consistently found signatures of alkenes and polyenes. Polyethylene glycol falls into that category, used for the lipid nanoparticle encapsulation for the supposed mRNA in the COVID 19 shots.

One of the most important technical reactions of alkenes is their conversion to high molecular weight compounds or polymers.[128] A polymer is defined as a long-chain molecule with recurring structural units.

These are all building blocks of hydrogel. Vinyl is a functional group found in polyvinyl alcohol which is also a hydrogel building block.

Poly (vinyl alcohol) hydrogels have a long and successful history of applications in biomedicine. Historically, these matrices were developed to be nondegradable, limiting their utility to applications as permanent implants.[129]

Our findings continue to be entirely consistent and a warning to humanity.

Blood Clot Analysis from Living and Deceased Individuals – Preliminary Chemical Solubility Testing – Part 3

JULY 10, 2023[130]

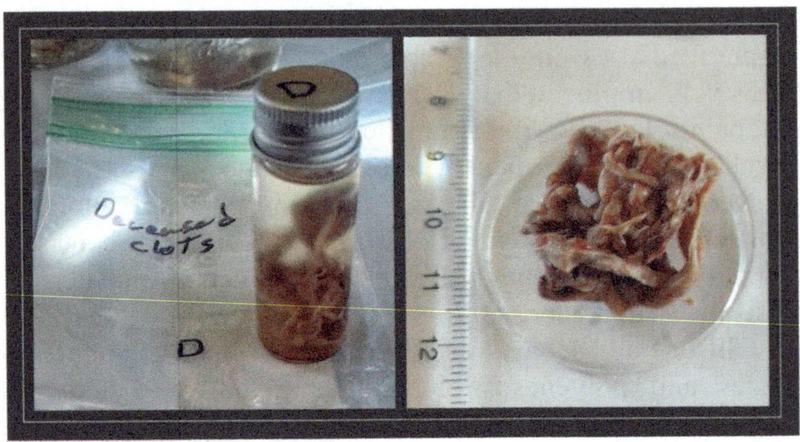

Figure 66. Clot from deceased individual. Carnicom Institute.[131]

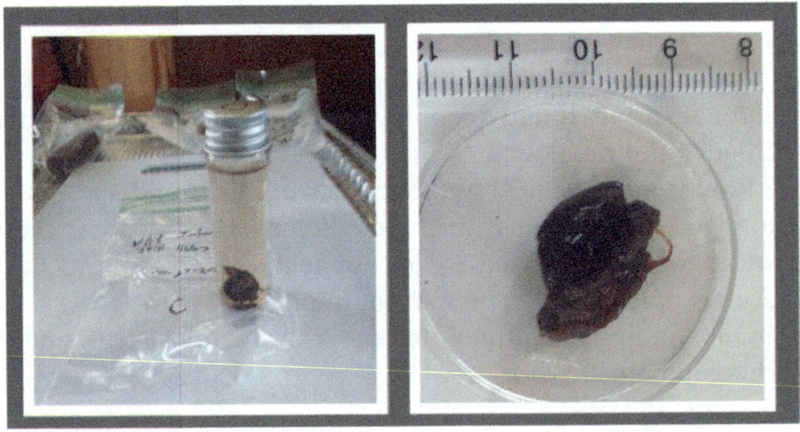

Figure 67. Clot from vaccine injured individual. Carnicom Institute.[132]

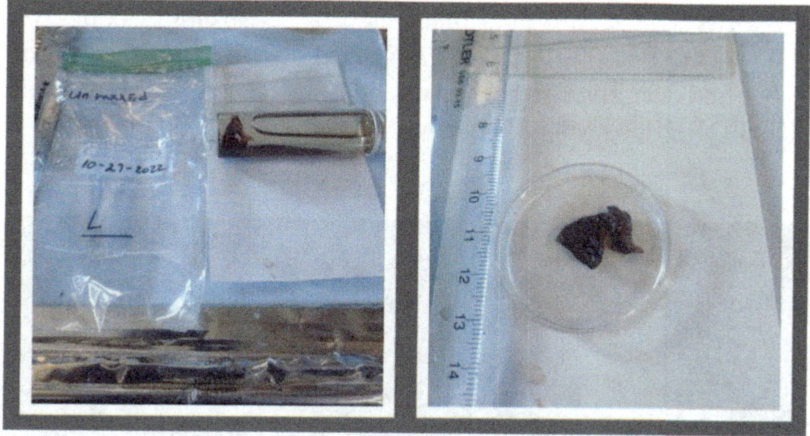

Figure 68. Clot from unvaccinated individual. Carnicom Institute.[133]

In this paper we show the preliminary data of clot solubility testing with different caustic chemical reagents. We have previously reported on microscopy and near infrared spectroscopy involving these same clot samples comparing a deceased individual and COVID 19 vaccinated and unvaccinated living individuals.

Because protein polymers are a rubber-like substance, we used the following reagents in our solubility testing:

1. Strong sulfuric acid
2. Strong sodium hydroxide (lye)
3. Acetone
4. Alcohol
5. Toluene
6. Methylene chloride (stripper)
7. Petrol
8. NN-diethyl-meta-toluamide (DEET)
9. PIB, PEA, PIBA (fuel injector cleaner)

WARNING: The solvents listed here are extremely dangerous AND TOXIC FOR HUMANS. These experiments are performed strictly for solubility testing. These substances are NOT FOR HUMAN CONSUMPTION.

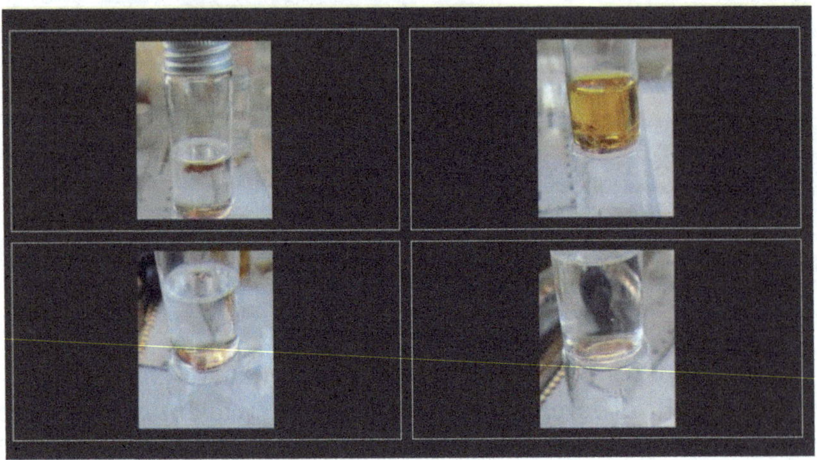

Figure 69. Clots in different reagents. Carnicom Institute.[134]

All of our solubility tests, except sodium hydroxide, failed completely within a window of 72 hours.

Sodium hydroxide (lye) shows the possibility of a slight reaction within the same time window; however, it is highly toxic and should NEVER be consumed by humans.

More exhaustive studies, especially in respect to time frames, will be conducted in the future.

In my medical assessment, it appears that we must do everything we can to prevent the biosynthetic materials from forming structure, rather than trying to dissolve these rubbery clots once they have assembled in the body.

Analysis of Symptomatic Health Findings in COVID 19 Unvaccinated Individual Shows Hydrogel Signatures Matching Deceased Clots and Complete Absence of Water

AUGUST 01, 2023[135]

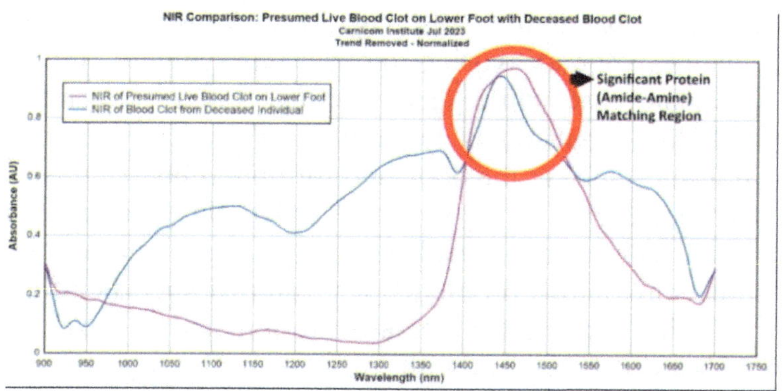

Figure 70. Comparison of NIR live blood clot (red) and deceased clot (blue). Match in the polyamide region (red circle) indicating same chemical. Carnicom Institute.[136]

In this particular research, we correlated clinical symptoms with NIR spectroscopy findings. Throughout this chapter, we have been discussing the correlation between the post COVID bioweapon era findings and the environmental geoengineering projects of synthetic biological spraying affecting people with Morgellons. We have shown, in previous experiments, chemical NIR functional grouping between deceased, unvaccinated, and vaccinated clot signatures. We have also identified extensive overlap in vaccinated and unvaccinated blood samples.

The Carnicom Institute Morgellons Research Project involved a questionnaire sent to 1000 people who were asked to describe any symptoms associated with Morgellons disease.[137] It became clear from this survey that people had every organ system involved. We have since found a huge overlap between COVID 19 vaccine injury, shedding, and long COVID symptoms with the suffering of Morgellons victims. In particular: chronic fatigue, brain fog, shortness of breath with mucus production, anxiety, blurry vision, ringing in the ears, headaches, circulatory problems and palpitations, joint stiffness, digestive problems, strange sensations under the skin, and more—all have shown significant overlap.

It seems that individuals with Morgellons who have had skin changes are endeavoring to expel this synthetic organism. We postulate that while these victims suffer tremendously, possibly this expulsion is favorable, rather than keeping the synthetic substance in the body and forming rubbery clots.

Here I describe a case report of a COVID 19 unvaccinated individual with several health manifestations, including lower extremity circulatory problems, a presumed superficial blood clot, a nonhealing painful ulcerative lesion, and an eczematous skin rash around the ears with intermittent drainage persisting for years. Several other chronic symptoms involving motile nerve, motile joint, motile lung, urinary blockage (filaments present), chronic hearing, thyroid cyst, blood conditions, and circulatory leg and feet issues are a part of the multi-decade symptom history of this individual.

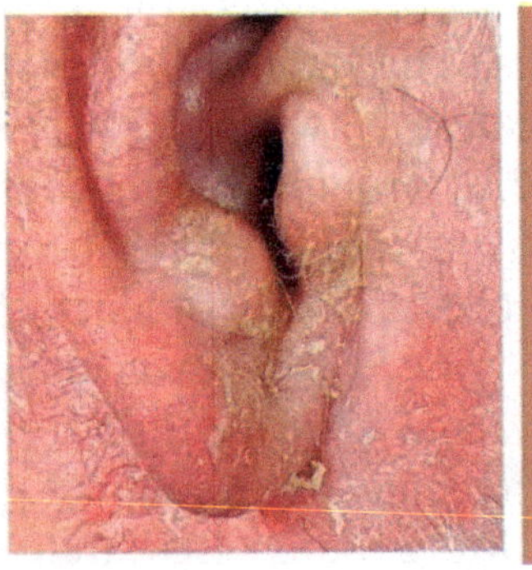

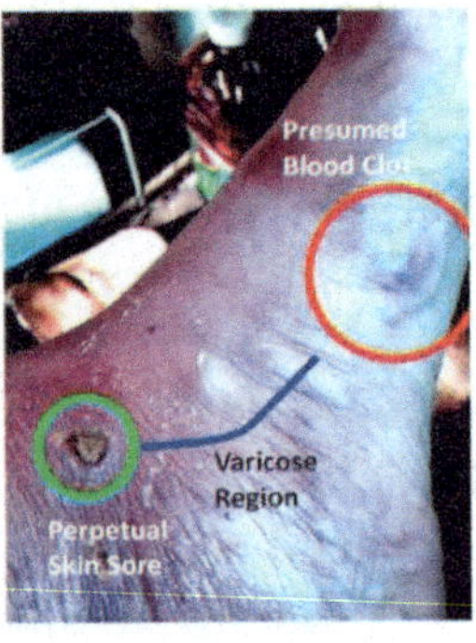

Figure 71. Scaly dry eczematous skin rash classically found in Morgellons victims and evidence of peripheral vascular disease with presumed blood clot and painful nonhealing skin ulcer. Carnicom Institute.[138]

These symptoms have been described in people affected with Morgellons/Cross Domain Bacteria. The affected individual's live blood analysis looked seemingly normal. However, when applying a low-level electrical current, the blood transformed into a CDB filament network.[139]

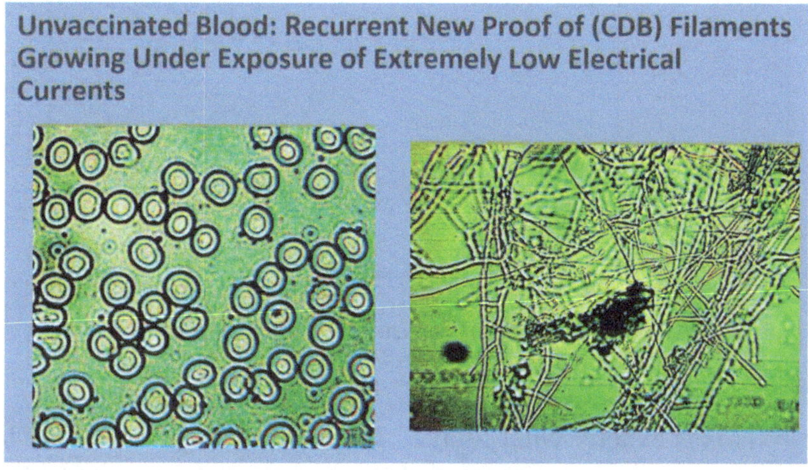

Figure 72. Left: COVID 19 unvaccinated blood. Right: Same blood exposed to low-level electrical current for 2 hours. Carnicom Institute.[140]

Clifford and I have shown that these CDB filaments express chemical functional groups of hydrogel, including alkenes and polyenes, which is what polyethylene glycol is (the component of lipid nanoparticle technology found in COVID 19 shots), polyamides, and polyvinyl—all constitute signatures of inorganic hydrogels.[141] By utilizing near infrared spectroscopy, we can now analyze many different tissues and materials and look for chemical matches.

First, with the individual mentioned above, we analyzed the affected skin adjacent to the leg ulcer and found dominant methyl groups, polyamides, and the lack of water. This is highly significant, since polymer hydrogels use the substrate of the cells to create a rubbery clot devoid of cells.

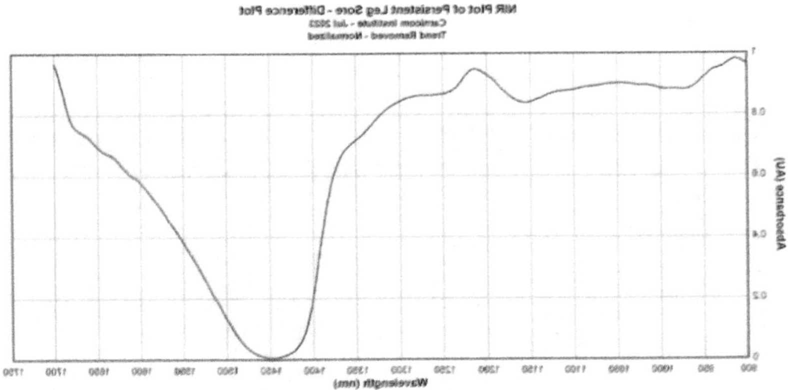

Figure 73. NIR difference plot of persistent leg sore. Carnicom Institute.[142]

This is exactly what I have been documenting via darkfield microscopy in unvaccinated live blood, showing how the substrate of the blood is being used to create hydrogel clots.[143] We have shown, via NIR spectroscopy, that these synthetic CDB filaments steal methyl groups from the body.

Second, we compared the region that appeared to have a superficial blood clot on the leg with the chemical signatures of the deceased rubbery clot received from Richard Hirschman. We found a significant match in the amide-amine protein region. You can see this plotted above in Figure 73. This is significant, because amide-amine cross-linked hydrogels made from polyethylene glycol are described in the literature.[144]

Within that literature, a new method for the rapid preparation of chemically cross-linked hydrogels, based on a multi-arm polyethylene glycol (PEG) bearing potassium acyl trifluoroborate (KAT) functional groups with multi-dentate amines, is described. These scaffolds, prepared in aqueous buffer, give strong, transparent hydrogels.

These findings have also been confirmed by the analysis of Dr. Hildegarde Staninger, who discovered a brain chip in a meningioma, as well as nanotechnological devices in nasal passages.[145] Dr. Staninger documented long-chain polyamide polymers, confirming our findings. She also validated our discoveries of halogen, polyethylene glycol (polyene), and silicone via Raman spectroscopy, Micro-Fourier transform infrared (FTIR) spectroscopy, scanning electron microscopy (SEM), and energy-dispersive X-ray spectroscopy (EDS) findings. These are non-destructive analytical techniques used for the study of microscale chemical composition. All of Dr. Staninger's analyses match our findings.

Below is a chart of our original NIR work on CDB isolate from COVID 19 unvaccinated blood:

Functional Group	Summary Group	Reference Peak(nm)	Peak Measurement(nm)	Peak Rating (0.5(LO) - 3 (HI))	Delta (nm)(absolute value)	Rank by Weight
CH Methyl, CH3I (Methyl Iodine)	Methyl - Halogen	1661	1661	3	0	3.00
CH Methyl, CH3Cl (Methyl Chlorine)	Methyl - Halogen	1661	1661	3	0	3.00
Methylene, Aliphatic	Methylene	938	938	2	0	2.00
Vinyl & Vinylidene CH2=C(CH3)-CH=CH2	Vinyl	1630	1629	3	1	1.50
CH3 Methyl RC(CH3)3 or RCH(CH3)2	Methyl	1396	1397	2	1	1.00
Polyamide	Polyamide - NH	1515	1516	2	1	1.00
C-H Vinylidene ass. w/ (CH2=C<)	Vinyl	1631	1629	3	2	1.00
CH Methyl ROHCH3 Alcohol	Methyl - Alcohol	1664	1661	3	3	0.75
Alkenes, Polyenes	Alkenes, Polyenes	1170	1172	2	2	0.67
CH Methylene, Aliphatic Hydrocarbon	Methylene	1395	1397	2	2	0.67
Methyl CH3	Methyl	908	911	2	3	0.50
Aromatic Amine	Aromatic	1456	1455	1	1	0.50
CH Methyl Bromine CH3Br	Methyl - Halogen	1655	1661	3	6	0.43
Methyl Aliphatic CH3	Methyl	915	911	2	4	0.40
NH or NH2 Amide/Protein	Amide - Protein - NH	1520	1516	2	4	0.40
NH Secondary Amine as R-NH-R	Amide - Protein - NH	1520	1516	2	4	0.40
CH Methyl Nitro CH3NO2	Methyl	1654	1661	3	7	0.38
OH from Water		979	981	1	2	0.33
OH from Water		1453	1455	1	2	0.33
NH Amide Amide/Protein	Amide - Protein - NH	1570	1572	1	2	0.33
NH Bonded - Polyamide	Polyamide - NH	1570	1572	1	2	0.33
OH Alkyl Alcohol	Alchohol	962	956	2	6	0.29
CH Aromatic Alkyl	Aromatic	1671	1661	3	10	0.27
Si-O from Silicone	Silicone - Oxygen	1452	1455	1	3	0.25
Methylene CH2	Methylene	930	938	2	8	0.22
Polymeric Alcohol	Alcohol	1450	1455	1	5	0.17
Carbonyl Group	Carbonyl	1450	1455	1	5	0.17
OH from Tertiary Alcohols -C-OH	Alcohol	1006	1008	0.5	2	0.17
SH	Sulfur Hydrogen	1308	1326	3	18	0.16
Aliphatic Hydrocarbon CH	Methylene	1225	1233	1	8	0.11
SH	Sulfur Hydrogen	1270	1255	1	15	0.06
Akyl Aromatic ArCH	Aromatic	1130	1120	0.5	10	0.05

Figure 74. NIR spectroscopy of CDB isolate of COVID 19 unvaccinated blood. Polyamides, vinyl, polyenes (like polyethylene glycol), silicone, and methyl groups found. Dr. Ana Mihalcea and Clifford Carnicom.[146]

Clifford and I performed near infrared spectroscopy on healthy adjacent skin and the persistent leg ulcer mentioned above and created a difference plot. This was to analyze the chemical difference between the two. The results, yet again, revealed methyl groups and the lack of absorbance at 1450 nm—showing the complete absence of water in the tissue.

The skin adjacent to the leg ulcer showed dominant NIR signatures of polyamines, vinyl (polyvinyl alcohol, a hydrogel plastic), and alkenes (such as polyethylene glycol).

The NIR spectroscopy of the skin affected around the ear again showed the complete lack of water—you can see the huge dip at 1450 nm in the graph below. The skin had literally become like plastic, a very painful condition as Morgellons victims can attest. There no longer is healthy skin function due to this complete lack of water.

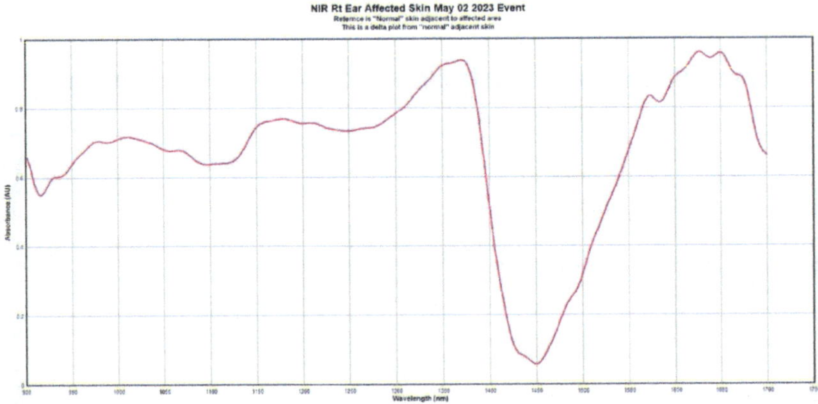

Figure 75. NIR of right ear skin. Carnicom Institute.[147]

In summary, we analyzed a COVID 19 unvaccinated individual with seemingly normal live blood analysis upon visual inspection; however, significant transformation of the blood became apparent under low-level electrical current. And we found an NIR signature match between the superficial blood clot in a living person and a deceased rubbery clot that showed hydrogel polyamine protein polymer. This again provides proof of previous analysis comparing a deceased rubbery clot with COVID 19 vaccinated and unvaccinated clots.[148,149,150]

We also analyzed skin abnormalities expressed as an eczematous rash that showed a complete lack of water, as well as adjacent polyamide hydrogel signatures—which is how polymer hydrogels self-assemble in human tissue, thereby replacing healthy tissue. These findings are entirely consistent with all our previous research.

The Danger in the Air – Rainwater Analysis Research by Dr. Geanina Hagimă Shows Magnetic Nanoparticles and Filaments

AUGUST 21, 2023[151]

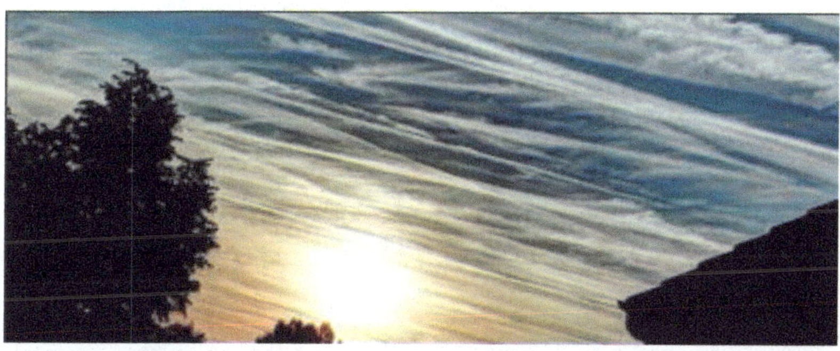

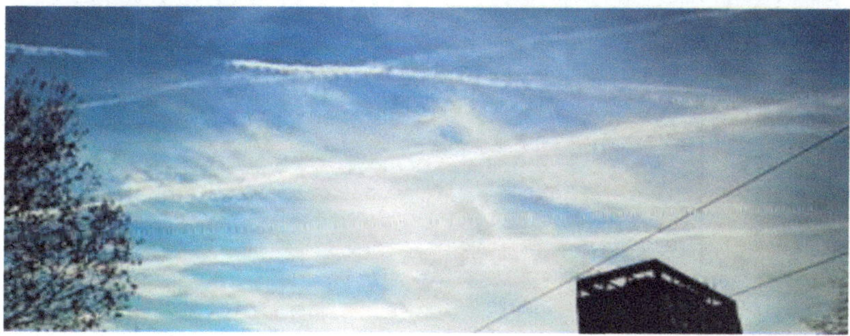

Figure 76. Chemtrails in the sky. Dr. Geanina Hagimă.[152]

My Romanian colleague, Dr. Geanina Hagimă, emailed me in early summer, 2023, regarding her findings of magnetic nanoparticles in rainwater. She published her findings through *ActiveNews* in Romania.[153]

In a video recording, Dr. Hagimă captured rainwater and showed how the particulate matter was magnetic.[154] This needs to be considered, as we know that many people after a COVID 19 bioweapon injection have become magnetic. This may also be accelerated by inhaling magnetic smart dust.

The laboratory analysis of Dr. Hagimă's rainwater sediment showed barium, strontium, aluminum, iron, copper, zinc, calcium, nickel, and arsenic.

Elemente		Concentratii*
Minerale [mg/L]	Na	1.824
	Mg	0.584
	K	0.530
	Ca	2.271
Metale grele [µg/L]	Al	**20.554**
	Cr	0.089
	Mn	0.795
	Fe	**11.392**
	Co	0.020
	Ni	2.551
	Cu	5.101
	Zn	**5.516**
Metale toxice [µg/L]	As	**0.111**
	Cd	**<0.001**
	Sn	0.0012
	Hg	**<0.001**
	Pb	0.177
Pamanturi rare [µg/L]	Sc	<0.001
	La	0.006
	Ce	0.017
	Pr	0.003
	Nd	<0.001
	Sm	<0.001
	Eu	0.001
	Gd	<0.001
	Tb	0.001
	Dy	<0.001
	Ho	<0.001
	Er	<0.001
	Tm	<0.001
	Yb	<0.001
	Lu	0.0001
Elemente critic tehnologice [µg/L]	Te	<0.001
	Ge	<0.001
	Ga	0.010
	In	0.033
	Nb	0.022
	Ta	0.0017
Elemente din grupa platinei [µg/L]	Pt	<0.001
	Pd	<0.001
	Os	<0.001
	Ir	<0.001
	Ru	<0.001
Metale alcaline, alcalino-pamantoase [µg/L]	Li	**0.206**
	Cs	**<0.001**
	Rb	<0.001
	Be	0.111
	Ba	**3.732**
	Sr	**4.757**
Metale de tranzitie, post-tranzitie [µg/L]	Zr	<0.001
	Hf	<0.001
	W	0.032
	Au	0.003
	Ag	**<0.001**
	Re	<0.001
	Ti	3.169
	V	0.186
	Mo	<0.001
	Bi	0.040
	Tl	<0.001

Figure 77. Metals analysis of rainwater shows many elements including toxic metals such as aluminum, barium, and strontium. Dr. Geanina Hagimă.[155]

Dr. Hagimă knew that graphene oxide was magnetic, and she wanted to see if this was in rainwater. She then conducted electron microscopy and energy-dispersive x-ray spectroscopy on the sample. Her research revealed fibers containing carbon, silicon, aluminum, and iron. She deducted that these are carbon silicon nanotubes, as described in her articles published on my Substack.[156,157,158]

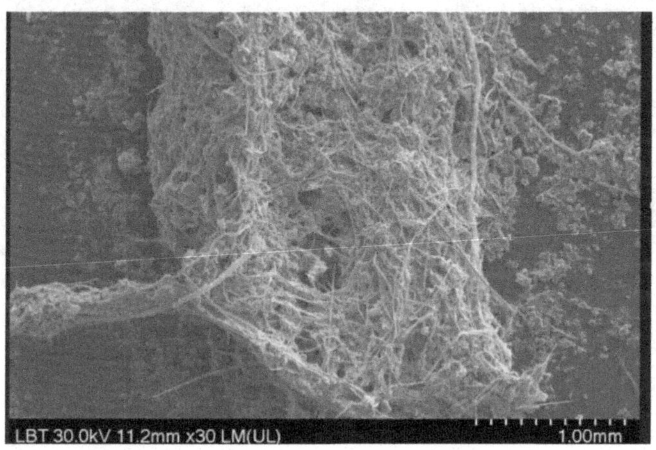

Figure 78. Electron microscopy shows filaments in rainwater. Dr. Geanina Hagimă.[159]

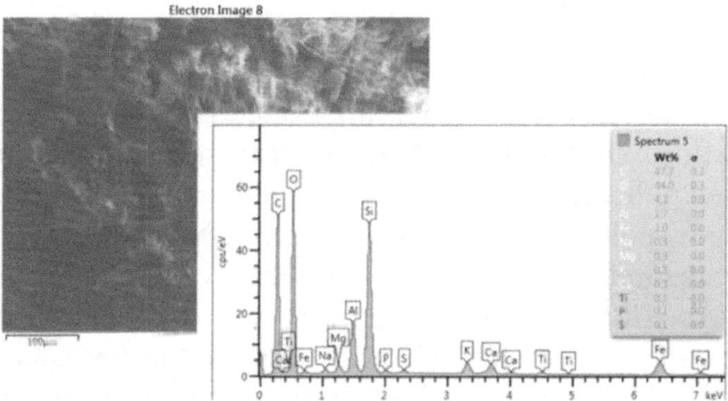

Figure 79. Mass spectroscopy of filaments shows multiple elements including titanium, aluminum, silicone, and iron. Dr. Geanina Hagimă.[160]

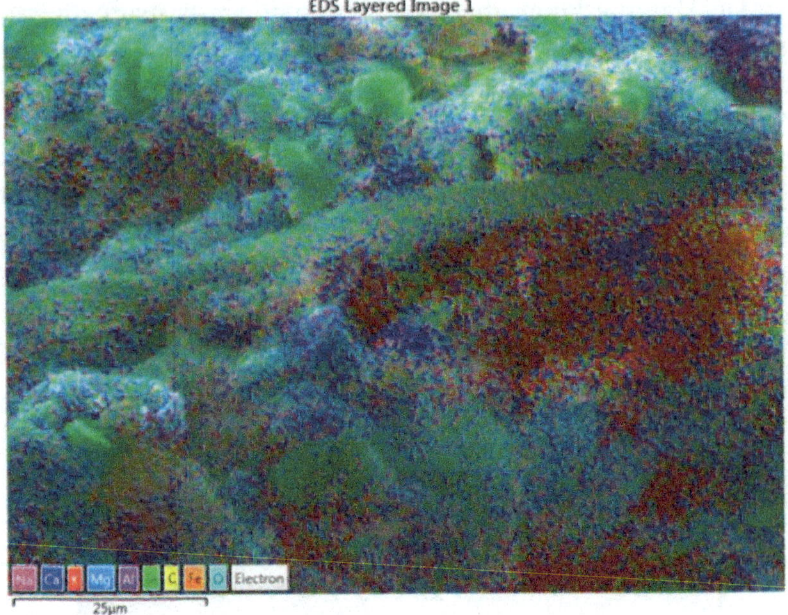

Figure 80. Energy-dispersive X-ray spectroscopy rainwater sample. Dr. Geanina Hagimă.[161]

Dr. Hagimă explains that these silicon carbon fibers contribute to sickening of the population causing respiratory problems and cancers.

I sent Dr. Hagimă's research to Clifford Carnicom since he had also done work on rainwater analysis. He found her results entirely consistent with his research since 1998.

Clifford shared these thoughts with me: "Metals are not supposed to be in rainwater in any significant amounts. But our rain is now polluted so that they are there. None of these metals should theoretically be there, but theory is another matter nowadays. There are some expectations of differences between rural and urban locations, this is an important factor. Cambridge University published books on atmospheric chemistry of rainwater, rural areas should be pretty much clean as a whistle. Urban areas will have some expected pollution, but never anything justified with these metals, such as aluminum, iron, calcium, silicon (metalloid), magnesium, etc. However, none of these findings are any surprise to me. I have found them in my own work years ago."

Below are some of Clifford's findings:

Element	Measured Mean Redox Voltage (Absolute Value)	Actual Redox Voltage (Absolute Value)
Titanium (Ti)	1.63, 1.32, 1.24	1.63, 1.31, 1.23
Aluminum (Al)	1.67	1.66
Barium (Ba)	2.90	2.90
Strontium (Sr)	2.90	2.89
Magnesium (Mg)	2.66, 2.35	2.68, 2.37
Gallium (Ga)	.52, .65	.56, .65
Scandium (Sc)	2.56, 2.09	2.60, 2.08
Zirconium (Zr)	1.45	1.43

Standard Error of Measurement 0.013 V; n = 15
(No information regarding concentration or concentration ranking is provided here)

Figure 81. The demise of rainwater, 2016. Analyzed metals content of rainwater. Carnicom Institute.[162]

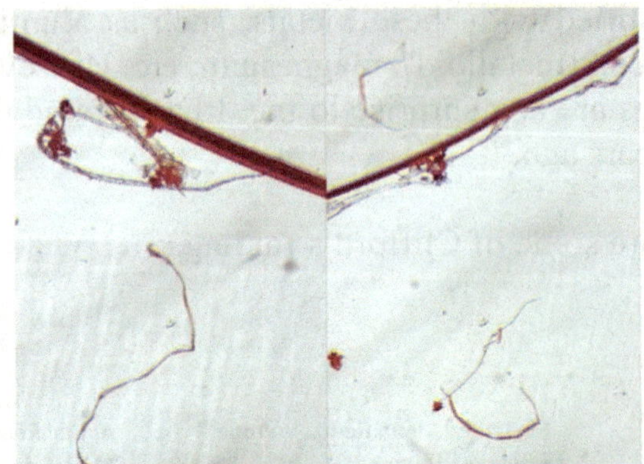

Low Power (~200x) of Biological Filaments Contained in
Residual Materials from Concentrated Rainwater Samples
(The colors of the filaments are a unique characteristic (commonly red and blue) and they exist as an aid to identification with low power microscopy)

Figure 82. Secondary rainwater analysis, 2015. This analysis looked at organic and inorganic components. Carnicom Institute.[163]

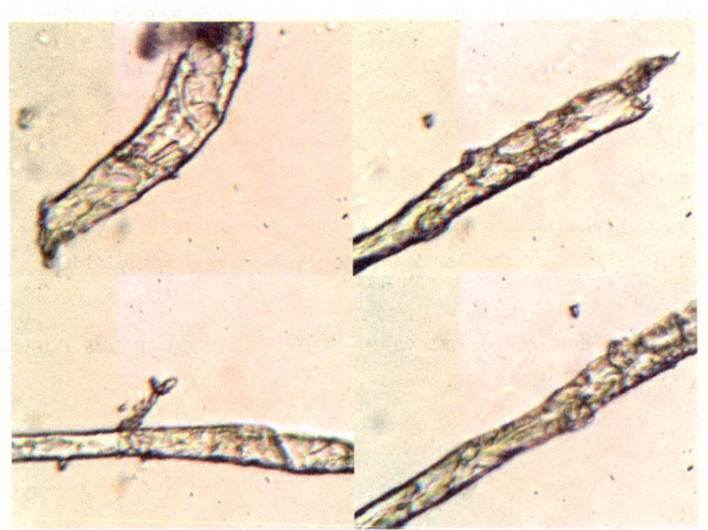

High Power (~5000x) of Biological Filaments Contained in
Residual Materials from Concentrated Rainwater Samples

Figure 83. Filaments in rainwater sample. Carnicom Institute.[164]

In 2015, Clifford began discussing possible toxic compounds to be found in rainwater.[165] At the time, he also found much higher aluminum levels than recommended by the EPA.[166] In his environmental filament metal analysis (see Figure 52), he showed that the filaments contain all of the same metals that were later identified in our COVID 19 research.[167]

Geoengineering is a crime against humanity and our biosphere. The spraying of millions of tons of nano particulate matter that is key to weather warfare—and other nefarious objectives like dimming the sun—needs to stop. Under the cover of a sham climate change agenda, these people are causing the destruction of our biosphere. High aluminum contents have been shown to ignite trees leading to massive wildfires. A global effort must come underway to ban all geoengineering operations.

ELF Fields Mind Controlling COVID 19 Injected Turning Them into Zombies – Confirms Contamination of Mankind's Blood with Nanotechnology

AUGUST 25, 2023[168]

I recently relistened to a lecture by Dr. Pierre Gilbert that confirms what Clifford and I have discovered. This lecture from 1995 is titled: *Dr. Pierre Gilbert Says Mandatory Vaccines Containing Liquid Crystals Will Turn Recipients into Zombies.* I include a brief quote of what he said:

"In the biological destruction there are the organized tempest on the magnetic field. What will follow is the contamination of the bloodstreams of mankind creating intentional infections. This will be enforced via laws that will make vaccinations mandatory. These vaccines will make possible to control people. The vaccines will have liquid crystals that will become hosted in the brain cells, which will become micro receivers of electromagnetic fields where waves of very low frequency will be sent. And through these low frequency waves people will be unable to think, you'll be turned into a Zombie. Don't think of this as a hypothesis… it has been done. Think of Ruanda."[169]

Do recall in an earlier segment we briefly discussed the extremely low frequency sensitivity of COVID 19 vaccinated blood being manipulated by HAARP.[170] In an interview with Maria Zeee, in August 2023, I explain in detail how the 4Hz ELF frequency can mind control the COVID 19 injected. It is not 5G that is controlling them, it is HAARP.[171]

Those liquid crystals mentioned by Dr. Gilbert are what I am finding in human blood, exactly as he predicted—the blood of mankind is contaminated. Infections can be induced via frequency fields that are externally manipulated. There is no virus or pathogen. There is, however, technology that can be remote controlled to sicken the host, as well as control them.[172]

CHAPTER 2

RUBBERY CLOTS

In this chapter, I have compiled Substack articles that relate to my research on rubbery clots. These are historical documents, as some of the questions I asked initially were then answered in my future research projects. I believe it is important to include some of the original findings as they are what prompted me to find answers and solutions.

Huge Rubbery Blood Clots in an Unvaccinated Individual – What Are They Made Of?

DECEMBER 21, 2022[1]

To my surprise one day, a subscriber to my Substack sent me a message asking for help on who she could contact to analyze blood clots. Until then, it was my understanding that even the embalmers had not been able to find willing scientists who would analyze what they were finding.

I am certainly concerned, after learning that an unvaccinated person can acquire such unusual blood clots, as documented in the case history below. Now, I do not exclude that it is possible because of the many live blood analyses that I have seen in the unvaccinated, showing significant clotting and these huge filaments, the same thing Mike Adams has found.[2]

My questions regarding this subject led me to post the information online, with the specific question of whether anyone knew a laboratory that could and would analyze these rubbery clots. It is my understanding the anonymous subscriber had already contacted some prominent doctors and been dismissed in her concern. She was informed that unvaccinated people do not get these rubbery clots. I would hope not—but I would certainly make sure that is true!

It has been my concern that if left undetected, these structures in the blood may grow, possibly via exposure to WIFI or other external energy sources, like magnetic or light fields, in particular UV light if the carbon is graphene. If I can see so many structures in one drop of blood, what else might be going on undetected in 6 liters?

In my practice, I have seen blood clots that look like pulmonary embolism in several unvaccinated individuals, after they were in contact with vaccinated people. An article I wrote several months prior mentioned my concerns about shedding as a possible source of this clotting phenomena.[3]

During the past few years, I have seen many unvaccinated women with severe menstrual abnormalities, including postmenopausal bleeding from shedding. Shedding is the known transmission of biological material from recently vaccinated individuals via their body fluids that can infect surrounding unvaccinated individuals and make them ill.

I have also seen a lot of people with elevated D-dimers, something that I discussed in my video presentation: *D-dimer Elevation in the Unvaccinated. A Marker of Shedding?*[4] which I recorded in the summer of 2022. Some of the assumptions made in that video are now outdated. I did not have a microscope at the time, and since then, my knowledge and research have evolved substantially. The reason that video is still relevant, is because it shows how many unvaccinated people had elevated D-dimers.

I wanted to know if these clots were a carbon-based polymer (hydrogel) combined with metals, such as Mike Adams has found in cadaver clots.[5] If it was, humanity was in deeper trouble then I even thought possible.

Below is the exchange I received from this anonymous Substack subscriber:

“I had an EBO2 (Extrancorporeal Blood Oxygenation and Ozonation) treatment. The doctor was able to get a vein, and a little bit of blood came out but then it stopped flowing, and she tried and tried and tried, but the blood would not flow. So she finally took the IV needle out of me, and with it this long, stringy, rubbery blood rope got pulled out. That’s what was blocking the blood from flowing. After a ton of effort, she finally found a vein that she was able to get some flow going, and we proceeded with the treatment. But by the end, the filter had a bunch of these wormy things in it. We’ve all seen this stuff being pulled out from dead people in those videos but it’s in me.

“I am unjabbed, and I don’t hang out with jabbed people—I avoid them, because I don’t want them shedding on me. I haven’t had sex or kissed any jabbed people. I see my jabbed family a few times a year, but beside that, my only expos[ur]e to jabbed people is in passing (grocery store, waiting room at the chiropractor office, etc). But even with that, I think this if from their shedding.

“Not to be graphic, but in 2021, when I saw my jabbed family for Easter, starting the next day for 3 months, I had tons of stuff coming out of my uterus—like menstrual blood but not liquid—just this weird clumpy stuff. Nothing worked until I had some intense energy work focusing on my reproductive system and then it finally stopped. I had no idea it could be in my veins. I take enzymes regularly—Serrapeptase, Nattokinase, Bromelain, etc. And I have been taking Ivermection daily for 11 months, plus all the other stuff that’s recommended. And I never had a nasal swab. But still, this!”

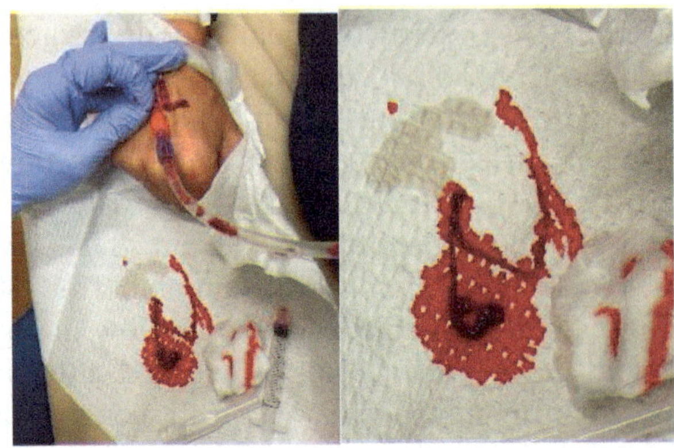

Figure 1. Left: Unusual clots seen in the tubing after starting IV access for EBOO treatment in COVID 19 unvaccinated individual. Right: Rubbery clots extracted from vein of anonymous Substack subscriber. AM Medical.[6]

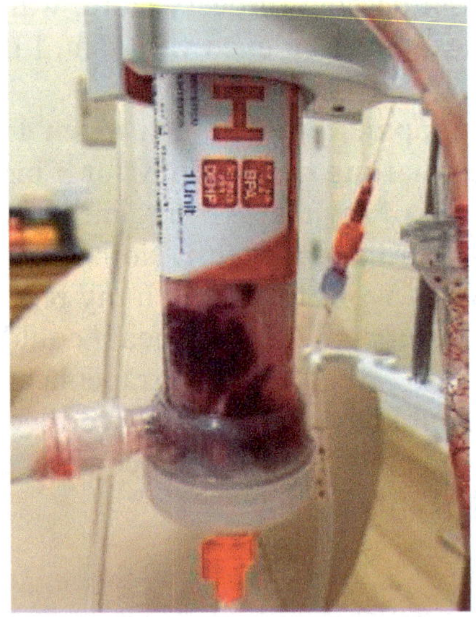

Figure 2. Rubbery clots within EBOO filter extracted from COVID 19 unvaccinated individual. Anonymous Substack subscriber. AM Medical.[7]

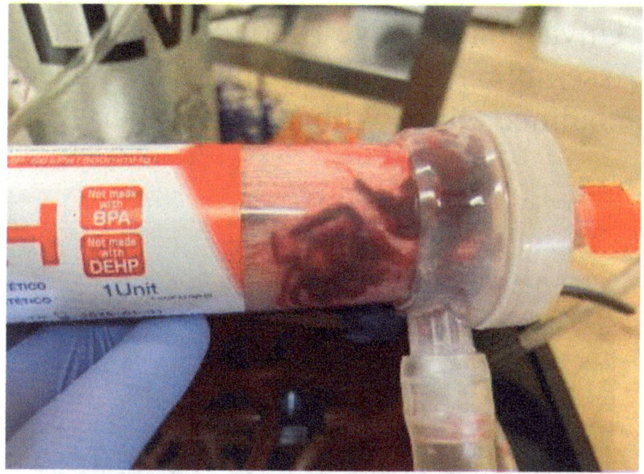

Figure 3. Rubbery clots within EBOO filter extracted from COVID 19 unvaccinated individual. Anonymous Substack subscriber. AM Medical.[8]

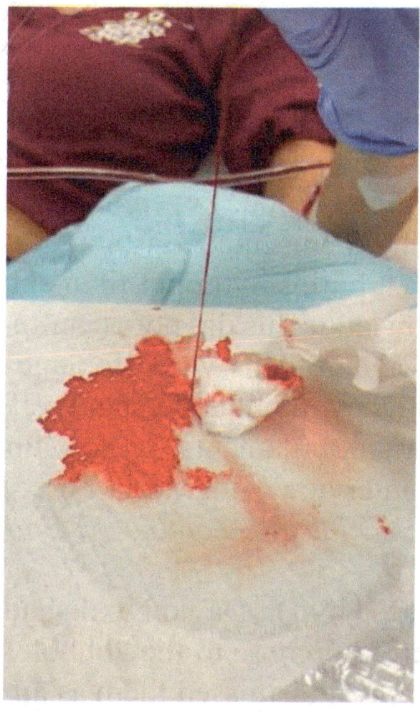

Figure 4. Long, stringy, rubbery clots extracted from COVID 19 unvaccinated individual. Anonymous Substack subscriber. AM Medical.[9]

Unvaccinated Live Blood Shows Same Self-Assembling Hydrogel Spheres as in Deceased Embalmed Blood with Huge Rubbery Clots

JUNE 19, 2023[10]

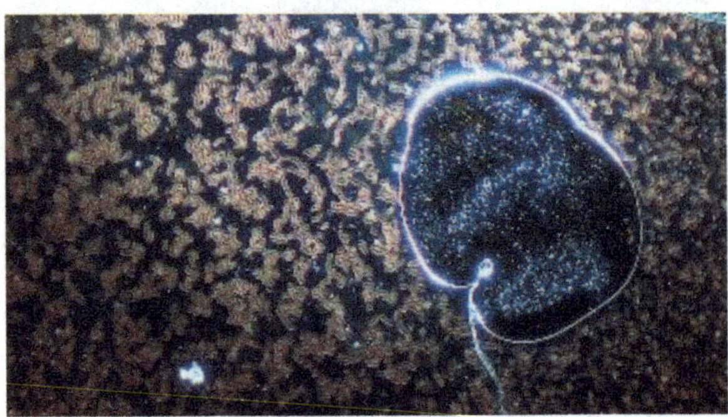

Figure 5. COVID 19 unvaccinated blood shows particle filled sphere and hydrogel filament growing out of it. Magnification 100x. AM Medical.[11]

In the image above, I captured the self-assembling process occurring in embalmed blood. I even took video footage of the speres containing light emitting, conscious, artificial, intelligent nanotechnology that builds hydrogel filaments in the blood. To the best of my knowledge this did not occur in humanity's blood prior to the COVID era. This video footage ***is imperative for everyone to see***, so they might understand self-assembly and the genesis of these strange filaments we now find in blood. To do so, please see my interview with Maria Zeee, *Biden's Universal Nanotechnology Vaccine & "Zombie" Blood*, available on my Substack.[12]

I was first alerted by Dr. David Nixon and engineer Shimon Yanowitz that there was more to the "bubbles" we were seeing in blood. Initially, I just dismissed them as air trapped under the slide cover. But I soon realized they were right, and in looking at embalmed blood samples I saw this clearly.

Around that time, I had an unvaccinated couple come to my office. The lady was experiencing extreme fatigue, unresolved by visits to many functional doctors. I looked at her blood and was astounded by what I saw. In Figure 5 above, you can see a huge, blue, hydrogel nanotechnology filament growing out of a sphere. This is at 100x magnification. When blue like this, it's self-assembled nanotech. Nothing else.

In that blood drop, you can see the same light emitting small, "intelligent" spheres responsible for interacting and building these filaments. It is as if the spheres are mathematically fractal. Smaller light spheres accumulate to create larger ones, but the individual small ones can give information for filament growth. These looked exactly like what I had seen in the embalmed blood. After seeing such anomalies in a person's blood who had been dead for eight months, as mentioned in Chapter 1, I no longer dismissed these classic "blinking lights" as some sort of food or bacteria… they are technology, and they change from blue to red to yellow light. This is even occurring in a live, COVID 19 unvaccinated person!

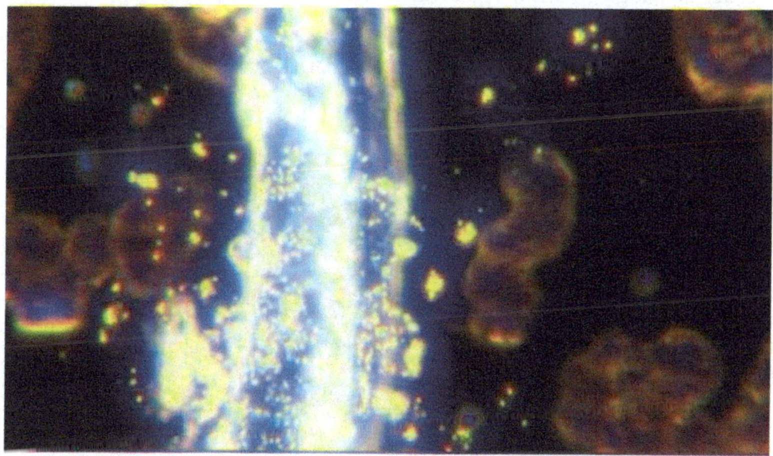

Figure 6. COVID 19 unvaccinated blood shows hydrogel filaments and surrounding quantum dot microrobots involved in self-assembly. Magnification 2000x. AM Medical.[13]

I kept the slide for a few days because I wanted to see what would happen to the filament and the sphere. In the images captured above and below (Figures 6 - 9), you can see the red blood cells are degrading, but the hydrogel filament is still clearly visible. The sphere has gotten larger and irregular. This filament is thousands of times larger than a red blood cell and could certainly cause problems like blood clots, heart attacks, and strokes.

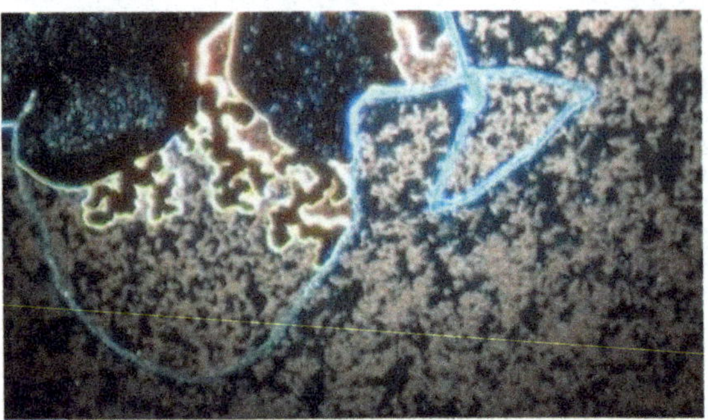

Figure 7. COVID 19 unvaccinated blood left to dry for several days shows large, blue, hydrogel filament and adjacent sphere from which it was constructed. Magnification 100x. AM Medical.[14]

In the area where a lot of red blood cells had died, you can clearly still see the light spheres:

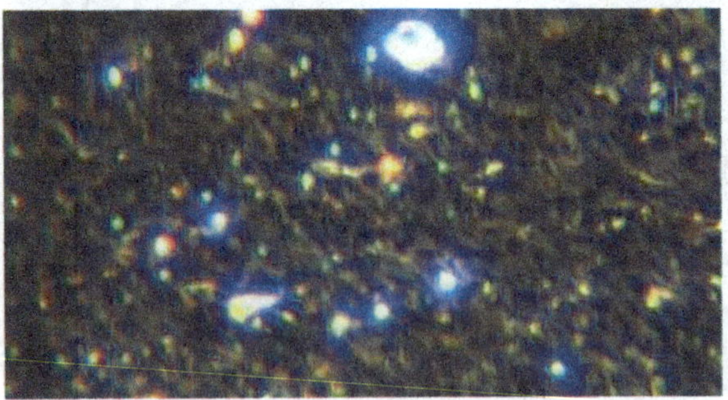

Figure 8. COVID 19 unvaccinated blood left to dry for several days shows many quantum dot microrobots emitting multicolored light and completely destroyed red blood cells. Magnification 100x. AM Medical.[15]

Below is a sphere with the same content. Recall this is exactly what I had seen in the embalmed blood:

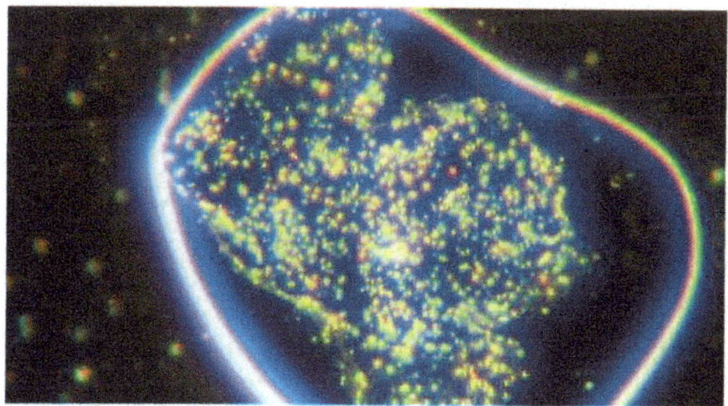

Figure 9. COVID 19 unvaccinated blood shows a large sphere with many multicolored lights emitting quantum dot microrobots. Magnification 100x. AM Medical.[16]

The blood of this woman's partner looked similar. Identical blue filaments with many smaller spheres attached (Figures 10 - 11). Seeing this similarity made me think about mutual shedding, because you do not see such specific blue filaments that often and this large. The fact that both partners had them made me aware they could be reinfecting each other with this material.

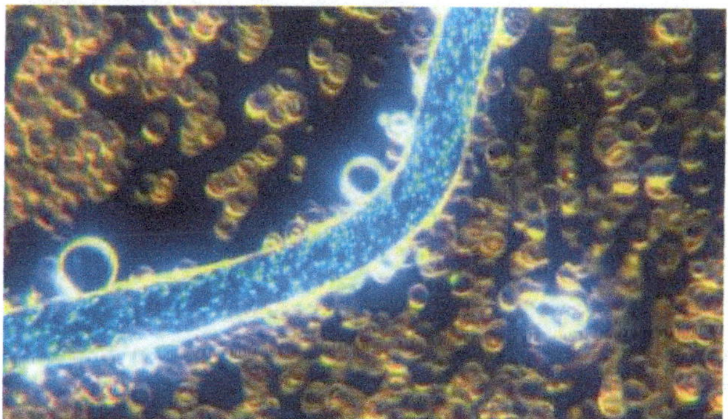

Figure 10. COVID 19 unvaccinated blood shows large, blue, self-assembly nanotechnology filament. Magnification 100x. AM Medical.[17]

The partner had many blue filaments which is unusual—if I find blue filaments it is usually just one:

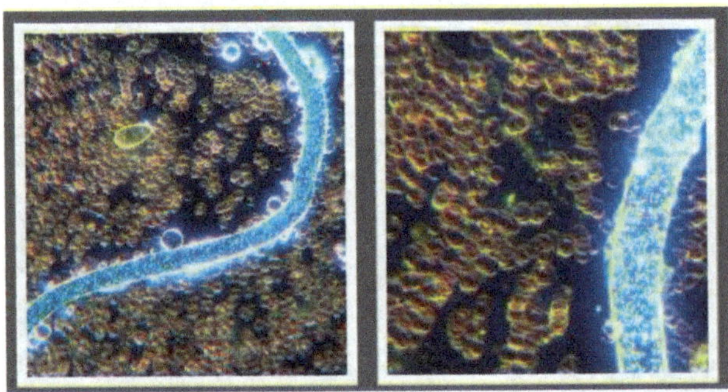

Figure 11. COVID 19 unvaccinated blood shows large, blue, self-assembly nanotechnology filaments. Magnification 100x on the left and 200x on the right. AM Medical.[18]

Again, below is what I also found in embalmed blood—spherical blinking lights and these spheres that kept growing and self-assembling. These images are available as video footage on my Substack for those who are interested.[19]

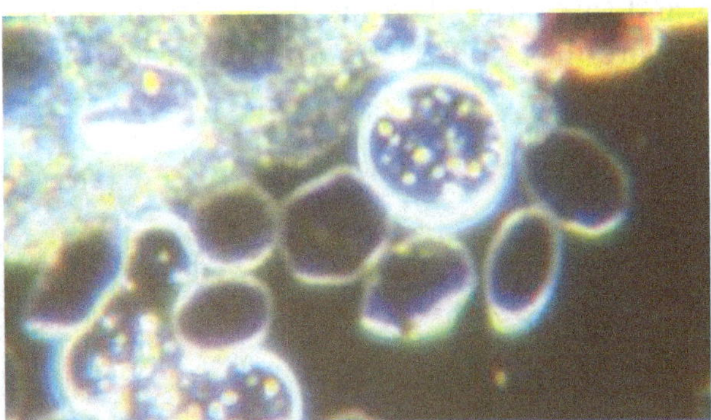

Figure 12. Embalmed blood of someone who died with the rubbery clots eight months prior. Sample sent to me by embalmer Richard Hirschman. Deformed red blood cells seen and spheres that contain multicolored quantum dot microrobots. Magnification 4000x oil objective. Red blood cells are 5-7 micrometers in size. These robots are estimated approx. in the 500 nm size range. AM Medical.[20]

Below is what I found in another unvaccinated person's blood. Look familiar?

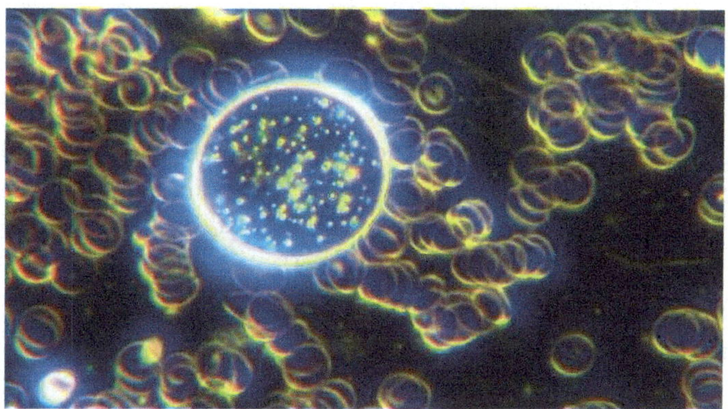

Figure 13. COVID 19 unvaccinated blood shows the same spherical structure with blinking quantum dot microrobots surrounded by red blood cells. AM Medical.[21]

Figure 14 shows a blood sample from yet another individual who felt like he was dying when he came to see me. You can clearly see spheres with substrate and the filaments being formed:

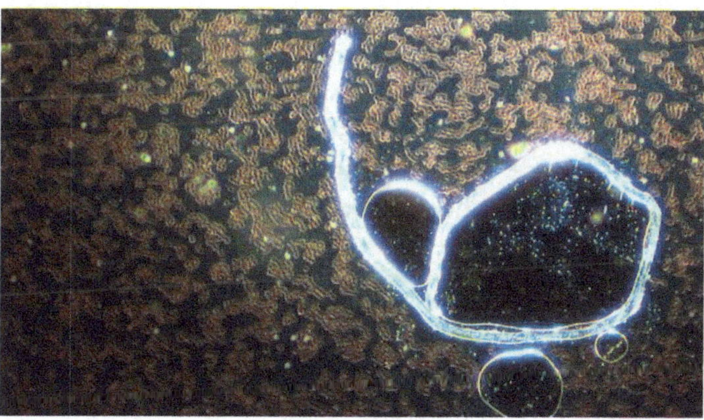

Figure 14. COVID 19 unvaccinated blood shows a spherical structure with blinking quantum dot microrobots building hydrogel filament, surrounded by red blood cells in rouleaux coin-stacking formation. AM Medical.[22]

It is evident to me now that these spheres are what create the hydrogel filaments and provide the substrate to self-assemble them.

Please study these images and contemplate this for yourself. Looking back, I realize that for months I had been dismissing these formations as air bubbles caught by the cover slip, never considering they might be something artificial invading the human blood stream. But they are, in fact, nanotechnology substrates for self-assembly—in essence poisoning the host.

There is no difference in the self-assembly spheres from a deceased individual with huge rubbery clots and a COVID 19 unvaccinated individual whose blood is contaminated from shedding. The findings are identical. The spheres appear to provide the building materials for the self-assembly of the hydrogel filaments you see in my photographs.

Imagine, if this is what I found and continue to find in just one drop of blood, how much is there in the whole body? This technology grows and grows and does not stop! Even in someone long dead!

These filaments can cause heart attacks, strokes, and many other health problems.

I emphasize that it is important to obtain a live blood analysis from someone who knows what they are looking at. I say that because I have seen live blood practitioners falsely claim people have clean blood—while they are filled with these filaments. Another claim is these are holograms. I assure you they are not. Please find someone who knows about nanotech and understands what they are seeing.

Rubbery Clot Formation Shown in Living C19 Unvaccinated Person – Hydrogel Replacing Blood

JULY 21, 2023[23]

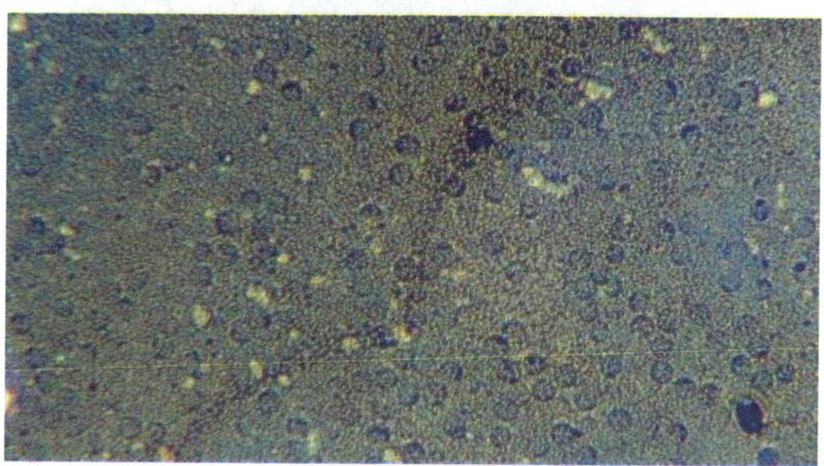

Figure 15. COVID 19 unvaccinated live blood analysis shows hydrogel sheets that have used red blood as a substrate and created rubbery clots. Darkfield microscopy 200x. AM Medical.[24]

In previous articles, I have shown the correlation between the amount of hydrogel seen and the formation of rubbery clots from the polymerized protein hydrogel CDB in blood.[25]

In one example, an unvaccinated individual who lives with someone vaccinated became symptomatic through C19 "vaccine" shedding. They have been suffering ever since from symptoms of fatigue, malaise, emotional stress, nausea, and more. Their blood showed self-assembly of the polymer mesh network, and many quantum dot, light-emitting structures coordinating self-assembly. The hydrogel had become a solid sheet of material.

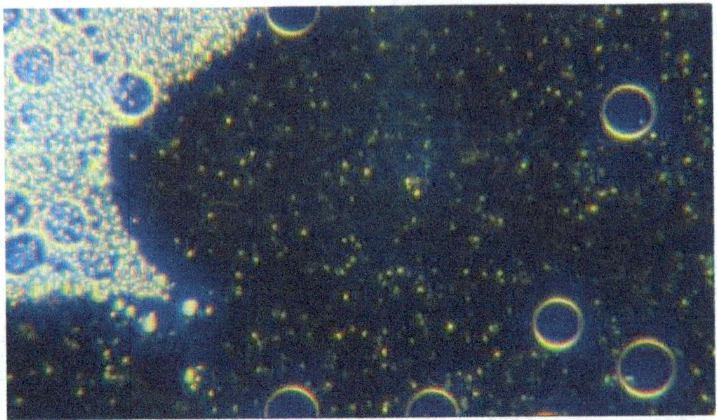

Figure 16. COVID 19 unvaccinated live blood analysis shows hydrogel sheets that have used red blood as a substrate and created rubbery clots. Darkfield microscopy 400x. AM Medical.[26]

The image below reveals the extent of the hydrogel polymer found in one drop of their blood. This was seen within minutes. One can see ongoing building activity within the sheet of dimensional network:

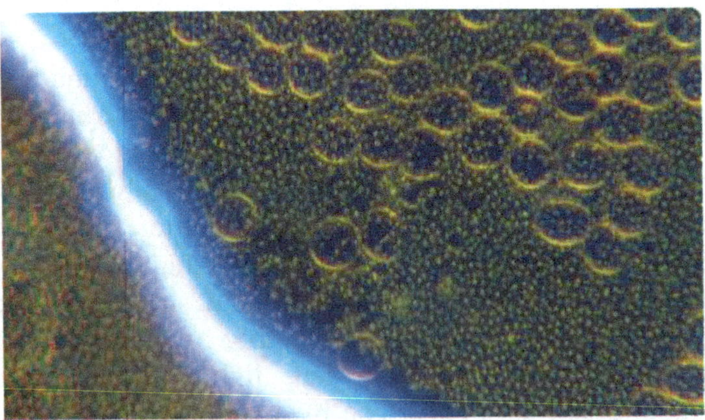

Figure 17. COVID 19 unvaccinated live blood analysis shows hydrogel sheets that have used red blood as a substrate and created rubbery clots. Darkfield microscopy 400x. AM Medical.[27]

Since those early days of COVID 19 research, I have often observed, under the microscope, the construction of hydrogel via nanotechnology in human blood. On video, and as captured in the photograph below, one can see how the edges of the hydrogel are being built in a coordinated effort by these artificial, intelligent nanorobots. Noone can say that the slide cover was contaminated as I was filming an active process. When taken slightly out of focus, one can see the optical communication coordination between individual self-assembling quantum dots.

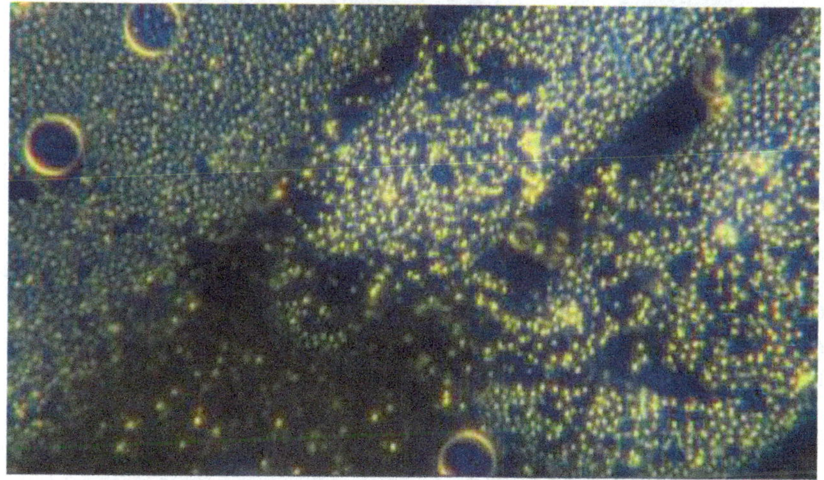

Figure 18. COVID 19 unvaccinated live blood analysis shows hydrogel sheets that have used red blood as a substrate and created rubbery clots. This process was video filmed. Darkfield microscopy 400x. AM Medical.[28]

My colleague, Clifford Carnicom, confirmed my findings in his analysis of a deceased individual's rubbery clot, and COVID 19 vaccinated and unvaccinated clots, and showed they are all the same.[29]

Below is an image of blood from another unvaccinated individual who was very careful about exposure to COVID 19 vaccinated people, but then spent a week with COVID 19 injected relatives. This is the worst live blood analysis this individual has had. One can clearly see vast networks of self-assembling hydrogel:

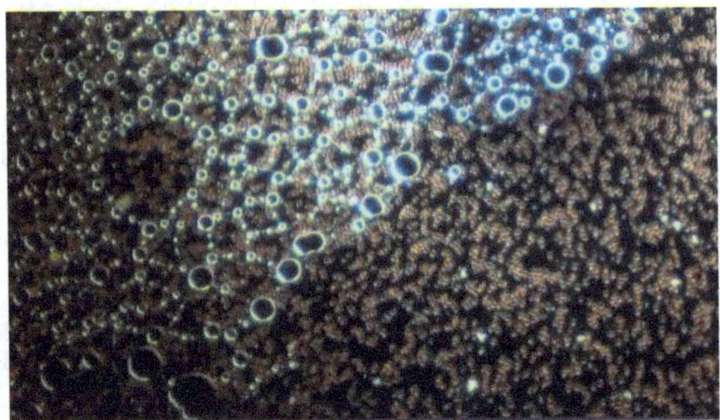

Figure 19. COVID 19 unvaccinated live blood analysis shows hydrogel mesh network transforming the blood. Darkfield microscopy 400x. AM Medical.[30]

You can see microscopically, in Figure 20, an earlier stage of the dense polymer network I have shown above that is clearly on the way to creating these rubbery clots and replacing the blood. This patient was asymptomatic:

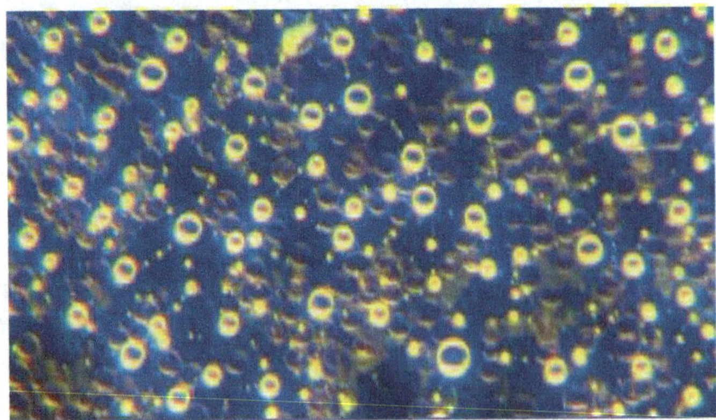

Figure 20. COVID 19 unvaccinated live blood analysis shows hydrogel mesh network transforming the blood. Darkfield microscopy 2000x.
AM Medical.[31]

Much of the blood is being replaced by the network construction sites in this series of images taken over a brief period from the one blood sample.

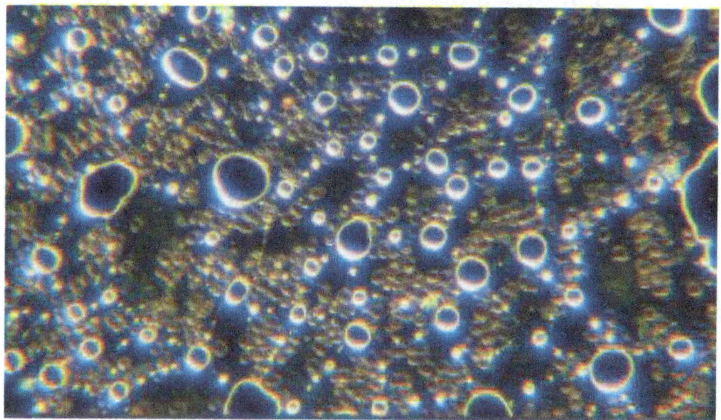

Figure 21. COVID 19 unvaccinated live blood analysis shows hydrogel mesh network transforming the blood. Darkfield microscopy 400x. AM Medical.[32]

In the image below you can see self-assembly polyacrylonitrile polymer networks formed in water. This is a polymer that creates a mesh network just as I have seen in the live blood above:[33]

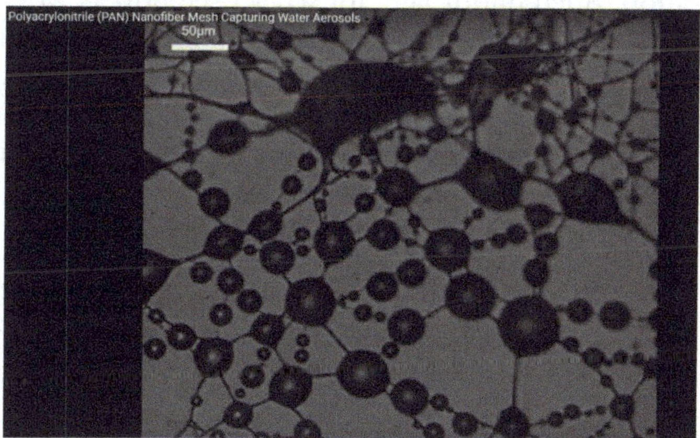

Figure 22. Polyacylonitrile (PAN) nanofiber mesh capturing water aerosols. SciTech Daily.[34]

I continue to sound the alarm on these extremely worrisome findings. People ask me all the time to be careful as I may get targeted by the corrupt FDA, medical boards, fake media, and other government agencies who have knowingly contributed to this genocide.

My answer is the same: I am witnessing and documenting the mechanism of genocide that most people are not talking about, and that means not enough scientists are actively finding answers. We are running out of time. This is an immediate threat to the survival of all of humanity and must be addressed. I do not understand why doctors and scientists around the world will not stand up and do their own research on this—and why human beings everywhere are not revolting against their corrupt healthcare systems and governments and asking for immediate answers. Right now, the digital currency system is being rolled out. Surveillance under the skin has already happened and this self-assembling polymer, along with self-assembling quantum dots, are part of that technology, making your biometric data accessible, as well as remote mind control possible.

Humankind will not survive this if people do not address the problem. This process is rapidly accelerating and evolving. I am postulating that there has been some sort of frequency acceleration rolled out of late, for what I see now is worse than ever before. Watch the videos available on my Substack and see for yourself.[35] These videos documenting live blood analysis of COVID 19 unvaccinated people leave no question about the reality of nanotechnology and synthetic biology shedding as well as environmental contamination via geoengineering.

If we are to survive, WE MUST ACT NOW.

Rubbery Clot Development in C19 Unvaccinated Individual with Previous Deep Vein Thrombosis and Massive Pulmonary Emboli

OCTOBER 19, 2023[36]

I have long been warning about the hydrogel rubbery clots affecting COVID 19 unvaccinated people and shown images of how the blood develops a hydrogel layer within 4 hours of being drawn after allowing it to sit. I have also been warning that the spike protein story is simply not enough to explain what is happening with humanity's blood. This blood contamination is greatly accelerating due to the amount of nanotechnology seen in COVID 19 bioweapon shedding, geoengineering, and food contamination, to name a few sources. Colleagues in multiple continents around the world have confirmed an alarming uptick of synthetic biology and nanotechnology findings in the blood.[37,38,39,40]

Mainstream scientists and doctors have also ignored the scientific findings that the spike protein sequence encodes for hydrogel at pH 7, not amyloid. They continue to speak of amyloid being a contributing factor to what is seen in COVID 19 injected individuals—not rubbery hydrogel plastics engineered as synthetic biology, which is what it is. Most are ignoring the shedding issue altogether.

Here I continue my examples by describing a case report of a 63-year-old COVID 19 unvaccinated male who presented with a deep vein thrombosis in January 2022. He was treated with Eliquis® (made by Pfizer). The patient had a follow up ultrasound three months later which showed resolution of the clot at the time. All hypercoagulable workup was negative, and he showed no genetic or lifestyle predisposition to clotting. He tapered off Eliquis® after six months. The patient works in the healthcare field and is constantly exposed to COVID 19 vaccinated individuals. He has a history of having had "COVID."

In September 2022, he presented with acute shortness of breath. In the hospital, he was found to have bilateral extensive deep vein thrombosis and massive, multiple pulmonary emboli with extensive lung infarction. He was restarted on Eliquis®. The patient also started Nattokinase 20.000 units, Lumbrokinase, and Serrapeptase. A year later he was symptomatically improved, but still complaining about fatigue, brain fog, and some shortness of breath with exertion. He came to me for a second opinion.

An initial live blood analysis showed extensive nanotechnology and hydrogel contamination with polymer mesh network development as well as rouleaux formation.

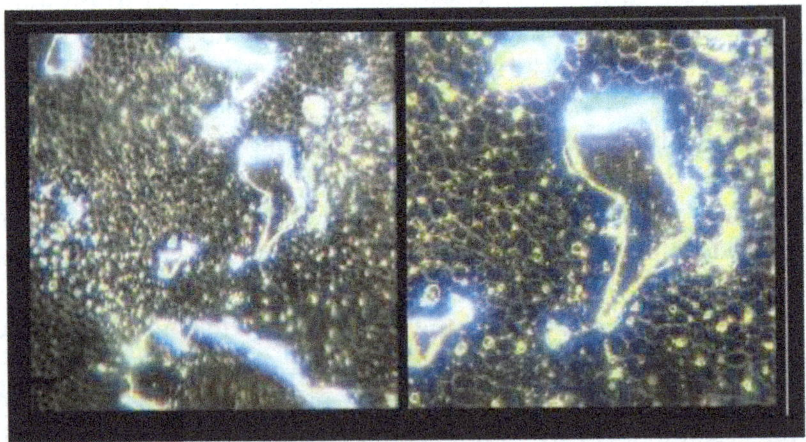

Figure 23. Extensive transformation of blood into clots is seen with red blood cells used as a substrate. Note the red blood cells are dead. Left magnification 100x. Right magnification 200x. AM Medical.[41]

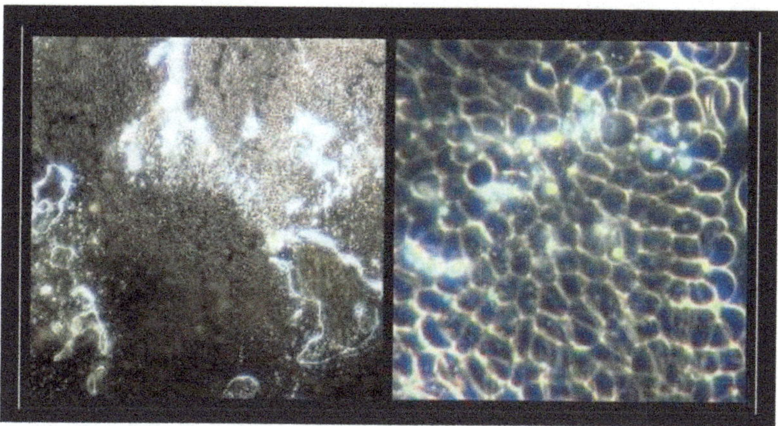

Figure 24. Extensive transformation of blood into clots is seen with red blood cells used as a substrate. Note the red blood cells are dead. Left magnification 100x. Right magnification 400x. AM Medical.[42]

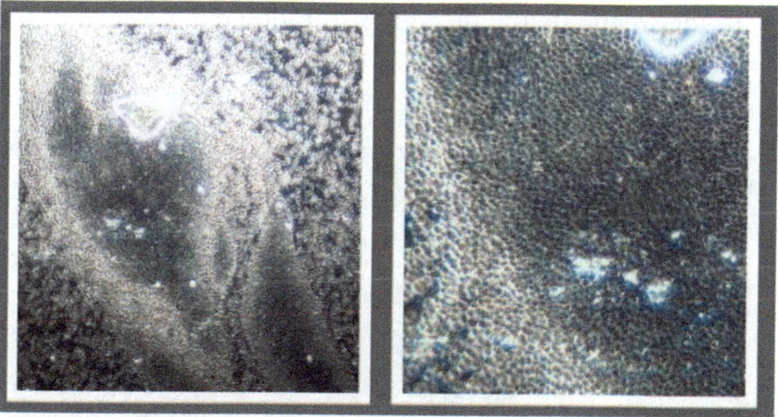

Figure 25. Extensive transformation of blood into clots is seen with red blood cells used as a substrate – seen as darkened areas. Note the red blood cells are dead. Left magnification 100x. Right magnification 200x. AM Medical.[43]

Many hydrogel filaments were seen in the blood as well as extensive rouleaux formation.

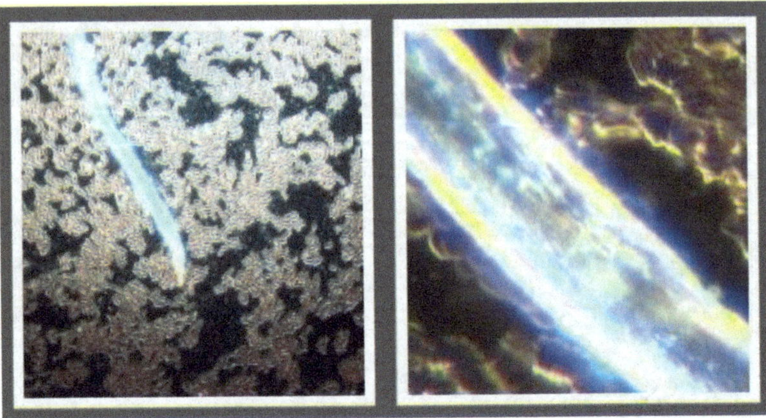

Figure 26. Hydrogel polymer filaments seen with abnormal rouleaux stacking of red blood. Left magnification 100x. Right magnification 400x. AM Medical.[44]

In the image below the sluggish blood can be seen as well as microrobots:

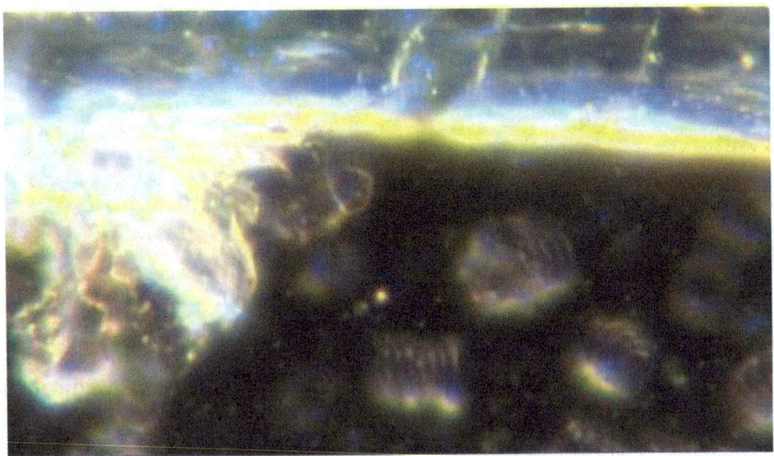

Figure 27. Hydrogel polymer filaments seen with abnormal rouleaux stacking of red blood. Microrobots seen (blue dots). Magnification 200x. AM Medical.[45]

I had drawn 30 cc of blood for this patient, who also is a doctor. I gave him the syringe that had been left overnight in my office during which time his blood had clotted. He inspected the clot himself with another physician colleague as shown in this image:

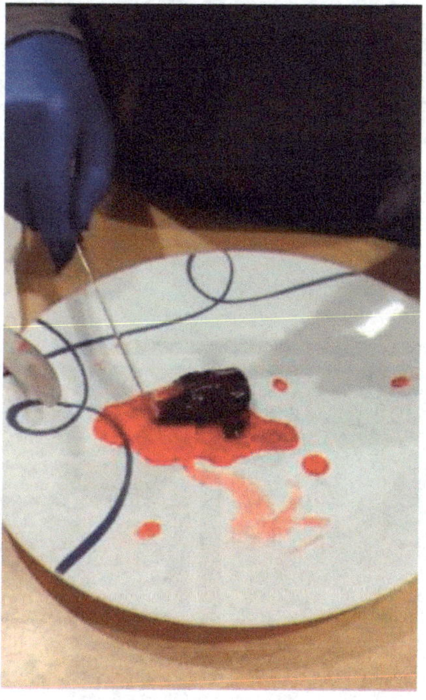

Figure 28. Rubbery blood clot inspection. AM Medical.[46]

Subsequently, the patient followed my treatment protocol which was the following: day one EDTA Chelation and glutathione; second day high dose vitamin C; third day EDTA Chelation and glutathione. He also received intravenous Plaquex®. Several anti-aging peptides were also given daily. He symptomatically improved and had more energy. A follow up, live blood analysis on the third day showed clean blood.

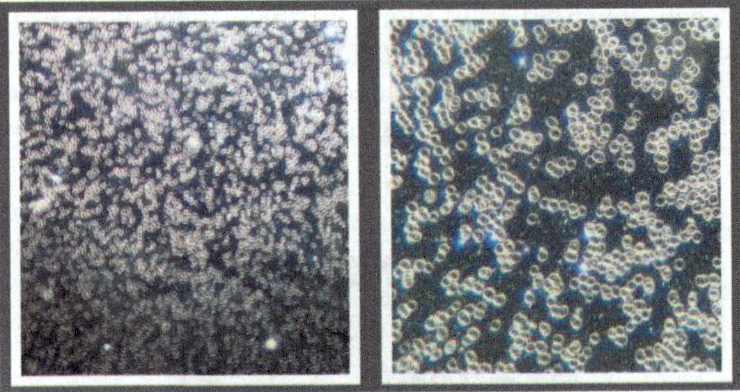

Figure 29. Darkfield live blood analysis post treatment shows clean blood much improved. Left magnification 100x. Right magnification 200x. AM Medical.[47]

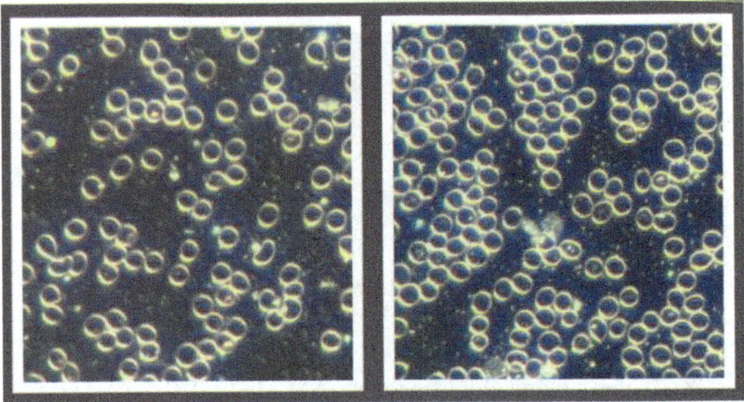

Figure 30. Darkfield live blood analysis post treatment shows clean blood further improved. Left magnification 400x. Right magnification 400x. AM Medical.[48]

A video of this gentleman's blood after treatment is available on my Substack. It shows excellent flow, no rouleaux, and no hydrogel construction sites.[49]

I have seen many cases of COVID 19 unvaccinated individuals with life threatening blood clots who continued to have recurrence of the clots even while on Eliquis®. This includes heart attacks and strokes as well as extensive deep vein thrombosis. I have previously shown that Eliquis® does not prevent clotting, but EDTA and vitamin C in high doses do, once the blood is cleaned. I am again sounding the alarm to clinicians that mainstream blood thinners do not prevent the rubbery clot formation that is now affecting the COVID 19 unvaccinated through shedding. Live blood analysis, then testing the blood by letting it sit for four hours or overnight and watching for hydrogel formation, must be done to find out if therapies are effective.

Thank you to my patient/colleague who allowed me to share this case history. Seeing is believing. May this information wake up more doctors so that we can adequately prevent patients from experiencing these potentially life-threatening, rubbery hydrogel, clot intrusions.

Same Self-Replicating Nanotechnology Spheres Seen in C19 Unvaccinated Blood as in Deceased Embalmed C19 Vaccinated Blood

NOVEMBER 15, 2023[50]

My microscopy of long, rubbery clots found in the embalmed blood of an individual who had died 8 months earlier should be familiar to everyone by now. The same rubbery clots were even featured in the documentary *Died Suddenly.*[51]

The spheres that I filmed continued to replicate—and in the image below you can see how those spheres are developing. Recorded on video, I observed the spheres at 4000x magnification. Clearly light-emitting microrobots were seen.

Considering the size of the surrounding red blood cells they are estimated to be several hundred nanometers in size.

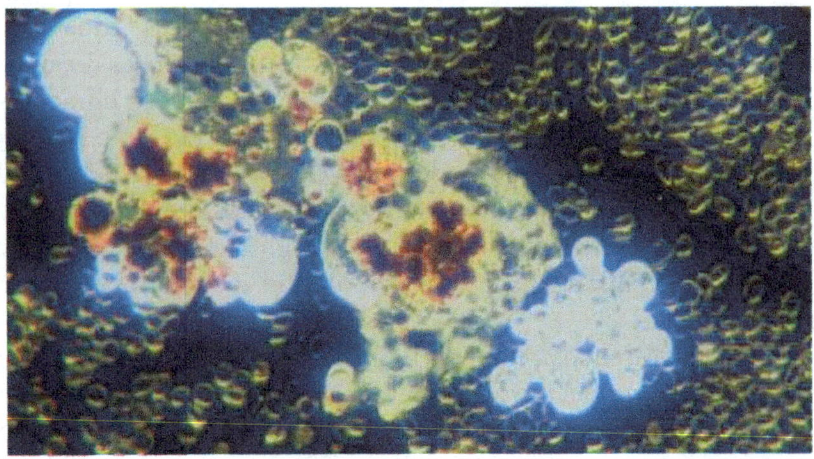

Figure 31. Embalmed blood of individual who died with rubbery clots eight months prior shows self-replicating nanotechnology. Magnification 400x. AM Medical.[52]

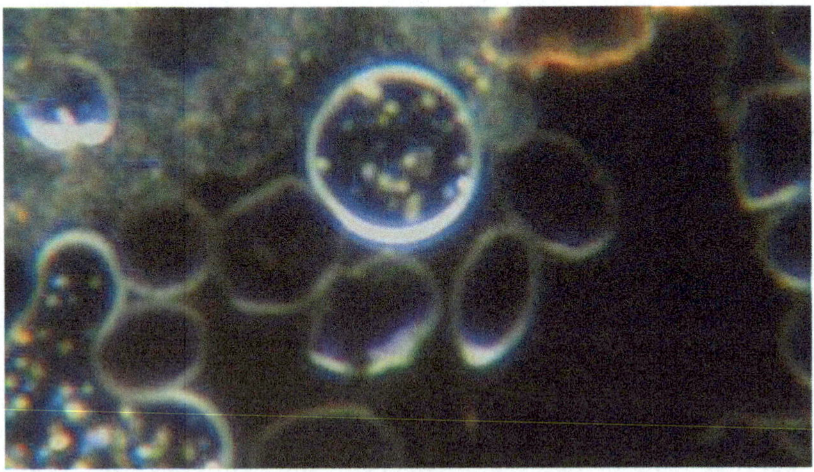

Figure 32. Embalmed blood with self-replicating nanotechnology oil objective magnification 4000x. AM Medical.[53]

I have revealed in many interviews and publications how these spheres contain nano- and microrobots that are emitting light in different frequencies and colors—as quantum dot, polymer coated, bidirectional biosensors would do—having photographed them multiple times in COVID 19 unvaccinated blood. I have also shown how these spheres construct the filaments we see in both vaccinated and unvaccinated blood.

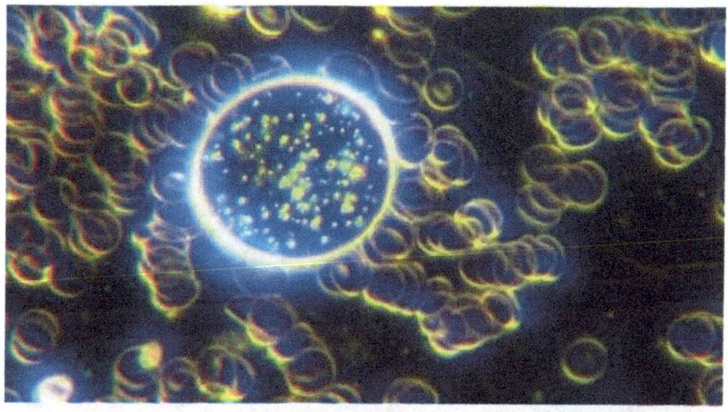

Figure 33. COVID 19 unvaccinated blood sphere filled with nanotechnology. AM Medical.[54]

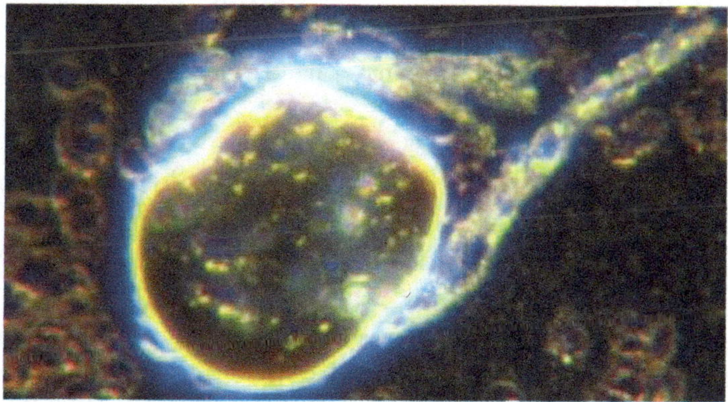

Figure 34. COVID 19 unvaccinated blood sphere filled with nanotechnology constructing hydrogel polymer filament. AM Medical.[55]

I have a lot of conversations with people on this topic. Still, many are in denial. Doctors do not believe in nanotechnology and deny its existence. Supposedly, people are still not ready to hear about nanotechnology that has self-disseminated worldwide via shedding and is now causing the rubbery clots seen everywhere. We have proven that. They are made of a rubber-like material, a polymer that has self-assembled.

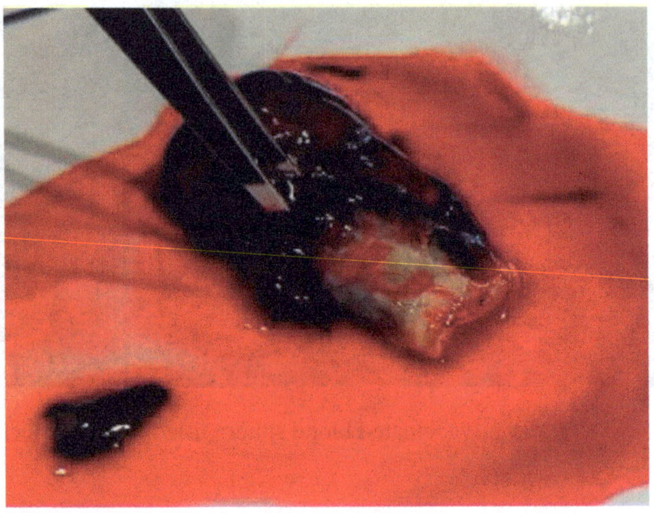

Figure 35. Rubbery clot development in COVID 19 unvaccinated individual with previous deep vein thrombosis and massive pulmonary emboli – while on Eliquis®, Nattokinase, Lumbrokinase, and Serrapeptase. AM Medical.[56]

My question is when will the denying doctors, scientists, politicians, attorneys, and media decide people are ready to know about this and start discussing the issue? When they are dead?

To include another interesting case study, below is a live blood analysis from an individual who, after air travel, started having upper respiratory tract symptoms suggestive of "COVID." I have discussed elsewhere that acute COVID symptoms correlate with significant replication of the hydrogel filaments and excessive rouleaux formation. Therapeutic dose Ivermectin quickly resolved the symptoms. However, through live blood analysis one can see that Ivermectin helps resolve the rouleaux but does not diminish microrobots or hydrogel production.

The individual then had a follow up live blood analysis a week later where I filmed how the blood was being transformed by the same familiar spheres filled with nanotechnology. The blood was loaded with these spheres. You could see the movement and optical light emissions. Red blood cells surrounding this were in severe oxidative stress—they were dying. Shown in the image below, this is the same magnification as the deceased COVID 19 vaccinated blood shown in Figures 31 – 32. While the nanorobots are tiny, you can easily see them under the microscope and on video emitting light and moving.

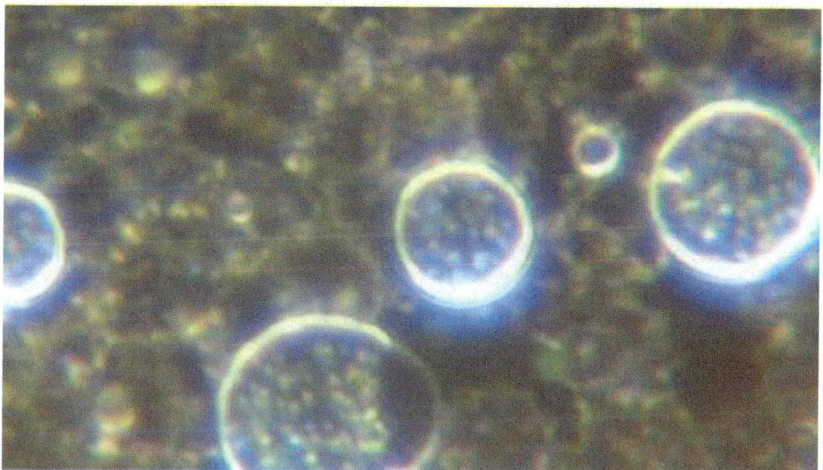

Figure 36. COVID 19 unvaccinated blood shows multiple spheres filled with nanotechnology. Surrounding red blood cells are in extreme oxidative distress. Magnification 4000x – oil objective. AM Medical.[57]

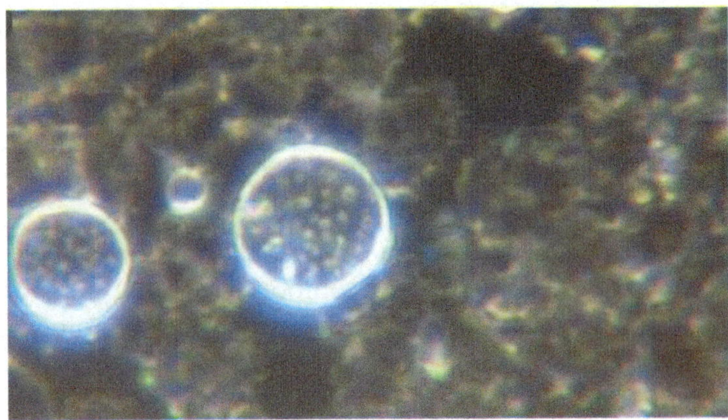

Figure 37. COVID 19 unvaccinated blood shows multiple spheres filled with nanotechnology. Surrounding red blood cells are in extreme oxidative distress. Magnification 4000x. AM Medical.[58]

Next is the same blood, different sample, with many of these small spheres somewhere between 5-10 micron in size, but they can become much larger. The blood is being transformed into a polymer mesh network:

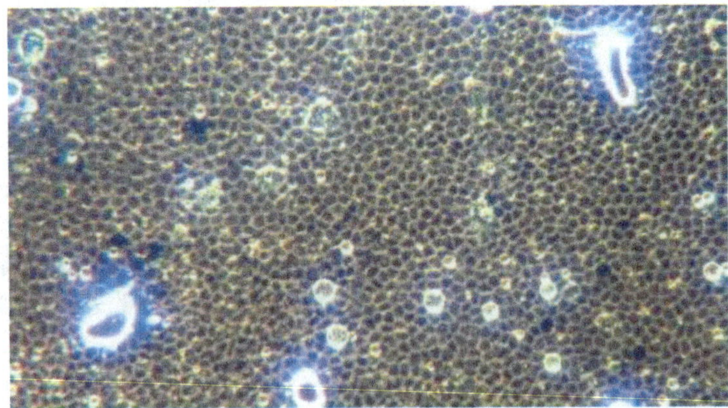

Figure 38. COVID 19 unvaccinated blood shows multiple spheres filled with nanotechnology. The surrounding red blood cells are being transformed into rubbery clots. Magnification 200x. AM Medical.[59]

These spheres in the blood are not air bubbles. They are hydrogel nanotechnology construction sites. You can see in the image below many spheres that are perfectly round interconnecting and extracting the life out of the red blood cells:

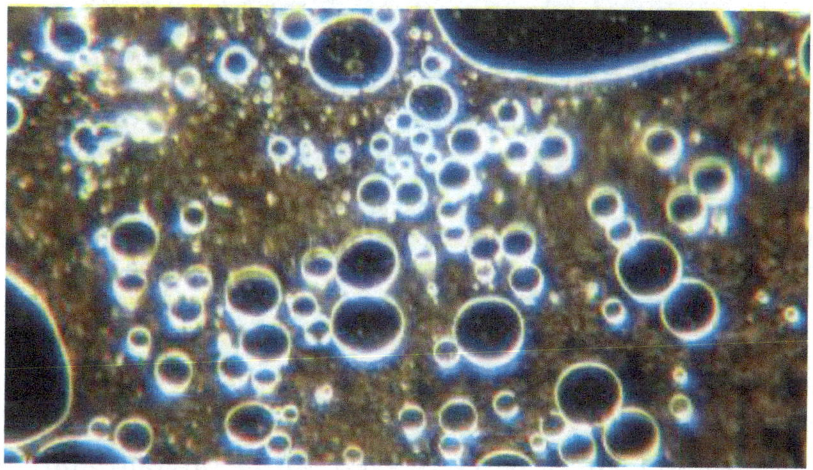

Figure 39. COVID 19 unvaccinated blood shows multiple spheres. The surrounding red blood cells are being transformed into rubbery clots. Magnification 200x. AM Medical.[60]

These impacted blood cells clearly show oxidative stress as they are being transformed under the coordinated effort of microrobots. Microrobots can be recognized by the blinking lights coordinating smaller nanorobots. If you think about one red blood cell being approximately 5-7 micrometers, some of the very small swarming nanobots are estimated at around 500 nanometers. Watch the blinking lights, those are robots.

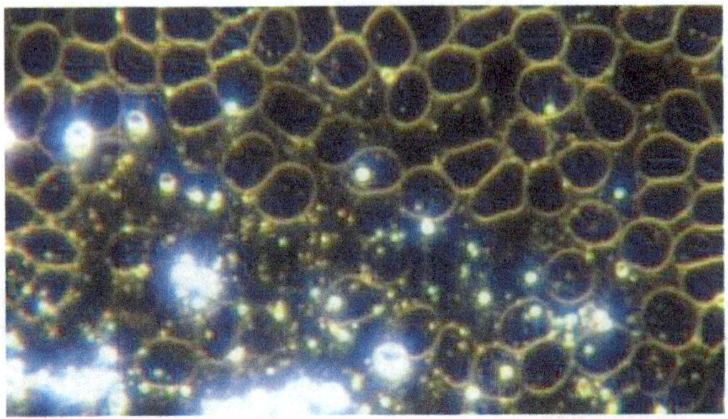

Figure 40. COVID 19 unvaccinated blood shows multiple blinking lights that are destroying the red blood cells. Small spheres filled with self-assembly nanotechnology also visible. Magnification 2000x. AM Medical.[61]

Torsion Spectroscopy of C19 Vaccinated Deceased Clots – Dr. Wojtkowiak Confirms Prion-Like Protein Cannot be Dissolved with Conventional Blood Thinners

DECEMBER 14, 2023[62]

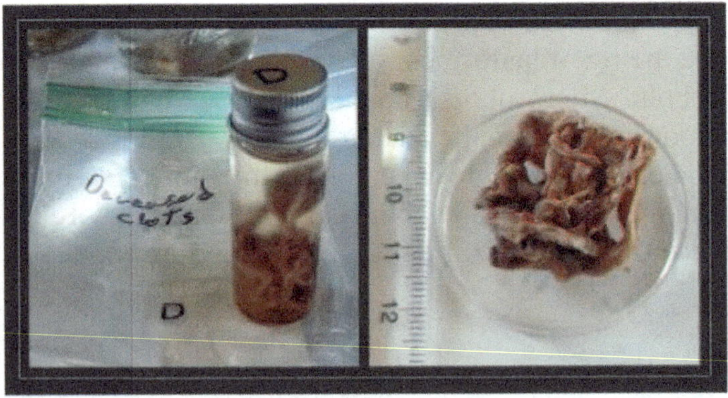

Figure 41. Photos of clots from blood clot analysis of deceased individual COVID 19 injected. AM Medical.[63]

In conclusion to this chapter, I am so honored to publish the original research outlined below by the brilliant Dr. Diana Wojtkowiak. She has a master's degree in chemistry and a doctorate in molecular biology. For twenty years she has conducted research in molecular biology and biotechnology. I was introduced to her, after which she sent me an email that she had conducted torsion spectroscopy on the clots that Clifford Carnicom and I had analyzed. The clots had been sent to me by the embalmer, Richard Hirschman.

Dr. Wojtkowiak has analyzed injectable medications and has found filament structures, graphene, and metals in vaccines, insulin, heparin, and other injectable medications. I have replicated her work with my own microscopy findings, showing significant contamination in vaccines, medications, and insulin.

Dr. Wojtkowiak's recent torsion spectroscopy work has provided revolutionary information on how the COVID 19 injection affects the antimatter aspect of the injected, changing them at the most fundamental level.[64,65]

Here is her message in regard to her paper:

Dear Ana,

I am sending you my results of spectral analysis of clots from your article. I am not sure if the foto (fig.1) shows clots from individual vaccinated or unvaccinated. The research was made for checking if the share of the expected signal in blood will be sufficient for identification known effects of vaccines. It cost me a few days of work, but it is a gift for you as an expression of sympathy. You can use this information as you wish.

Diana Wojtkowiak
Gdansk, 13 December 2023

Below is from Dr. Wojtkowiak's research paper. I did not post all the individual measurements that were included, only the summary graphs.

> In the study, I used my new torsion field particle spectroscope (fig. 4) with signal separation in the torsion field produced by two copper electrodes connected to a DC voltage. The signal taken directly from the image, directed between the deflecting electrodes, is then amplified with a radionic amplifier, and fed into a water bottle. Later the range of radiation taken every 0,5 degree is determined by the kinesiological type method with an accuracy of 5%. In the spectrum there are some multi-isotopic elements, that is why I present a comparison with these elements in the table and in the graph of Fig. 2. Because this is new spectroscope, I had to re-examine a few reference elements for this measurement.

Natural isotopic composition of copper, zinc and selenium:
^{63}Cu 69.1%, ^{65}Cu 30.9%.
^{64}Zn 48.89%, ^{66}Zn 27.81%, ^{67}Zn 4.11%, ^{68}Zn 18.57%, ^{70}Zn 0.62%.
^{74}Se 0.87%, ^{76}Se 9.02%, ^{77}Se 7.58%, ^{78}Se 23.52%, ^{80}Se 49.82%, ^{82}Se 9.19%.

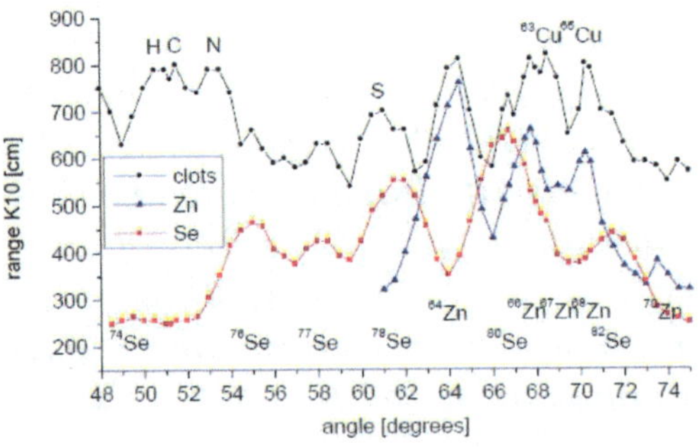

Fig. 2. Torsion field particle signal spectrum taken from foto of clots Markings: H – hydrogen, C – carbon, N – nitrogen, S – sulphur, Cu – copper, Zn – zinc, Se – selenium. Horizontal axis: the angle of the deflected beam with respect to the normal for the undeflected beam measured in degrees. Vertical axis: K10 Category radiation range from samples at the output of the spectroscope, in cm.

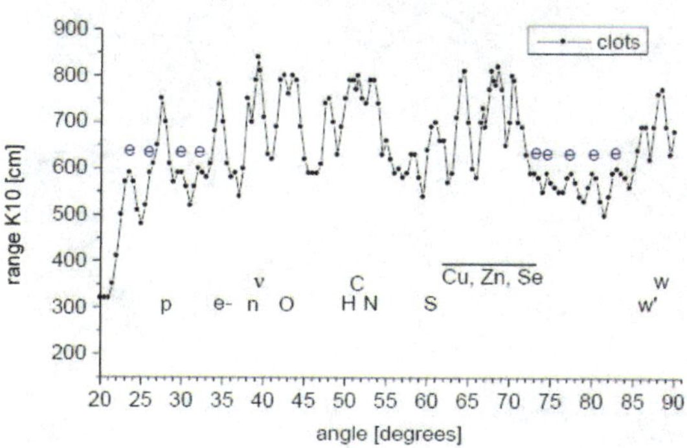

Fig. 3. Torsion field particle signal spectrum taken from foto of clots Markings: p – protons, e- – electrons, n – neutrons, v – neutrinos, O – oxygen, H – hydrogen, C – carbon, N – nitrogen, S – sulphur, Cu – copper, Zn – zinc, Se – selenium, w – WIMPs, w' - WIMPS with some information, e – signal from aromatic amino acid rings. Horizontal axis: the angle of the deflected beam with respect to the normal for the undeflected beam measured in degrees. Vertical axis: K10 Category radiation range from samples at the output of the spectroscope, in cm.

From this spectrum, it is evident that the signal of prion-like proteins predominates in clots. The characteristic signals for prion-like proteins revealed are copper, zinc, selenium, sulfur, elementary particles from the prion-led nuclear reaction: protons, electrons, neutrons, neutrons, WIMPs, and the pattern of aromatic amino acid system characteristic of each prion-like protein. We know that prion-like proteins tend to form pseudocrystals in the form of fibers with even macroscopic dimensions. They are very resistant to acids, alkalis, and detergents, so normal methods of dissolving clots, as in a blood clotting cascade, are useless.

Figure 42. Torsion spectroscopy on rubbery clots. Dr. Diana Wojtkowiak.[66]

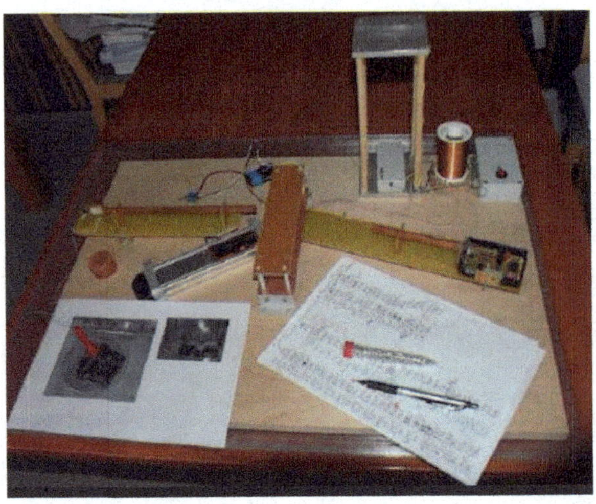

Figure 43. The torsion field particles spectroscope. Dr. Diana Wojtkowiak.[67]

The spectral analysis Dr. Wojtkowiak performed on the deceased clots shows a prion-like protein. Clifford Carnicom and I identified polyamide proteins via near-infrared spectroscopy. The same polyamide proteins were identified in Morgellons filaments and mesogen brain chips analyzed by Dr. Hildegarde Staninger.[68] Polyamide proteins are polymers used in the manufacturing of nylon and they create extremely strong filaments. Dr. Wojtkowiak's spectroscopy found carbon, oxygen, nitrogen, and sulfur, which are the building blocks of polyamides/prion proteins. She also found copper, zinc, and selenium in the clots. I have discussed at length my observation that the biosensor/microrobots create with the hydrogel polymers the long filaments we see in the blood. The technology uses building blocks from the body to self-assemble itself. I also showed the microrobots/biosensors creating and building the clots. These particular nanoparticles are used for biosensing applications.[69,70,71]

The polyamide proteins that have been identified, and that Dr. Wojtkowiak calls prion-like proteins, are part of polymer manufacturing. They have been identified chemically in humans under the term "microplastics" and have been found to be building blocks of mesogen brain chips for human control, as analyzed by Dr. Staninger.[72]

Here is the chemical explanation of polyamide polymers:

> A polyamide is a polymer in which the individual units are held together by amide linkages. For example, nylon 66 is obtained from the monomers 1,6-hexanediamine, and hexanedioic acid. On one end, the product molecule has a carboxylic acid group, which can undergo a condensation reaction with another 1,6-hexanediamine molecule. On the other end there is an amine group, which can react with another hexanedioic acid molecule. Such continuous condensation reactions lead to the formation of a nylon 66 polymer strand, the repeating unit of which is also shown above.
>
> The "66" in nylon 66 stands for the six carbon atoms in each of the monomer molecules. Other nylons have different numbers of carbon atoms in the monomer molecules, such as nylon 510, which has 5 carbon atoms in the diamine (1,5-pentanediamine) and 10 carbon atoms in the diacid (decanedioic acid).
>
> Nylon makes extremely strong threads and fibers because in addition to London dispersion forces and dipole-dipole attractions, there are hydrogen bonds between the polymer chains. Specifically, a hydrogen bond can form between a N-H in one strand and a carbonyl O lone pair in a neighboring strand.[73]

Dr. Wojtkowiak confirms what I have been warning anyone who will listen: that conventional blood thinners, which work on the clotting cascade, are useless for the dissolution of these self-assembling nanotechnology polymers. Prions are self-perpetuating protein structures (polymerized protein) that typically take the form of amyloid/hydrogel aggregates. Polyamides polymers are used for drug delivery.[74]

CHAPTER 3

FLUORESCENCE PHENOMENON

In this chapter, a compilation of the research regarding glowing faces and fluorescent filaments is presented. This is correlated with the findings of other scientific groups that analyzed the COVID 19 injections and found fluorescent elements.

Fluorescent Filaments Coming Out of C19 Vaccinated Individual's Skin Glowing Under UV Light

JANUARY 27, 2024[1]

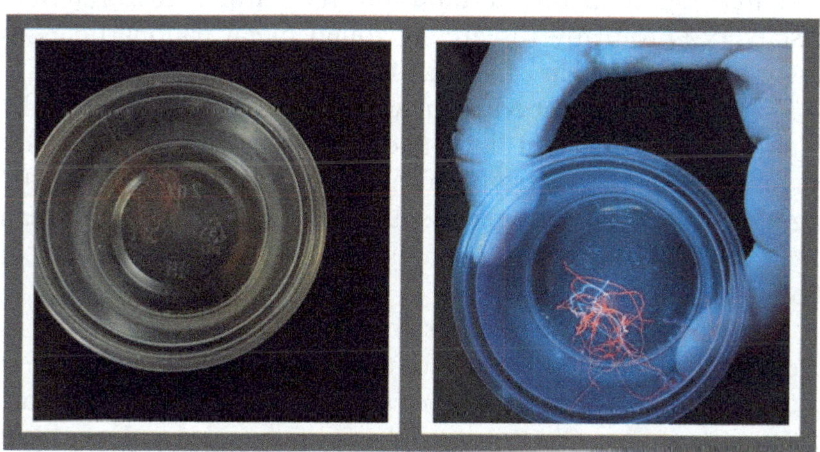

Figure 1. Filaments coming out of the skin of a COVID 19 injected individual are shown in regular light (left) and under UV light (right). AM Medical.[2]

In January 2024, I was visited in my clinic by Dr. Justin Coy, PhD, a former Department of Defense contractor who has been following and validating my research. He brought with him a filament sample and a UV flashlight—365 nm. Here I am documenting the darkfield microscopy of those polymer filaments and my experiments with UV light.

Justin was suspecting luciferase to be present in the filaments and asked me to take a look. Luciferase is used in molecular biology—the luciferase enzyme and a substrate (such as luciferin) are used to study gene regulation at the level of transcription. I did not think that was the mechanism causing the fluorescence of the polymers. That's because other mechanisms using metals to create fluorescence have been described in the literature. Clifford Caricom's analysis also showed huge amounts of metals in the filaments he analyzed that made this plausible.

Metal contamination has been found in the COVID 19 bioweapons and there have been research developments where bright orange proteins were fused with luciferase in biological systems—this remains a question for further research and discovery.[3] From my research, I found metal nanoparticles in Justin's filaments that can cause fluorescence.

We know that embedded quantum dot technology can make filaments emit different light, and filaments found in the blood have been shown to have birefringence. We also know that UV light can be used as an energy source by nanosensors which can embed themselves in what is called "Self-Assembly of Polymer."

Polymers have been described in the scientific literature as glowing when stretched.[4] Spider fossils have also been found to glow under UV light. In other chapters we further investigate polyamide spider silk. Polymer plastics even release fluorescent molecules to warn manufacturers of cracks.[5]

Below are different images of the same filament analyzed by me while observing how they change under normal light versus UV light.

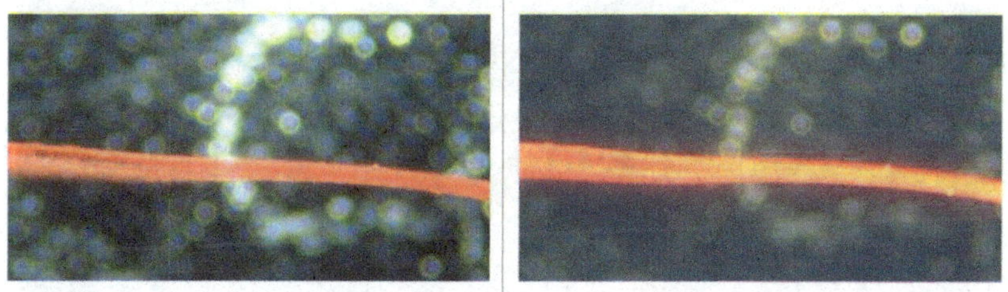

Figure 2. Darkfield microscopy on filament coming from skin: UV light off left, UV light on right. AM Medical.[6]

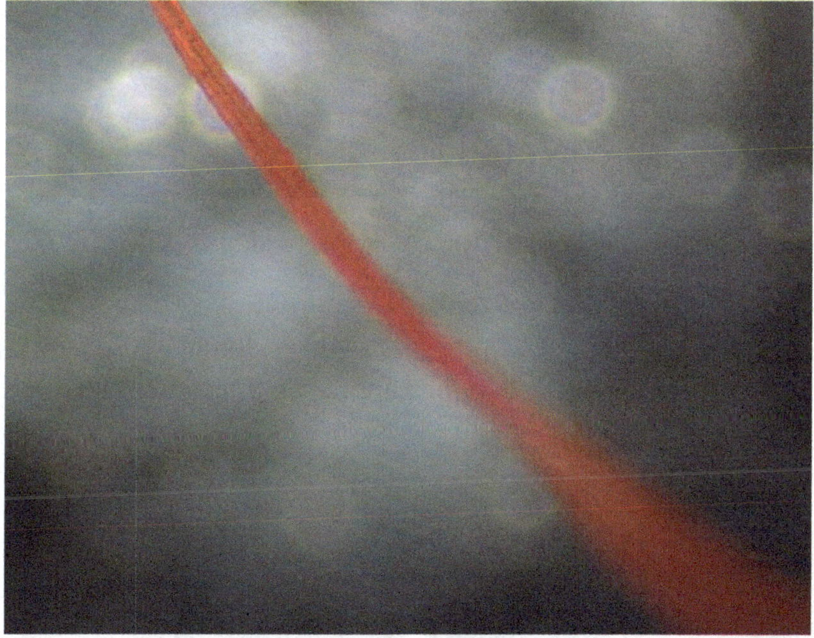

Figure 3. Filament under normal light. AM Medical.[7]

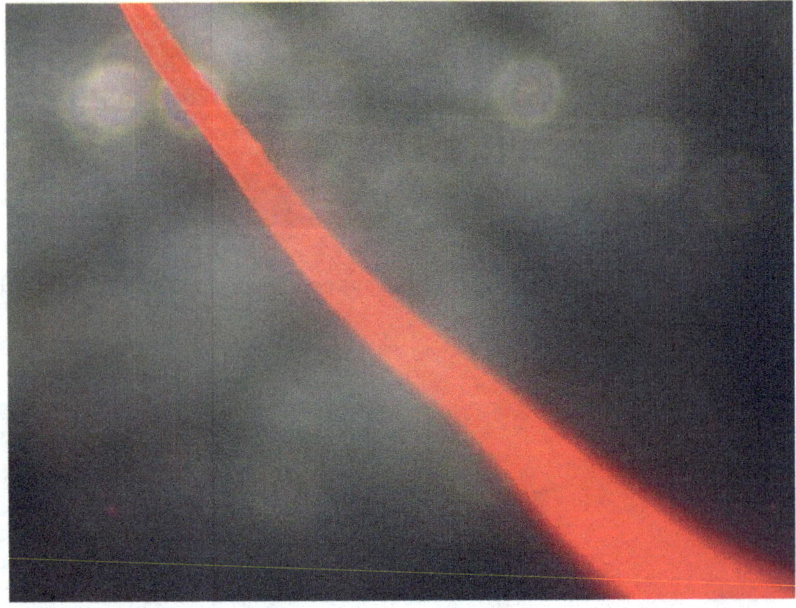

Figure 4. Fluorescent filament with UV light on. AM Medical.[8]

I then wanted to see if different aspects of the filament react differently to UV light, and they appear to. Some areas are more luminescent than others:

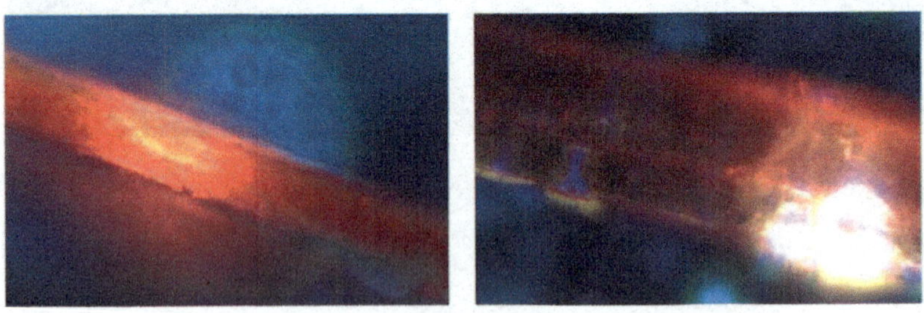

Figure 5. Fluorescent filament with UV light on, both pictures. AM Medical.[9]

Below you can see a closer view of this filament glowing under UV light, with a very specific region reacting to the UV light source:

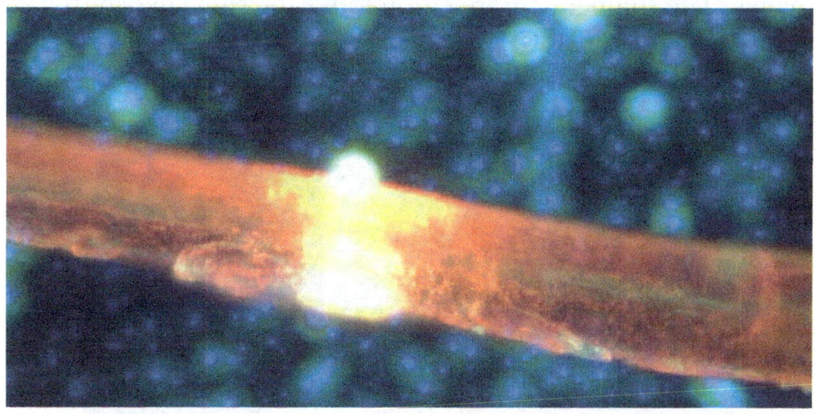

Figure 6. Fluorescent filament with UV light on. AM Medical.[10]

Out of this orange filament a white one came forth. Magnification of 2000x on the image to the right shows a central cavitation of the filament:

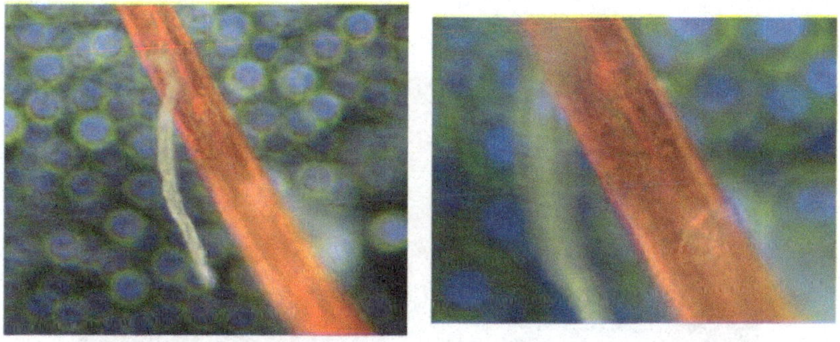

Figure 7. Fluorescent filament with UV light on. Left: Magnification approx. 400x. Right: Magnification 2000x. AM Medical.[11]

In Figure 8 below, one can compare this orange filament found on the skin to a self-assembling nanotechnology hydrogel filament I have seen in COVID 19 unvaccinated blood. Many visible quantum dot-like structures are seen embedded in both images. The filament composition looks the same except for the colors being different.

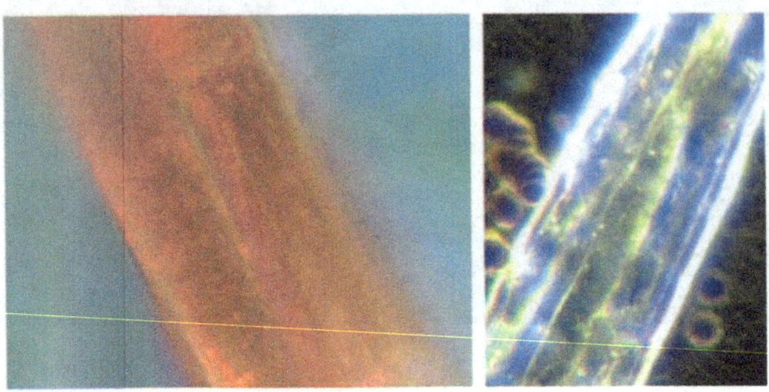

Figure 8. Left: Fluorescent filament with UV light on. Magnification 2000x. Right: Polymer filament in COVID 19 unvaccinated live blood shows same internal structure. Magnification 2000x. AM Medical.[12]

Here are different areas of the same skin filament that have enormous glow under UV light:

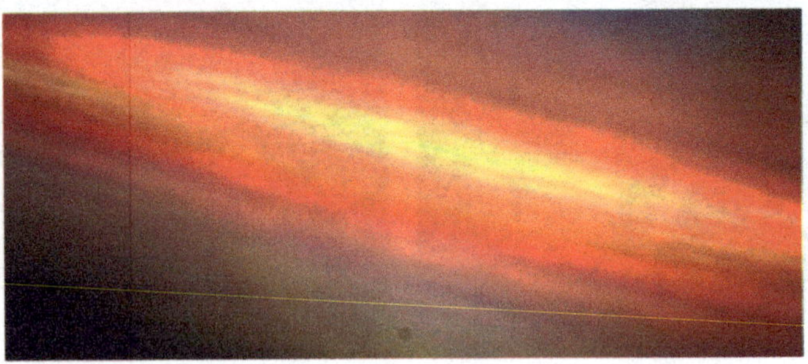

Figure 9. Fluorescent filament with UV light on. Magnification 2000x. AM Medical.[13]

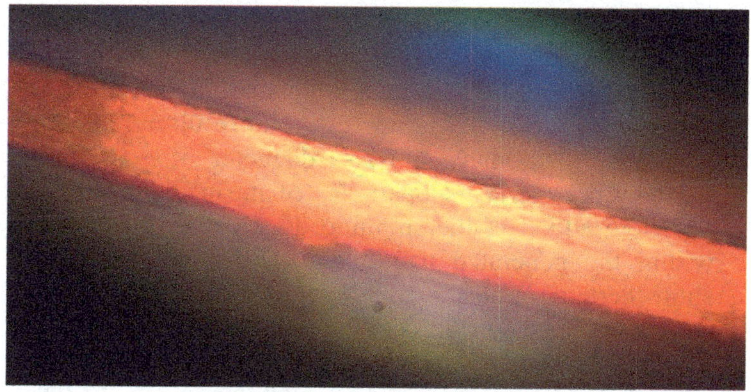

Figure 10. Fluorescent filament with UV light on. Magnification 2000x. AM Medical.[14]

Here is the same filament without UV light:

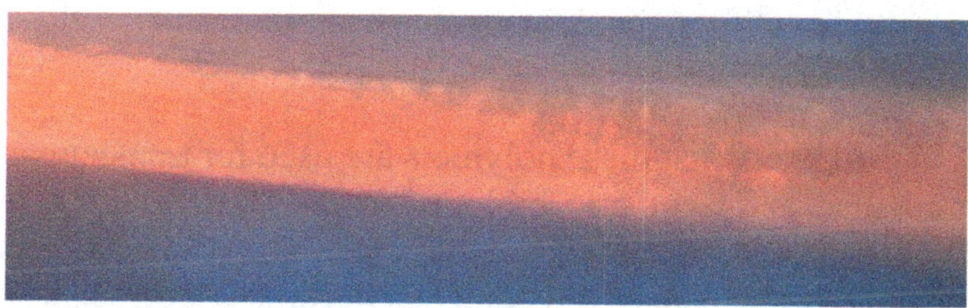

Figure 11. Filament under normal light. Magnification 2000x. AM Medical.[15]

I have been speaking about spider silk, which is a polyamide protein, and recently did microscopy on an environmental filament found.[16]

Below is the Abstract from an article published by *Spie.Digital Library* that explains how, if metals are introduced into these polymer nanofibers, fluorescence can be achieved:

> The work demonstrates an electrospun nano-composite of recombinant spider silk protein (rSSp)

> nanofibers with embedded cerium oxide (ceria) nanoparticles. RSSP (MaSp1) has been produced, extracted from goat milk, and fabricated into nanofibers using an electrospinning process. The resulting electro spun nanofibers have a mean diameter of ~50 nm. Furthermore, ceria nanoparticles of mean diameter 10 nm were added in the spinning dope to be embedded within the generated nanofibers. These nanoparticles show certain optical activity due to optical trivalent cerium ions, associated with formed oxygen vacancies. The formed nanocomposite shows promising mechanical properties such as the Young's modulus, elasticity (or elongation at break), and toughness. In addition, the electrospun mat becomes fluorescent with 520 nm emission upon exposure to UV light, due to excitation of the optically active ceria nanoparticles. Also, the formed nanocomposite shows a decay of its electric resistance over time upon exposure to cyclic loads at different humidity conditions. The synthesized nanocomposite can be utilized in different biomedical, textile, and sensing applications.[17]

We do know that these polymers are used for transhumanist surveillance and synthetic biology. In the description above, they simply used spider silk as an inspiration. However, I wish to emphasize that "the electrospun mat becomes fluorescent with 520 nm emission upon exposure to UV light, due to excitation of the optically active ceria nanoparticles." Please also note: "The synthesized nanocomposite can be utilized in different biomedical, textile, and sensing applications."

Below others describe how these polymers can wrap around nerves, muscles, and hearts and be the next generation tissue-electronic interface.

> Linking biological tissues with electronic devices is challenging owing to the softness of tissues and their arbitrary shapes and sizes. An innovative water-responsive, super contractile polymer film, inspired by

> spider silk, allows the construction of soft, stretchable, and shape-adaptive tissue-electronic interfaces.
>
> We designed water-responsive super contractile polymer films composed of poly (ethylene oxide) and poly (ethylene glycol)-α-cyclodextrin inclusion complex, which are initially dry, flexible, and stable under ambient conditions, contract by more than 50% of their original length within seconds (about 30% per second) after wetting and become soft (about 100 kPa) and stretchable (around 600%) hydrogel thin films thereafter. This super contraction is attributed to the aligned microporous hierarchical structures of the films, which also facilitate electronic integration. We used this film to fabricate shape-adaptive electrode arrays that simplify the implantation procedure through super contraction and conformally wrap around nerves, muscles and hearts of different sizes when wetted for in vivo nerve stimulation and electrophysiological signal recording. This study demonstrates that this water-responsive material can play an important part in shaping the next-generation tissue-electronics interfaces as well as broadening the biomedical application of shape-adaptive materials.[18]

After meeting with Justin Coy and analyzing the fluorescent skin filaments he brought me, I took a blood sample and applied UV light to see what would happen to the microrobots. As in my experiments with the 450 nm cold laser,[19] the robots appeared quite happy and seemed to absorb the extra energy—if you observe the robot's light emission it intensifies, and that is consistent with a recent Wireless Body Area Network (WBAN) article stating light is an energy source for biosensors.[20]

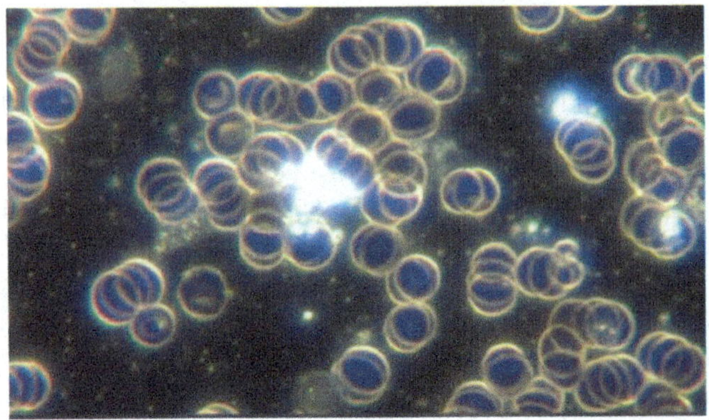

Figure 12. Microrobot aggregation in COVID 19 unvaccinated blood. AM Medical.[21]

Fluorescent Orange Face Tattoo Under UV Light in C19 Vaccinated and Eye of Horus Phenomenon – Are Humans' Limbic Systems Being Altered for Behavior Modification?

FEBRUARY 18, 2024[22]

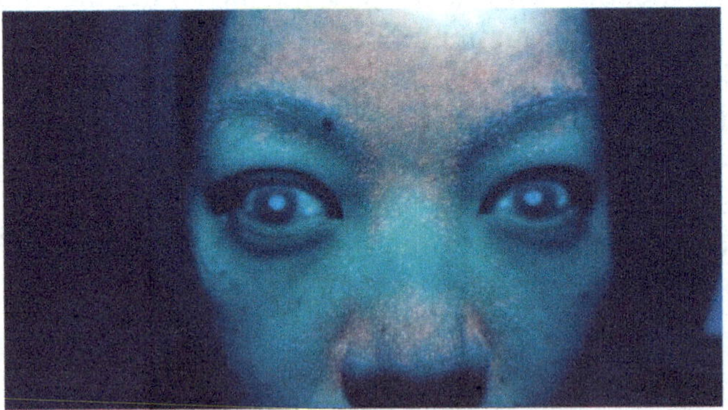

Figure 13. Individual after one Moderna COVID 19 injection and 3 PCR tests shows orange, fluorescent skin tattoo. In the white sclera are two fluorescent bright spots on both sides of the iris consistent with the Eye of Horus phenomenon. Justin Coy, PhD.[23]

As discussed, Dr. Justin Coy brought me filaments being expelled from individuals' skin, and he also provided images of their faces glowing orange, as seen in Figures 13 and 14.

I have briefly mentioned the research of Dr. Hildegarde Staninger regarding "The Eye of Horus Effect," where she utilized UV light to find self-assembling nanotechnology markers after aerial spraying of pheromone pesticides in California in 2008. I include the Abstract from an article on this research by Dr. Staninger:

> 'The Eye of Horus Effect' is coined after the W[e]dj[a]t or Eye of the Moon, and afterwards known as the Eye of Ra or Udjat. It is an ancient Egyptian symbol of protection and royal power from deities, in this case from Horus or Ra. The symbol is seen on images of Horus' mother, Isis, and on other deities associated with her. During the early months of 2008 in specific locations of the State of California aerial spraying of a biological pesticide designed to kill the Brown Moth through the use of pheromones. Field and clinical observations were made for ocular exposure the dye used to coat the nano or microspheres in the aerial spraying of this new and applied 'safer' pesticide. It was suspected that some kind of invisible fluorescent dye was applied to the microspheres. Random individuals consented to having their eyes exposed to UV-B light to observe any accumulation of this dye chemically known as fluorescein thiocyanate. Specific parts of the sclera were examined and revealed fluorescent 'highlighter yellow' pigmentation on various sections of the sclera and eye, which matched ancient Egyptian symbols for the Eye of Horus. These symbols were then matched to specific Ancient Egyptian measurement system, the Eye of Horus defining an Old Kingdom rounded off number one (1) = ½ + ¼ + 1/8 + 1/16 + 1/32 + 1/64, by throwing away 1/64th. The dye is used specifically in bionanotechnology studies to monitor cell receptor sites, such as the olfactory system and pheromones that cause fear. Currently, pheromone fear and infrared invisible dye

> marking is being applied to nonlethal weapon and riot control research and technologies.[24]

Below is another image of these fluorescent spots seen in the eyes after this nanotechnology pesticide deployment in 2008, as detected by Dr. Hildegarde Staninger:

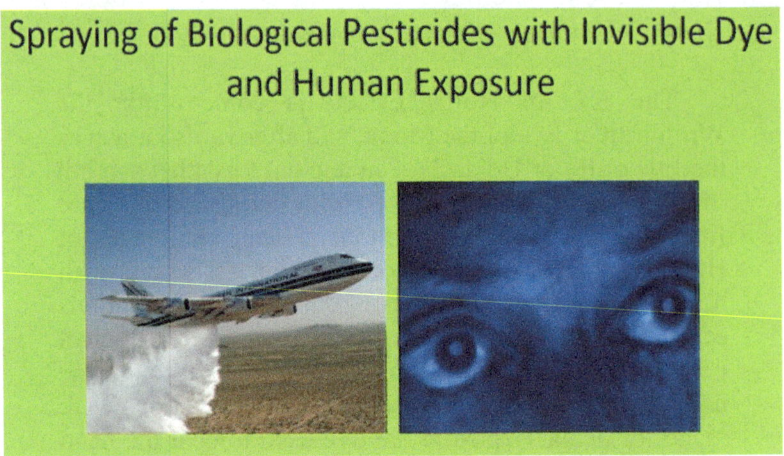

Figure 14. Left: Airplane spraying pesticides. Right: Eye of Horus Effect in a California resident. Glowing spots on both sides of the iris are seen. Dr. Hildegarde Staninger.[25]

As Dr. Staninger explained in her article, attacking the limbic system with self-assembly nanoparticles and potentially pheromones can affect memory, emotions, and was specifically suspected to cause fear.

In my interview with Dr. Coy, we discussed how many people could smell the COVID 19 vaccinated; they emit a very specific scent. I have had many patients complain to me that this scent is unpleasant.

The other interesting aspect of discovering the Eye of Horus markings in the C19 vaccinated, is that Clifford Carnicom and I had found the difference between the COVID 19 injected and uninjected is an extreme sensitivity to 4 Hz.[26]

The relevance is that the limbic system also controls the olfactory system—our sense of smell. Isn't it interesting how many people lost their sense of smell when the self-assembling nanoparticles they called "COVID" were aerosolized? Do you realize that is a way to emotionally manipulate people and affect their memory? The reason this connection is interesting is that the same phenomenon was found in 2008, when using pheromones during aerial pesticide spraying.

I include a portion of an article from *The Harvard Gazette – Science and Tech* that explains how the olfactory system works:

> Smell and memory seem to be so closely linked because of the brain's anatomy, said Harvard's Venkatesh Murthy, Raymond Leo Erikson Life Sciences Professor and chair of the Department of Molecular and Cellular Biology…
>
> Smells are handled by the olfactory bulb, the structure in the front of the brain that sends information to the other areas of the body's central command for further processing. Odors take a direct route to the limbic system, including the amygdala and the hippocampus, the regions related to emotion and memory. 'The olfactory signals very quickly get to the limbic system,' Murthy said.
>
> …For decades individuals and businesses have explored ways to harness the evocative power of smell. Think of the cologne or perfume worn by a former flame. And then there was AromaRama or Smell-O-Vision, brainchildren of the film industry of the 1950s that infused movie theaters with appropriate odors in an attempt [to] pull viewers deeper into a story—and the most recent update, the decade-old 4DX system, which incorporates special effects into movie theaters, such as shaking seats, wind, rain, as well as smells. Several years ago, Harvard scientist David Edwards worked on a new

> technology that would allow iPhones to share scents as well as photos and texts.
>
> ...[Dawn Goldworm, co-founder of 'olfactive branding company'] explained that smell is the only fully developed sense a fetus has in the womb, and it's the one that is the most developed in a child through the age of around 10 when sight takes over. And because 'smell and emotion are stored as one memory,' said Goldworm, childhood tends to be the period in which you create 'the basis for smells you will like and hate for the rest of your life.'[27]

I spoke about the fact that the military has weaponized pheromones in my interview with Justin Coy.[28] This next excerpt is from an article by David Hambling, published on *WIRED*:

> American military researchers are working to uncover and harness the most terrifying chemical imaginable: that most primal odor, the scent of fear. Pheromones are chemicals released by animals as signals to their own kind: for sex, for territorial marking, and more. They're often detected in the olfactory membranes. But there's more to pheromones than attraction. Many animals have an alarm pheromone which is used to signal danger; aphids, for example, use it to cause their fellow lice to flee.
>
> Now, the US Army is trying to track down and harness people's smell of fear. The military has backed a study on the 'Identification and Isolation of Human Alarm Pheromones,' which 'focused on the Preliminary Identification of Steroids of Interest in Human Fear Sweat.' The so-called 'skydiving protocol' was the researchers' method of choice.
>
> ...But what about offensive use? Pheromones are effective in minute quantities, so a wide area can be blanketed with just a few liters. Given sufficient concentration, would everyone exposed start suffering from an unidentifiable dread? The contagious aspect

> means that those affected would start churning out fear pheromone as well.
>
> On its own, the alarm pheromone probably would not do much. But given an external trigger, such as a loud noise, it could influence people to start stampeding like spooked cattle. Then again, the bee alarm pheromone triggers attack rather than flight, and the Viennese study suggested something similar may apply to humans—or are there multiple pheromones involved? Whatever is going on, this research is likely to uncover some novel and powerful ways of manipulating human behavior.
>
> Some in the military research complex have been down this road before. Remember the so-called 'Gay Bomb,' that would make enemy combatants irresistibly attracted to one another? Speaking of which, all those web sites advertising pheromones to make you irresistible to the opposite sex haven't actually got many decent studies to back them up, a topic I explored in last month's *Fortean Times* magazine.[29]

Here is another article, this time from *The Guardian,* in 2007, that talks about the US military weaponizing pheromones:

> What if it [the US air force] could release a chemical that would make an opposing army's soldiers think more about the physical attributes of their comrades in arms than the threat posed by the enemy? And thus the 'gay bomb' was born. Far from being the product of conspiracy theorists, documents released to a biological weapons watchdog in Austin, Texas confirm that the US military did investigate the idea. It was included in a CD-Rom produced by the US military in 2000 and submitted to the National Academy of Sciences in 2002. The documents show that $7.5m was requested to develop the weapon.
>
> The documents released to the Sunshine Project under a freedom of information request titled 'Harassing, Annoying and Bad Guy Identifying Chemicals' includes several proposals for the military use of chemicals that

> could be sprayed on to enemy positions. 'One distasteful but non-lethal example would be strong aphrodisiacs, especially if the chemical also caused homosexual behavior,' says the proposal from the Air Force's Wright Laboratory in Dayton, Ohio.[30]

Is there a cabal working to influence people's emotions and memories through the COVID 19 injection that is self-spreading via the limbic system? Could the "vaccine" be used for tracking—not just manifested as a MAC address phenomenon but also a facial tattoo? Is the scent emitted from the COVID 19 injected part of social engineering and manipulation of society? What are the pheromones emitted from the C19 injected programmed with? Is it fear? And is that contributing to the epidemic of anxiety and panic attacks that we see in both the COVID 19 injected and those unvaccinated who are affected by shedding?

Just as a reminder, nothing is visible on the face of a COVID 19 vaccinated individual until the 365 nm UV flashlight is turned on. This is when the orange facial tattoo is visible. As Dr. Coy explained, it will spread out, self-replicating over the entire forehead.

Below I show the filaments coming out of C19 vaccinated skin. One can detect them after a person takes a hot shower and then inspects the skin with a 365 nm UV flashlight. These filaments, just like Morgellons, are artificial intelligent synthetic life forms, sensitive and attracted to biophotons or any component of the human body, like hair. If these are shedding from the COVID 19 vaccinated, as has been shown in the research by Dr. Coy, and they are attracted to human skin, is that one way that shedding is transfecting to the C19 unvaccinated? If these filaments are airborne and then inhaled or transferred through touch, is that one of the mechanisms of shedding?

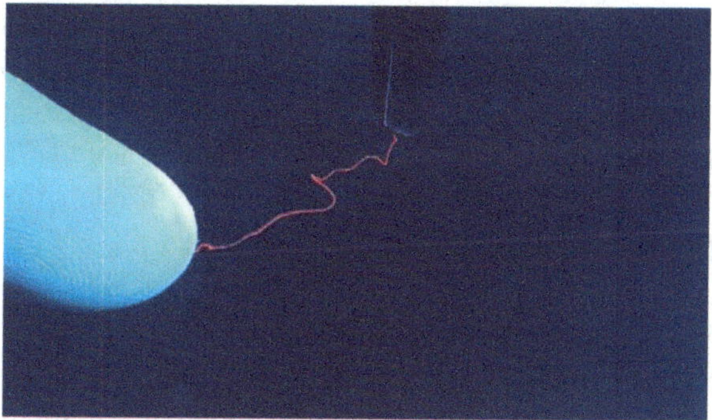

Figure 15. Fluorescent filament from COVID 19 vaccinated individual is attracted to finger. Dr. Justin Coy.[31]

If you recall, the Pfizer "vaccine" trial documents revealed that inhaling the air around a vaccinated person can cause an unvaccinated individual to become vaccinated. For reference, see that section from the trial documents below:

> 8.3.5.3. Occupational Exposure
> An occupational exposure occurs when a person receives unplanned direct contact with the study intervention, which may or may not lead to the occurrence of an AE [Adverse Event]. Such persons may include healthcare providers, family members, and other roles that are involved in the trial participant's care. The investigator must report occupational exposure to Pfizer Safety within 24 hours of the investigator's awareness, regardless of whether there is an associated SAE [Serious Adverse Event]. The information must be reported using the Vaccine SAE Report Form. Since the information does not pertain to a participant enrolled in the study, the information is not recorded on a CRF [Case Report Form]; however, a copy of the completed Vaccine SAE Report Form is maintained in the investigator site file.[32]

On page 69 of the Pfizer trial documents, we find the following validation of potential shedding to the unvaccinated:

A male family member or healthcare provider who has been exposed to the study intervention by inhalation or skin contact then exposes his female partner prior to or around the time of conception.

And further:

8.3.5.1. Exposure During Pregnancy
An EDP occurs if:

- Study intervention. is found to be pregnant while receiving or after discontinuing study intervention.
- A male participant who is receiving or has discontinued study intervention exposes a female partner prior to or around the time of conception.
- A female is found to be pregnant while being exposed or having been exposed to study intervention due to environmental exposure.

Below are examples of environmental exposure during pregnancy:

- A female family member or healthcare provider reports that she is pregnant after having been exposed to the study intervention by inhalation or skin contact.

And on page 67:

- The investigator must report EDP to Pfizer Safety within 24 hours of the investigator's awareness, irrespective of whether an SAE has occurred. The initial information submitted should include the anticipated date of delivery (see below for information related to termination of pregnancy).
- If EDP occurs in a participant or a participant's partner, the investigator must report this information to Pfizer Safety on the Vaccine SAE Report Form and an EDP Supplemental Form, regardless of

> whether an SAE has occurred. Details of the pregnancy will be collected after the start of study intervention and until 6 months after the last dose of study intervention.[33]

I have looked at many COVID 19 unvaccinated individuals under UV light using a 365 nm flashlight, and so far, some are completely clear, while others have an orange tattoo around their nose. Few have dots on their forehead, which is rare, and I have never seen the full, bright orange tattoo across the entire forehead like Dr. Coy has shown in numerous COVID 19 vaccinated individuals. In the scientific literature, the identification of fluorescent nanoparticles, specifically with glowing of the forehead, has been researched.

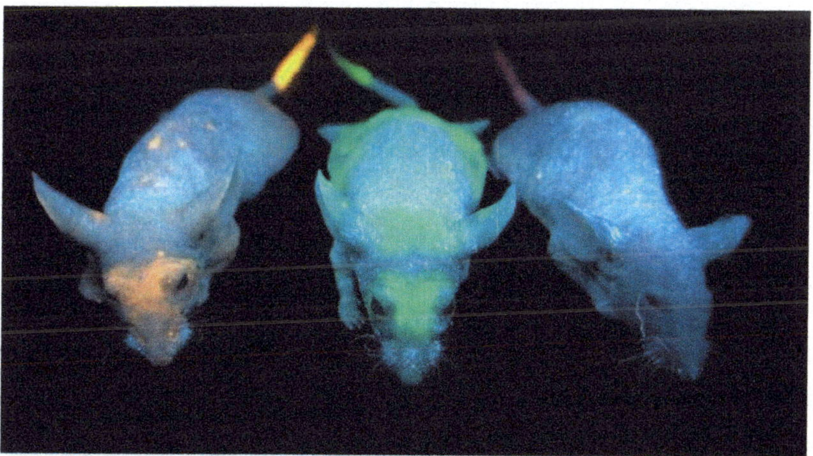

Figure 16. Research at the University of Toronto found the skin of mice became fluorescent after they were injected with nanoparticles called quantum dots. Cutting off a small piece of skin and running it through a machine provides a more precise measurement of nanoparticle exposure. Edward A. Sykes & Qin Dai/University of Toronto.[34]

According to *CBC News*, May 2014, "Canadian researchers have developed the first test for exposure to nanoparticles—new chemical technology found in a huge range of consumer products—that could potentially be used on humans.

"Warren Chan, a University of Toronto chemistry professor, and his team developed the skin test after noticing that some mice changed colour and others became fluorescent (that is, they glowed when light of certain colours were shone on them) after being exposed to increasing levels of different kinds of nanoparticles. The mice were being used in research to develop cancer treatments involving nanoparticles."[35]

C19 Uninjected Individuals Expelling Fluorescent Filaments Through Skin Similar to C19 Injected

MAY 31, 2024[36]

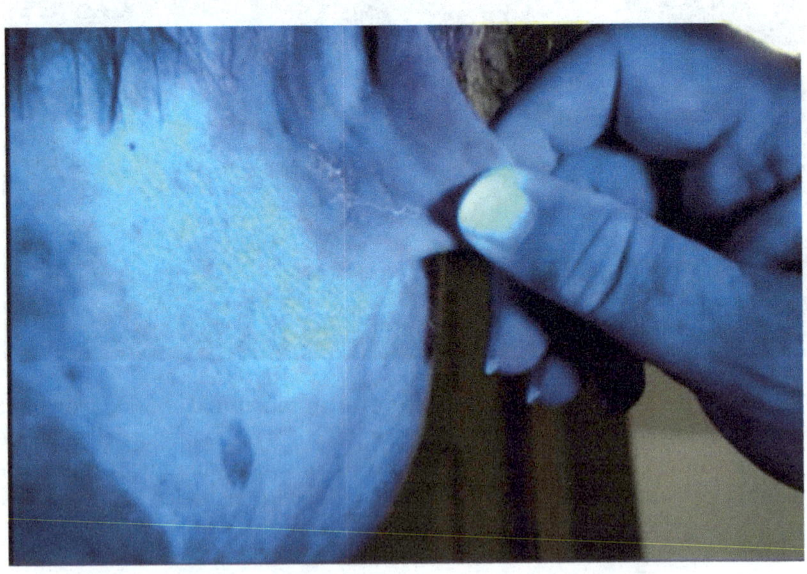

Figure 17. Fluorescent filament exiting behind the ear seen under UV light exposure in COVID 19 unvaccinated individual (patient A). AM Medical.[37]

After I had posted articles on my Substack about fluorescent filaments coming out of the COVID 19 injected and the orange tattoo glowing on the skin, some of my C19 uninjected patients who had been exposed to shedding, as well as environmental sources like breathing air contaminated by geoengineering, were investigating their skin. The image above (Figure 17) is from a video where you can see a fluorescent filament coming out from behind the ear of a patient (A).

The image below is a darkfield live blood analysis done previously with patient A showing filaments forming in the distressed blood:

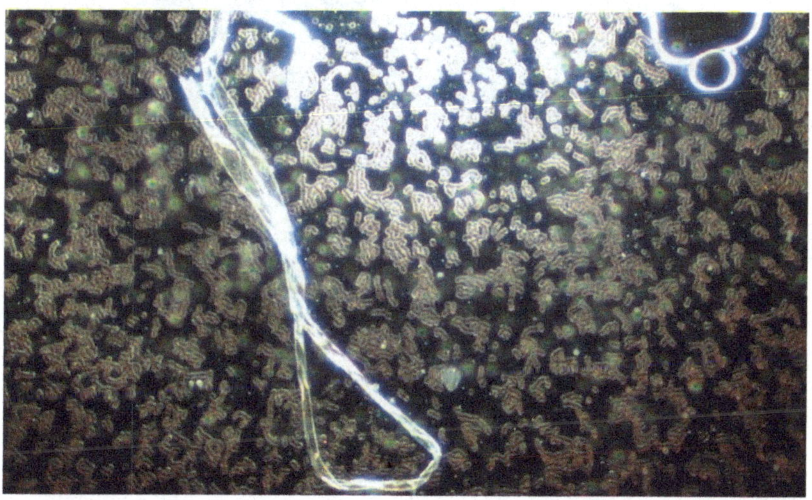

Figure 18. Earlier live blood analysis on the same COVID 19 unvaccinated individual (patient A) shows large polymer filament and rouleaux formation. AM Medical.[38]

In the next image, one can see UV light being shone on a fluorescent filament that is coming out of the skin of the same patient A on another spot of the body. The filament was observed reacting to the ambient energy field of the finger, trying to attach to it.

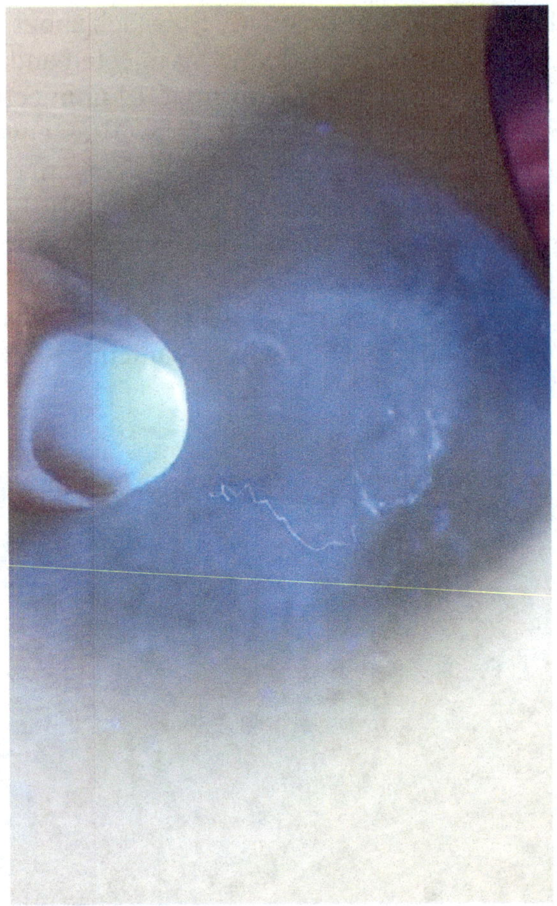

Figure 19. Fluorescent filament exiting the skin seen under UV light exposure in COVID 19 unvaccinated individual (patient A). AM Medical.[39]

In another COVID 19 uninjected patient (B), orange, fluorescent spots and fluorescent blue filaments were also observed coming out of the skin.

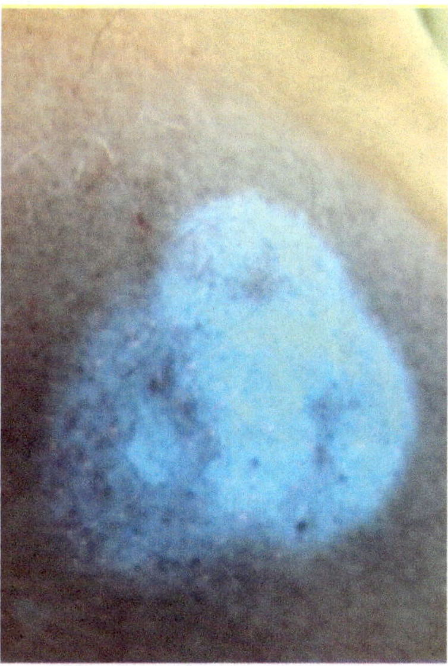

Figure 20. Fluorescent orange spots on skin of the chest seen under UV light exposure in COVID 19 unvaccinated individual (patient B). AM Medical.[40]

Patient B also had significant live blood contamination in a previous exam, as shown below:

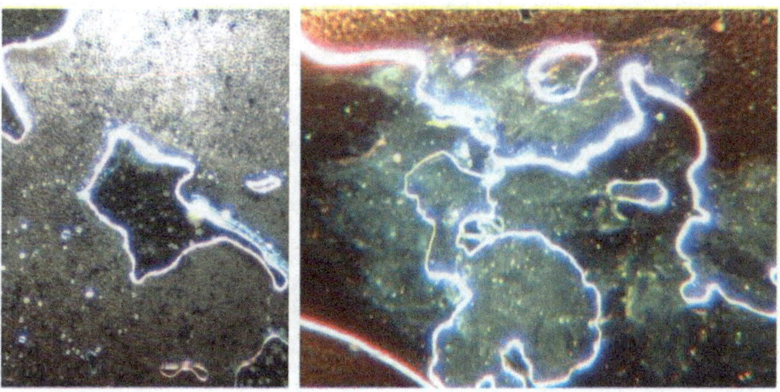

Figure 21. COVID 19 uninjected blood (patient B), construction sites building polymer filament on the left. Magnification 200x. Right: Large polymer construction. Magnification 200x. AM Medical.[41]

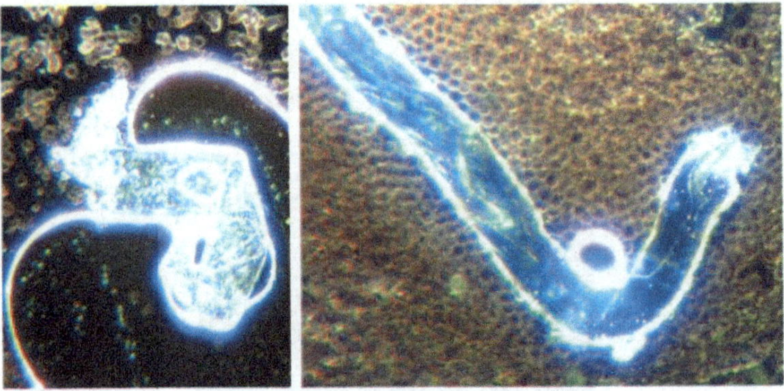

Figure 22. Left: COVID 19 unvaccinated blood (patient B), construction sites building polymer filament. Magnification 2000x. Right: Large polymer filament with red blood cells in severe oxidative distress. Magnification 2000x. AM Medical.[42]

I was given a sample of the filament that came out of patient A's skin. Without UV light the filament looks exactly as what we are seeing in the blood on the left of Figure 23 below. Then I turned on the UV light and you can see on the right the blue violet glow:

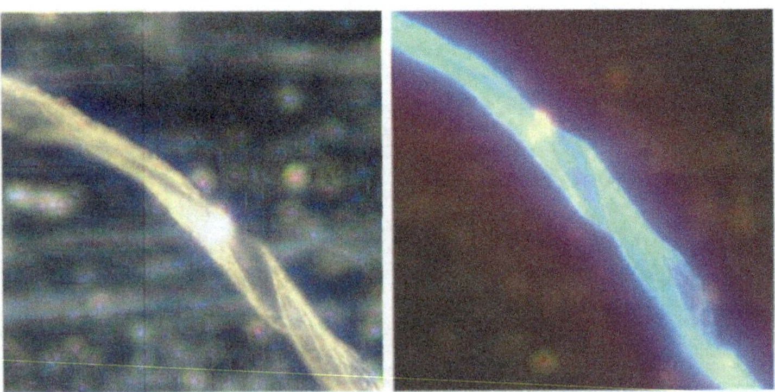

Figure 23. Left: Polymer filament from COVID 19 unvaccinated individual (patient A) under normal light. Right: Same filament with UV light on. Notice blue-violet glow. AM Medical.[43]

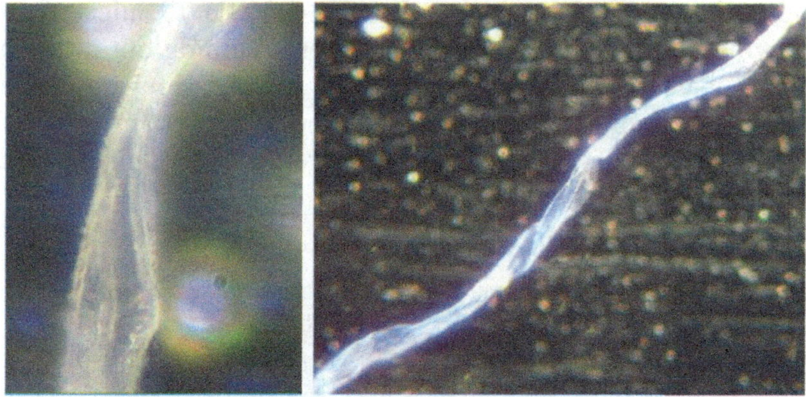

Figure 24. Left: Polymer filament from COVID 19 unvaccinated individual (patient A) under normal light. Magnification 400x. Right: Same filament with UV light on. Magnification 200x. AM Medical.[44]

I have had many other COVID 19 unvaccinated individuals without a history of Morgellons, report filaments were coming out of their skin. Strange, crawly sensations or intense itching can accompany this but does not have to happen. Extreme itching has also been reported to me in the area of the orange spots. Some people have no symptoms at all.

Fluorescent Filaments Coming Out of COVID 19 Unvaccinated Individuals and Orange Glowing Facial Spots – It's All Self-Assembly Nanotechnology

JUNE 03, 2024[45]

I have further analyzed the fluorescent blue filaments that have been shown to come out of C19 injected individuals as well as the fluorescent orange spots. Individually, researchers around the world sounded the alarm that the COVID 19 injected are glowing and have these strange filaments coming out of them. Unfortunately, I found the same thing is now occurring in the COVID 19 uninjected due to the poisonous bombardment of our atmosphere via geoengineering warfare that has contaminated our food and water supply.

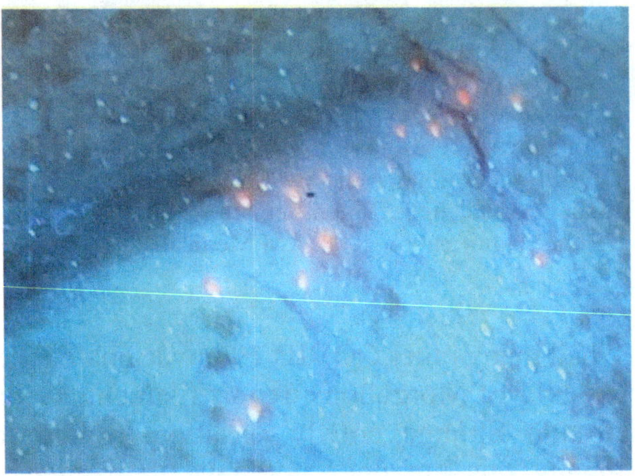

Figure 25. Nasal fold – fluorescent orange spots in COVID 19 unvaccinated individual. AM Medical.[46]

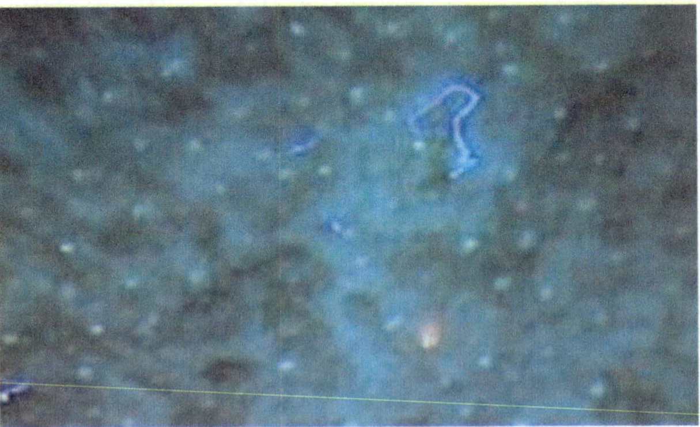

Figure 26. Fluorescent blue filament under UV light exiting the skin of COVID 19 unvaccinated individual. AM Medical.[47]

Below I offer further images of filaments from a COVID 19 uninjected patient at 2000x magnification. The same filament is depicted when the UV light is turned off, then on, off, and then on again. One can clearly see the filament's light emission and fluorescence under UV lighting.

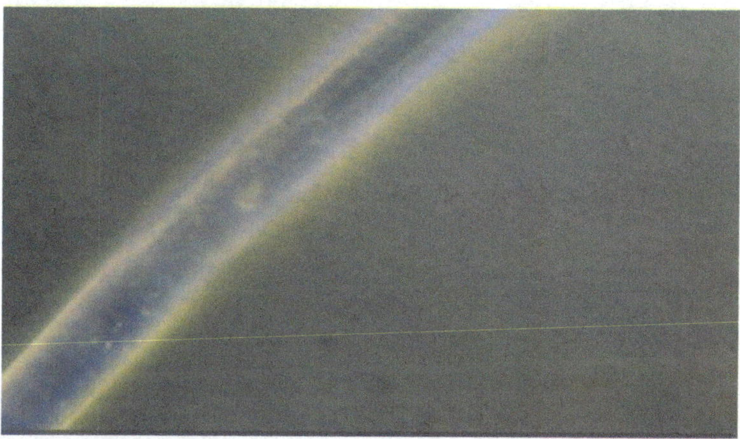

Figure 27. Filament from skin of COVID 19 unvaccinated individual in normal light. Magnification 2000x. AM Medical.[48]

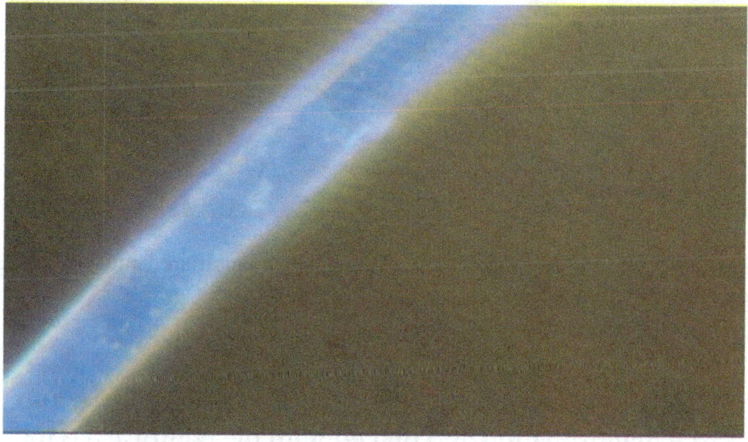

Figure 28. Filament from skin of COVID 19 unvaccinated individual under UV light. Magnification 2000x. AM Medical.[49]

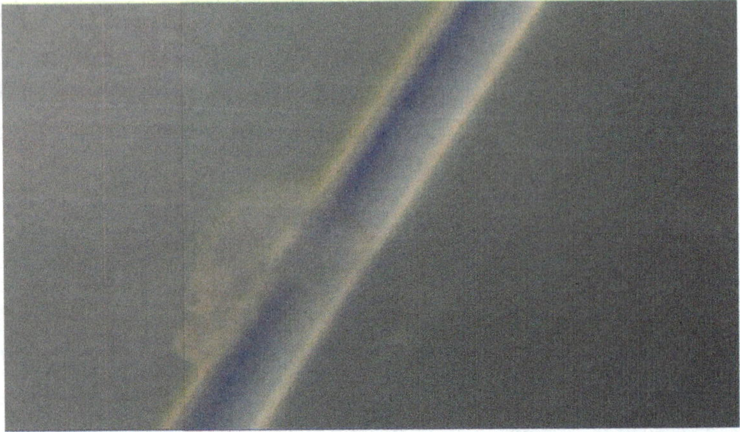

Figure 29. Filament from skin of COVID 19 unvaccinated individual again in normal light. Magnification 2000x. AM Medical.[50]

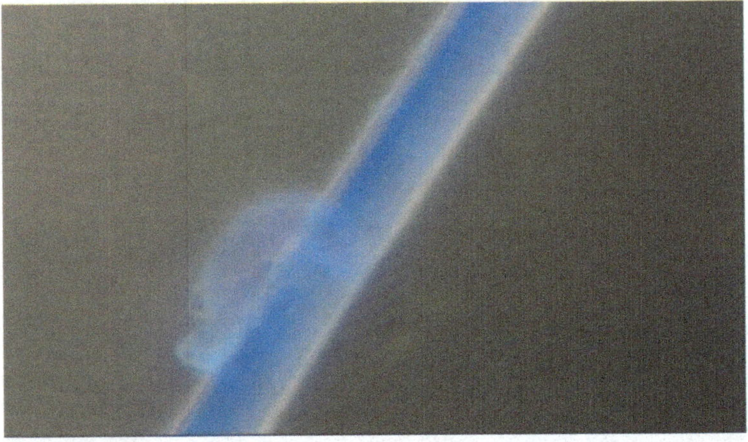

Figure 30. Filament from skin of COVID 19 unvaccinated individual again under UV light. Magnification 2000x. AM Medical.[51]

After these images were taken, I increased to 4000x oil objective magnification and played with the contrast. To me, the filaments look like artificial intelligence constructed of computer chips with elaborate electronic circuitry.

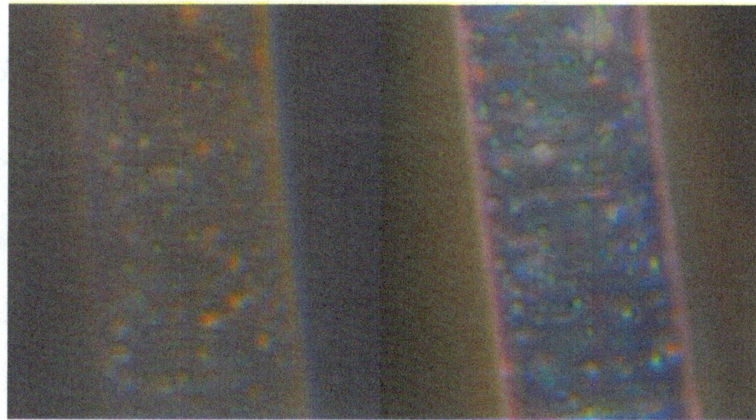

Figure 31. Filament from skin of COVID 19 unvaccinated individual. Left: Normal light. Right: UV light. Oil objective magnification 4000x. AM Medical.[52]

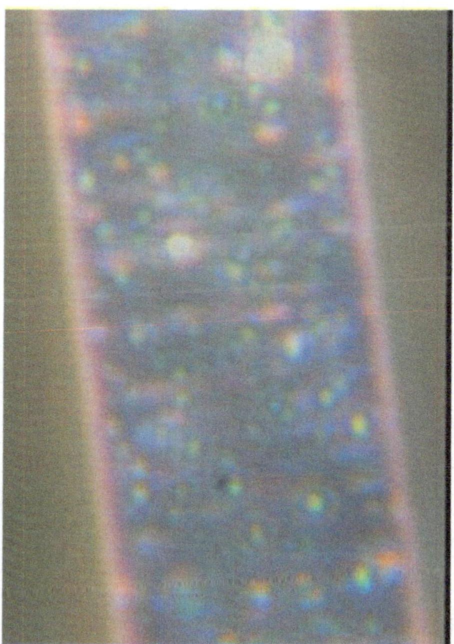

Figure 32. Higher contrast of filament from skin of COVID 19 unvaccinated individual under UV light. Oil objective magnification 4000x. AM Medical.[53]

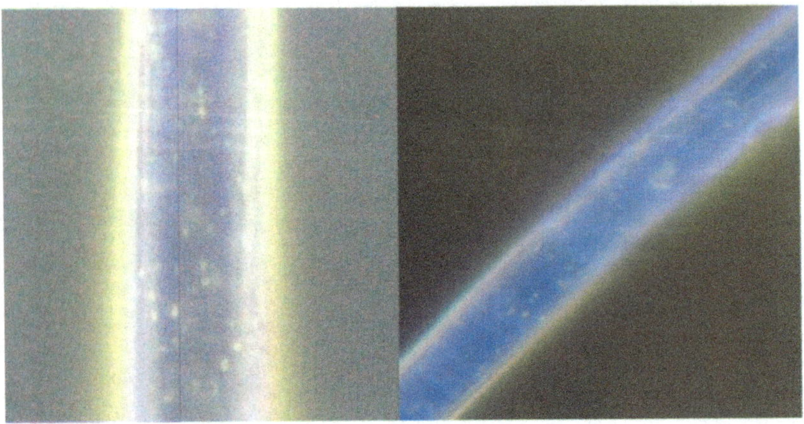

Figure 33. Filament from skin of COVID 19 unvaccinated individual. Left: Under normal light. Right: Under UV light. Magnification 2000x. AM Medical.[54]

Below is one of these orange spots scraped from the side of the nose of a C19 uninjected individual, as revealed under the microscope. Many people just dismiss this orange glow phenomenon because they have read somewhere that skin bacteria are fluorescent. Others dismiss the idea of nano- and microrobots and say they are chylomicrons. This looks like an advanced nanotechnology mesogen to me:

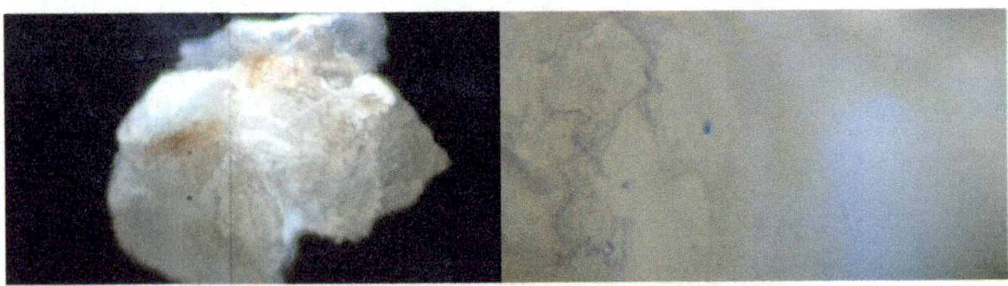

Figure 34. Nasal – orange, fluorescent mesogen from COVID 19 unvaccinated individual. Left: Magnification 100x. Right: Magnification 2000x. AM Medical.[55]

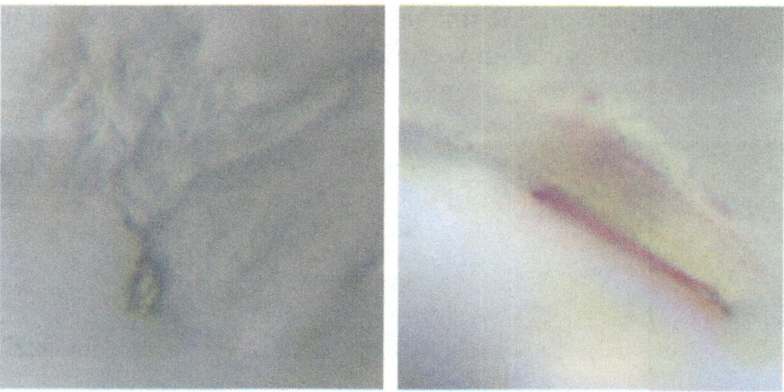

Figure 35. Nasal – fluorescent orange specimen from COVID 19 unvaccinated individual. Left: Polymer sheet. Right: Polymer sheet with red nanotechnology filaments. Magnification 2000x. AM Medical.[56]

These polymer sheets observed at high magnification look like the rubbery clots from a vaccine injured individual that I analyzed a year ago—a white plastic sheet that has fibers in multiple colors within it. The colored spots are different dyes. I have shown these also in geoengineered spider silk. The dyes are used for different nanotechnology functions.[57]

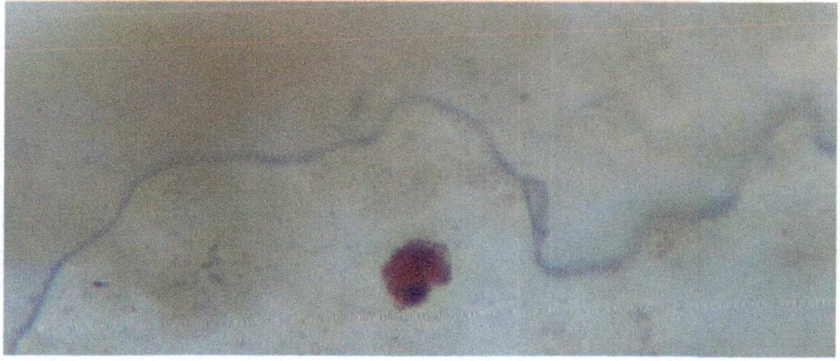

Figure 36. Nasal – fluorescent orange specimen from COVID 19 unvaccinated. Nanotechnology blue filaments and red dye mesogen.
AM Medical.[58]

For comparison, the images below show spider silk that has been sprayed via geoengineering:

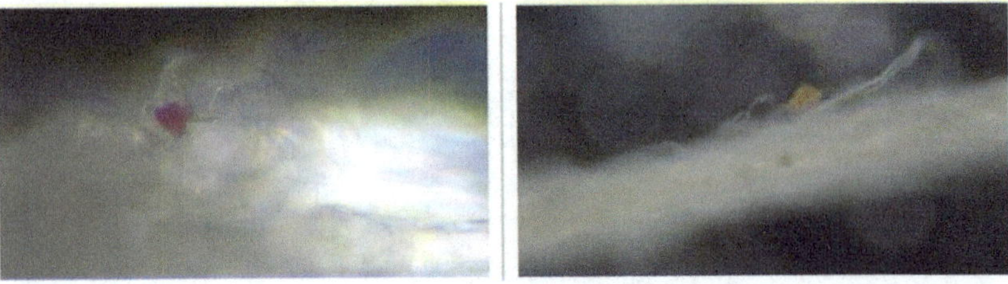

Figure 37. Darkfield microscopy of geoengineering that was chemically identified as spider silk. Red and yellow colored mesogens are seen. AM Medical.[59]

Analysis of rubbery clots found in a COVID 19 "vaccine" injured individual reveal a similar, plastic sheet-like appearance:

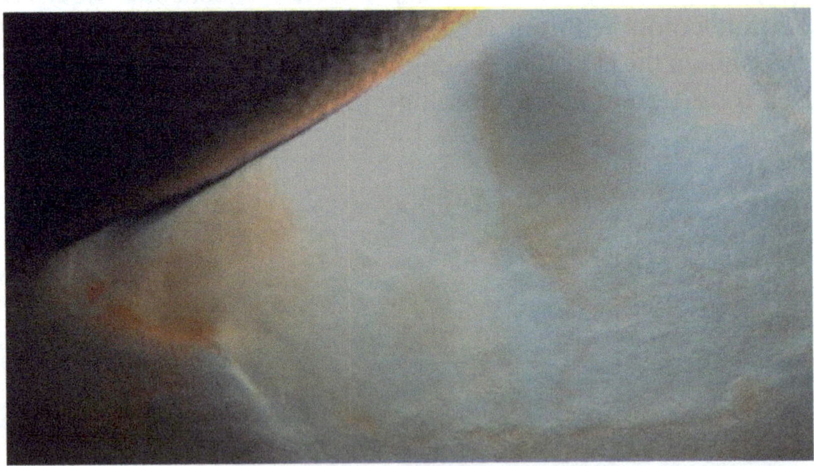

Figure 38. Plastic, sheet-like polymer in blood clot from COVID 19 injected, vaccine injured individual. AM Medical.[60]

This specimen is similar to a brain chip found in a targeted individual analyzed by Dr. Hildegarde Staninger in 2011. The chemical analysis revealed self-assembly, advanced nanotechnology components, including graphite, silicon, and sulfur.[61]

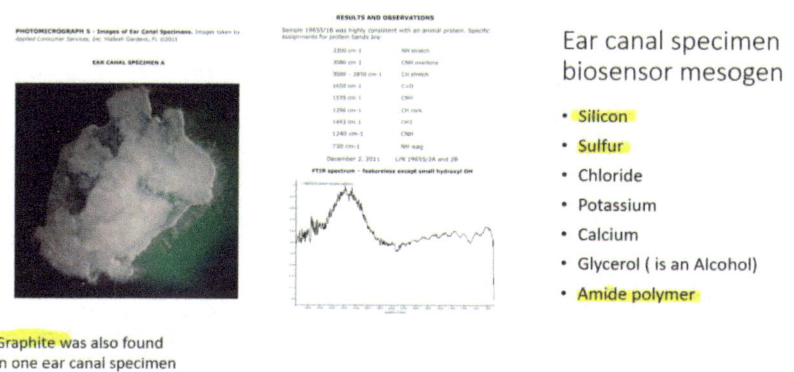

Figure 39. Ear canal biosensor mesogen chemical analysis. Dr. Hildegarde Staninger.[62]

To conclude, the fluorescent orange spots appearing since the COVID 19 "vaccine" roll out appear to be advanced nanotechnology mesogen with polymer sheets, similar to chemically analyzed nanoparticle specimens. The filaments are the same in construction as what I have seen repeatedly in human blood. Fluorescence is part of the self-assembling nanotechnology functionality and, in my opinion, introduced into humanity as part of the globalist transhumanist agenda.[63]

CHAPTER 4

COVID 19 BIOWEAPON AND CHILDHOOD "VACCINES"

Throughout the past couple of years, I have compiled articles written about analysis of the COVID 19 bioweapon contents, as well as other widely distributed "vaccines." This chapter encapsulates research from around the world. Additionally, I have evaluated many childhood "vaccines" using darkfield microscopy.

Nanotech in the Shots?

OCTOBER 02, 2022[1]

Life of the Blood, known as *LifeOfTheBlood*, is a group of anonymous researchers with microscopes residing in New Zealand, who have found remarkable abnormalities in the COVID 19 vials and in live blood analysis. These are not cholesterol crystals, as some doctors have falsely claimed when working to discredit our findings on self-assembling nanotechnology in the COVID 19 injections—a fact that has now been confirmed by researchers around the world. These microchip-like structures that have the complexity of an alien space station are not natural. And they most certainly are NOT ACCIDENTAL CONTAMINATION.

Please look at the live videos of their analysis posted on the link provided to their website.[2]

Below is one drop of New Zealand's Pfizer Comirnaty "vaccine" under a cover slip, after it was inadvertently heated lightly, then viewed later the same day through darkfield microscopy at low magnification and projected onto a TV monitor.

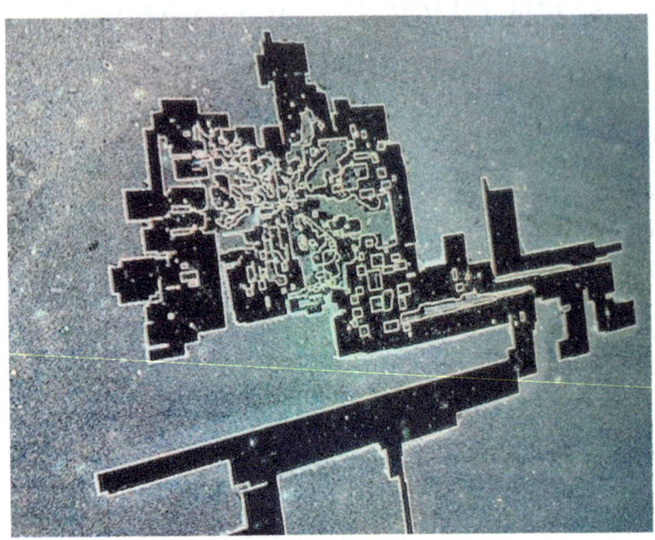

Figure 1. Self-assembly nanotechnology in Pfizer's COVID 19 Comirnaty injections. LifeOfTheBlood, New Zealand.[3]

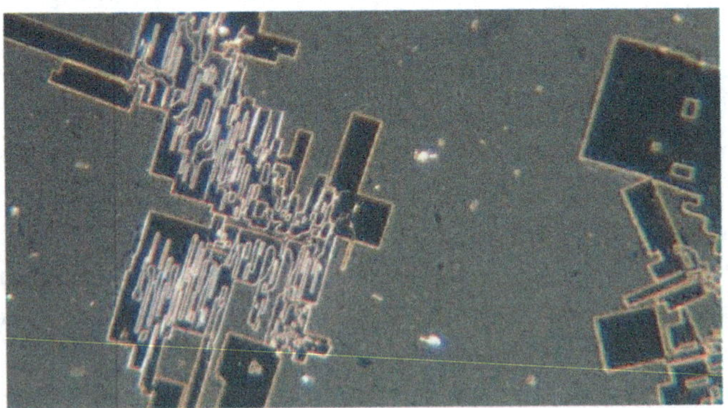

Figure 2. Self-assembly nanotechnology in Pfizer's COVID 19 Comirnaty injections. LifeOfTheBlood, New Zealand.[4]

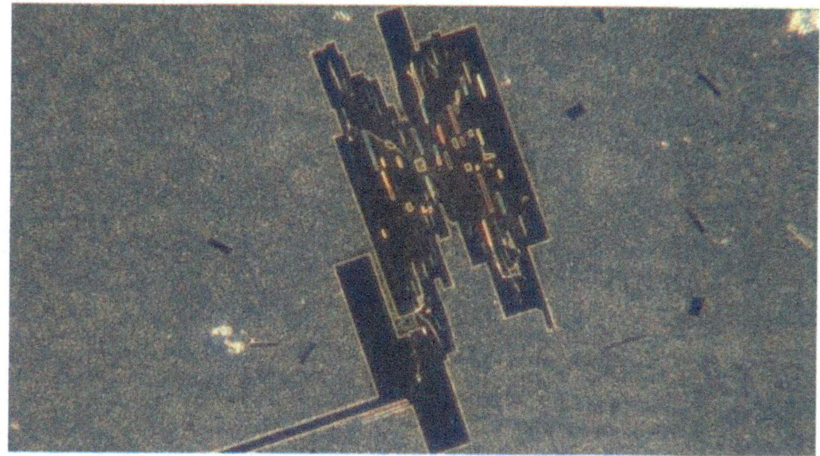

Figure 3. Self-assembly nanotechnology in Pfizer's COVID 19 Comirnaty injections. LifeOfTheBlood, New Zealand.[5]

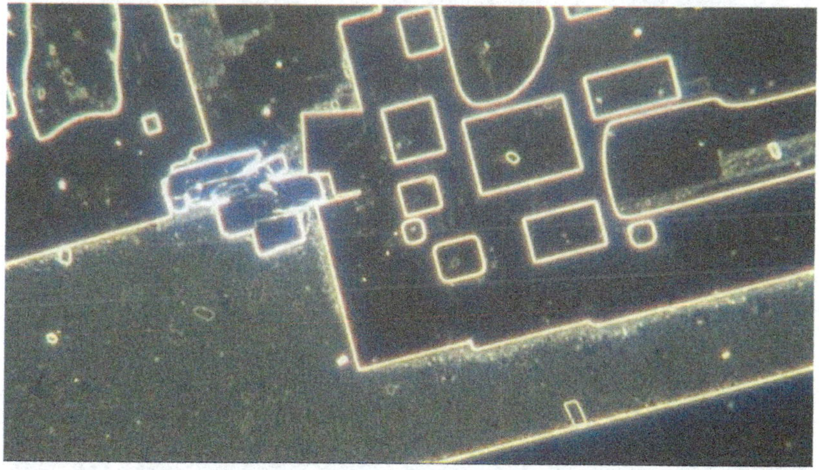

Figure 4. Self-assembly nanotechnology in Pfizer's COVID 19 Comirnaty injections. LifeOfTheBlood, New Zealand.[6]

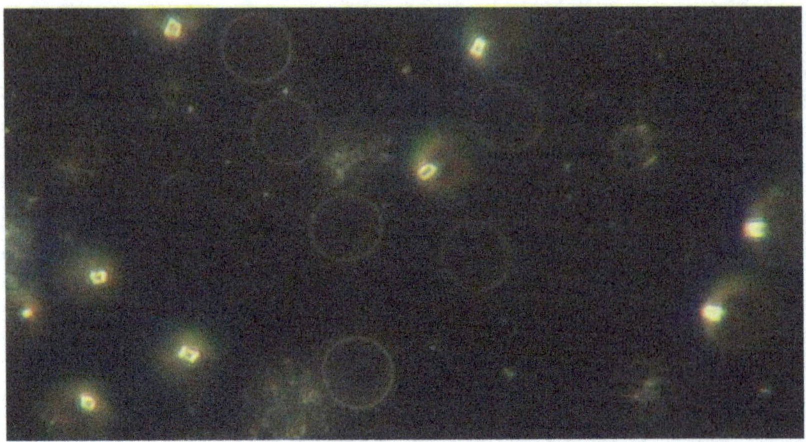

Figure 5. Square particles in Pfizer COVID 19 Comirnaty injected blood. LifeOfTheBlood, New Zealand.[7]

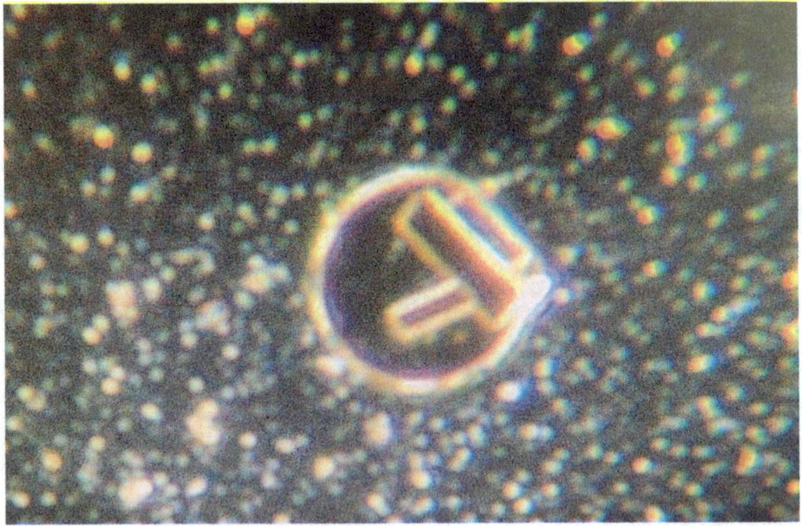

Figure 6. Unusual object in Pfizer COVID 19 Comirnaty injected blood. LifeOfTheBlood, New Zealand.[8]

LifeOfTheBlood's practitioner, a scientist with a background in medicine, mathematics, physics, and extensive phase contrast microscopy experience, says the following: "People who were injured by the Pfizer shot wanted help. Several doctors had come forward in other countries to report strange observations. Dr. Zandre Botha from South Africa showed the uniform strange round circles. La Quinta Columna showed what appeared to be microchips and other formations. Two other doctors talked about parasites and of all things, hydras!

"Having previously experienced how those of us that critically look at the vaccine situation are heavily infiltrated by persons wishing to divert and control the narrative, I thought, 'What is real?' 'What is put forth in order to lead questioners to look like fools?'

"Because of my previous extensive microscopy experience, learning to use a darkfield microscope didn't take a huge amount of education. I took a 12-week course on live blood analysis using the most sophisticated darkfield microscope and camera that my money could buy. It magnifies up to 4000x.

"After having a close look at the blood of dozens of vaccine injured people, patients started asking me about certain round and square bright yellow formations in their capillary blood as seen on the screen."[9]

The work of the New Zealand practitioner sheds additional light on the most dangerous bioweaponry ever to be cast upon humanity.

"Vaccine" Microscopy by Dr. Geanina Hagimă Shows Microrobots, Quantum Dots, and Microchip Development

OCTOBER 10, 2023[10]

Another fellow researcher, Dr. Geanina Hagimă, sent me her microscopy of multiple vaccines from Romania. Her methodology includes brightfield and darkfield microscopy. Her findings confirm what many scientists around the world, as compiled by Dr. David Hughes, have also found. I highly recommend watching my interview with Dr. Hughes and a review of the extensive evidence he has collected in his 133-page, scientific publication.[11]

Dr. Hagimă's findings are consistent with many international teams. The same microchips we have seen with COVID 19 injections have also been developed from the influenza "vaccine," commonly referred to as the "flu shot."

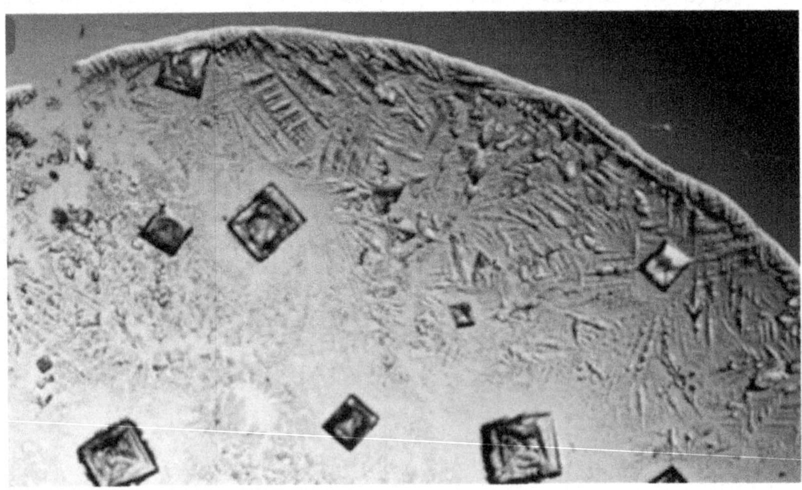

Figure 7. Microchips developed in dried influenza "vaccine." Brightfield microscopy. Dr. Geanina Hagimă.[12]

In the Moderna C19 "vaccine," many blinking lights can be seen:

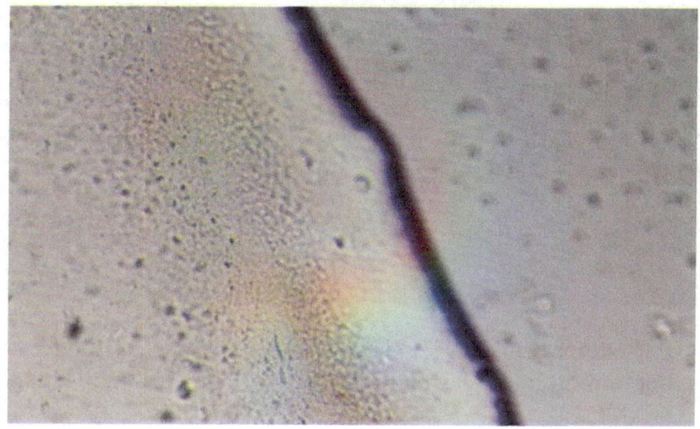

Figure 8. Moderna COVID 19 "vaccine" shows light-emitting particles. Brightfield microscopy. Dr. Geanina Hagimă.[13]

Brightfield shows large amounts of mobile nanotechnology (Figure 8). When switched to darkfield, multicolor light emissions are seen, consistent with quantum dot technology (Figures 9-11).

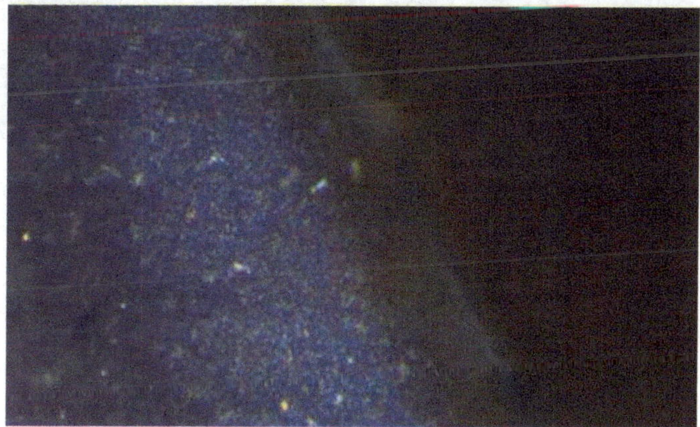

Figure 9. Moderna COVID 19 "vaccine" shows light-emitting particles that are quantum dot microrobots. Darkfield microscopy. Dr. Geanina Hagimă.[14]

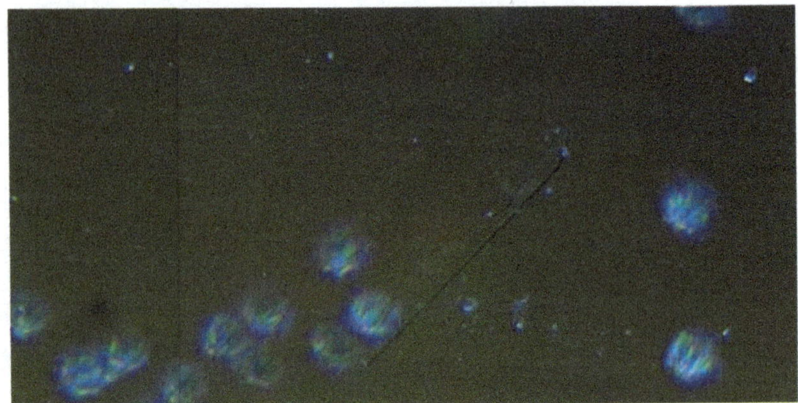

Figure 10. Moderna COVID 19 "vaccine" shows light-emitting particles – quantum dot microrobots. Darkfield microscopy. Dr. Geanina Hagimă.[15]

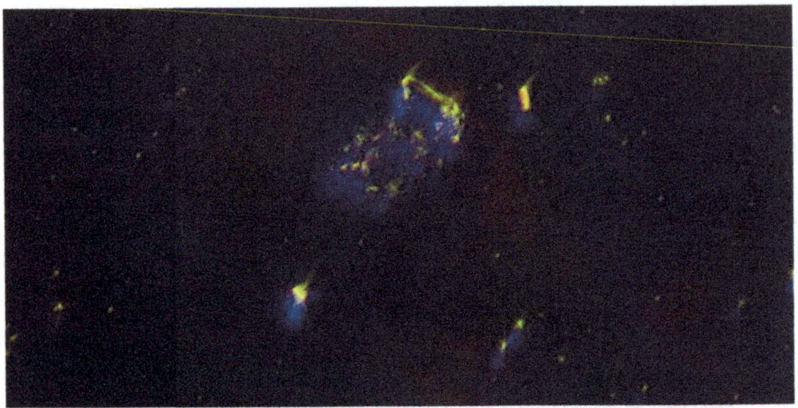

Figure 11. Moderna COVID 19 "vaccine" shows light-emitting particles. Darkfield microscopy. Dr. Geanina Hagimă.[16]

Motion of these self-assembling particles is visible in the video footage available on my Substack.[17] When switched to darkfield, clearly some of them are emitting blue light.

The Moderna "vaccine" under brightfield microscopy, and after 16 hours on the slide, shows spherical construction sites with the self-assembly of nanostructures. After 40 hours of observation, filament structures had developed, as seen below:

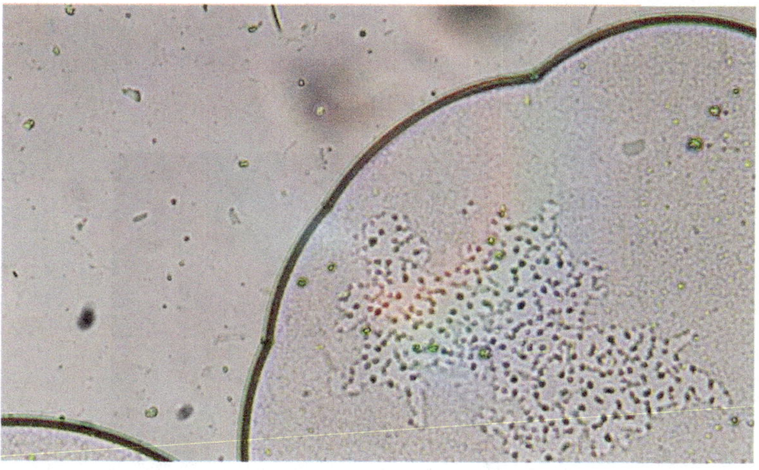

Figure 12. Moderna COVID 19 "vaccine" after 40 hours shows self-assembled filaments. Brightfield microscopy. Dr. Geanina Hagimă.[18]

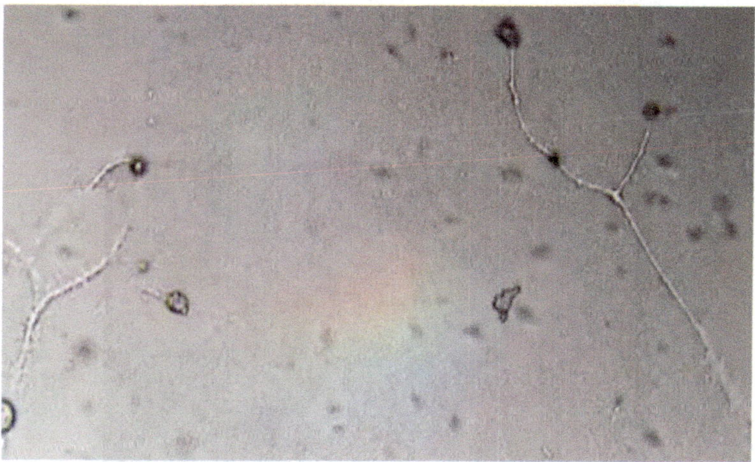

Figure 13. Moderna COVID 19 "vaccine" after 40 hours shows self-assembled filaments that look like antennas. Brightfield microscopy. Dr. Geanina Hagimă.[19]

The spherical structures with contents are seen on video with moving nanobots surrounding them. When observed in darkfield, again light-emitting quantum dots are seen.

Additionally, flower-like structures assemble. In Chapter 3 of *TransHuman – Volume 2: Overcoming the Global Depopulation Agenda*, regarding mesogen DNA biosensors, I explain that these are nanoantennas.

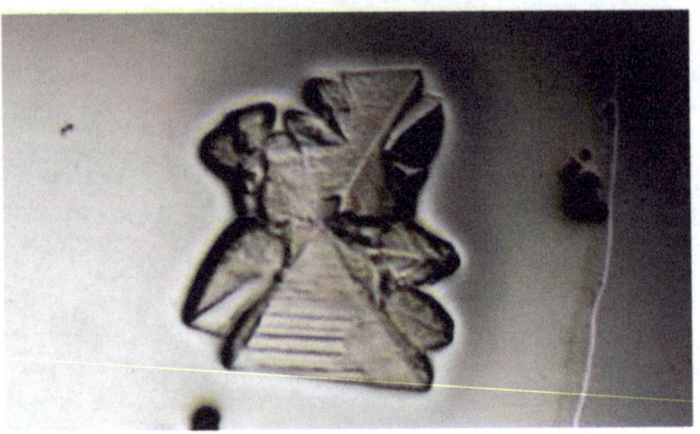

Figure 14. Moderna COVID 19 "vaccine" after 40 hours shows self-assembled flower-like crystals. Brightfield microscopy. Dr. Geanina Hagimă.[20]

This crystalline development we call microchips—again a fluorescence is seen using darkfield microscopy:

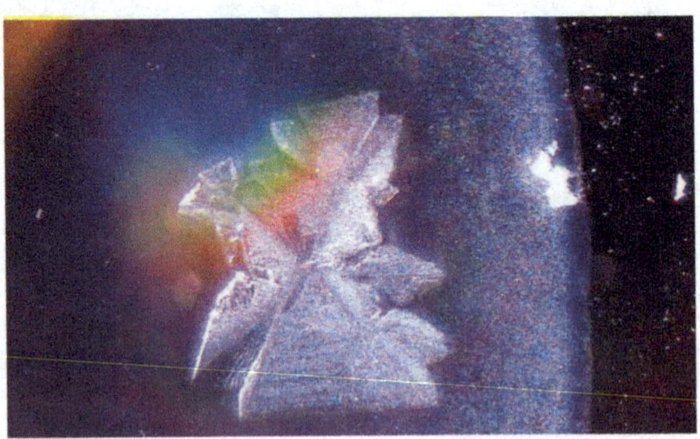

Figure 15. Moderna COVID 19 "vaccine" after 40 hours shows self-assembled flower-like crystals. Darkfield microscopy. Dr. Geanina Hagimă.[21]

Quantum dot structures seen in the background substrate and within these crystals themselves are consistent with the nanotechnology, and nano- and microrobots found in other "vaccine" bioweapon vials from Romania and elsewhere.

What is in the COVID 19 "Vaccines"? Evidence of a Global Crime Against Humanity

OCTOBER 16, 2022[22]

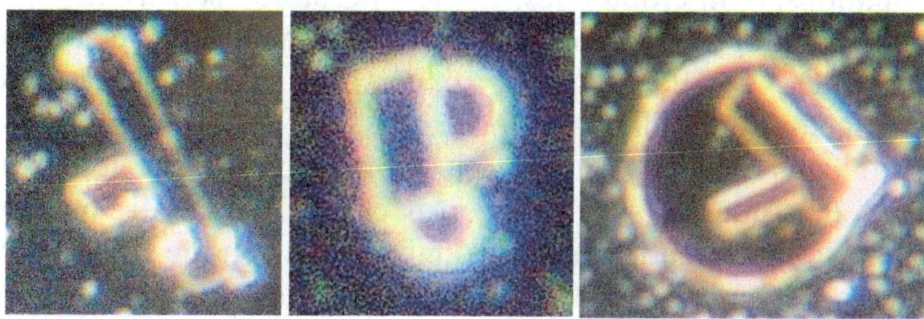

Figure 16. Pfizer COVID 19 Comirnaty injected blood. Darkfield microscopy. LifeOfTheBlood, New Zealand.[23]

Dr. David Hughes discusses, in his published paper, the worldwide findings of research scientists documenting self-assembling structures in COVID 19 injectables and correlating them with abnormal live blood analysis.[24] As a researcher who always had an interest in black projects, he rightfully asks the question why such enormous evidence of very disturbing findings is not leading to the immediate halting of the COVID 19 injectables?

Dr. Hughes writes: "Between July 2021 and August 2022, evidence of undisclosed ingredients in the COVID 19 'vaccines' was published by at least 26 researchers/research teams in 16 different countries across five continents using spectroscopic and microscopic analysis. Despite operating largely independently of one another, their findings are remarkably similar and highlight the clear and present danger that the world's population has been lied to regarding the contents of the COVID 19 'vaccines.'

"This raises grave questions about the true purpose of the dangerous experimental injections that have so far been shot into 5.33 billion people (over two thirds of the human race), including children, apparently without their informed consent regarding the contents. Surprise findings include sharp-edged geometric structures, fibrous or tube-like structures, crystalline formations, 'microbubbles,' and possible self-assembling nanotechnology. The blood of people who have received one or more COVID 19 'vaccines' appears, in case after case, to contain foreign bodies and to be seriously degraded, with red blood cells typically in rouleaux formation. Taken together, these 26 studies make a powerful case for the full force of scientific investigation to be brought to bear on the COVID 19 'vaccine' contents. If the findings of these 26 studies are confirmed, then the political implications are nothing short of revolutionary: a global crime against humanity has been committed, in which every government, every regulator, every establishment media organization, and all the professions have been complicit."[25]

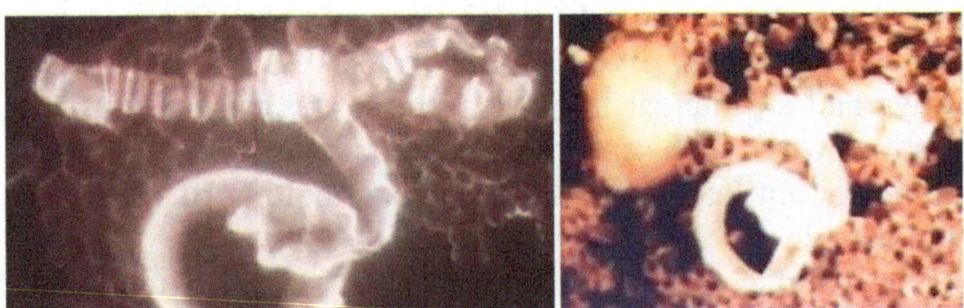

Figure 17. Live blood analysis of patients recently given the Johnson & Johnson "vaccine." Dr. Barbel Ghitalla.[26]

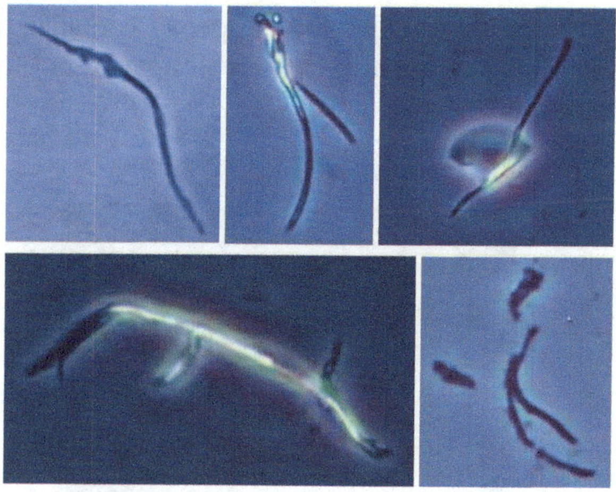

Figure 18. Anonymous Dr. John B analysis of Pfizer "vaccine."[27]

Graphene expert, Andreas Noack from Germany, who shortly after sounding the alarm on the toxicity of graphene hydroxide in the vaccine vials, died under suspicious circumstances, applied a magnet to the Pfizer sample:

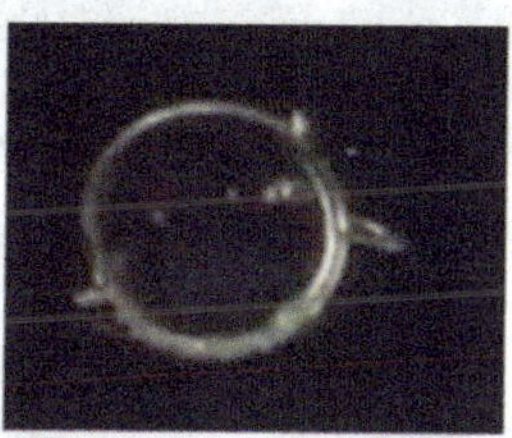

But look what happens when Noack applies a magnet to his sample. The structure lights up brilliantly, along with thousands of background specks:

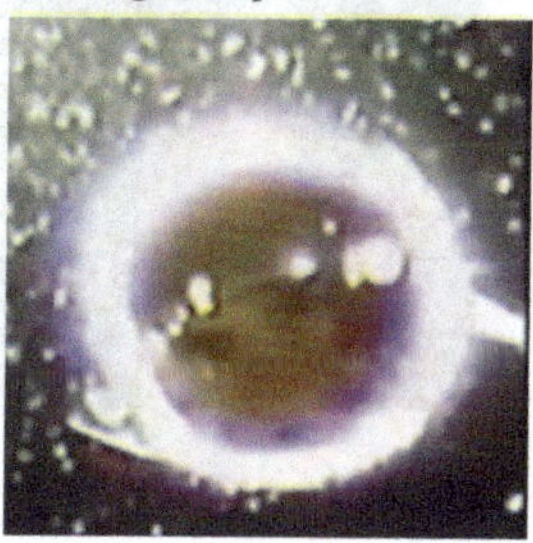

Figure 19. Sphere in Pfizer vial exposed to a magnet. Dr. Andreas Noack.[28]

Then, something unexpected happens. The structure lights up and suddenly grows an extremely long (2D?) "tail" along which energy appears to travel:

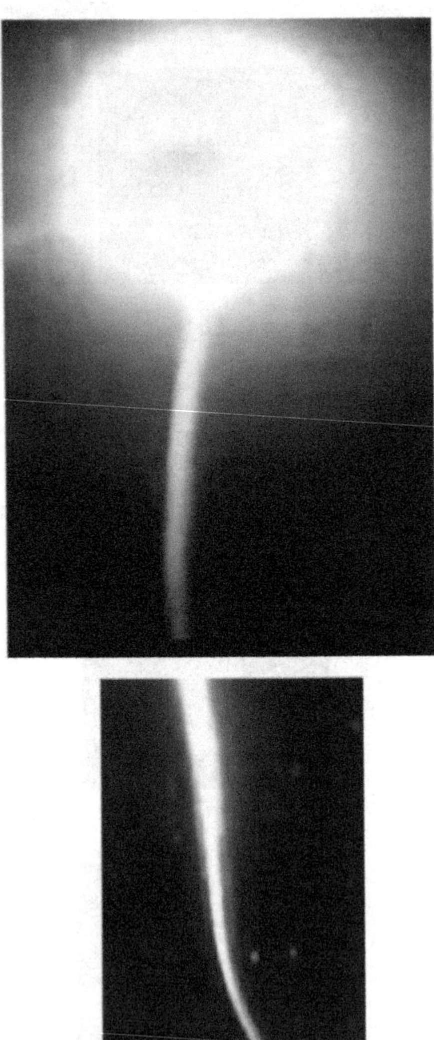

Figure 20. Sphere in Pfizer vial exposed to a magnet grows a long 2D tail. Dr. Andreas Noack.[29]

More images of these artificial structures were captured during the LifeOfTheBlood examination of the Pfizer vials:

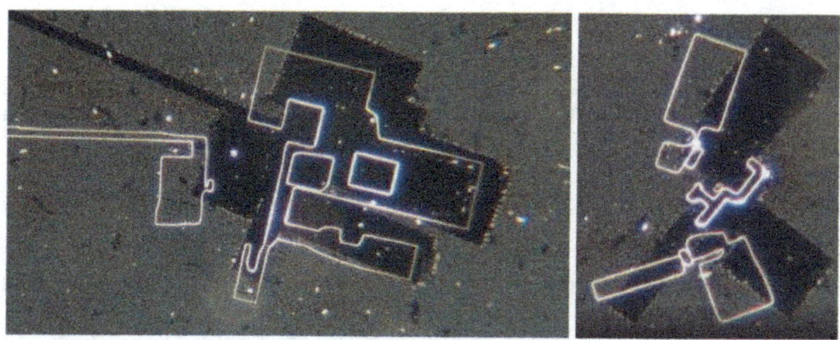

Here are some other examples of the complex substrate forming:

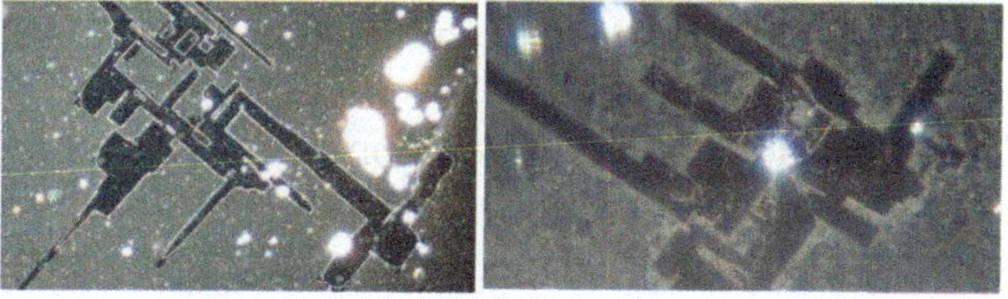

Figure 21. Multiple nanotechnological structures in COVID 19 Pfizer injections. LifeOfTheBlood, New Zealand.[30]

Dr. Hughes has collected studies from researchers around the world. His findings warrant immediate action: the halting worldwide of the COVID 19 injectables. These findings should be correlating evidence for every lawsuit in the world pertaining to crimes against humanity, as committed via these COVID 19 injections. They also warrant international attention by researchers, physicians, and scientists to evaluate and treat this microtechnology. No prominent vaccine injury protocol in the United States contains recommendations for detoxification of metals such as graphene via EDTA Chelation or other modalities. There is also little research in this area, since the only way to check for clearance of these structures is through live blood analysis, a modality that most allopathic physicians dismiss in the absence of any alternative solution.

Ivermectin does not detox the body of heavy metals that have been found in every "vaccine" regardless of manufacturer. Prominent doctors and scientists are completely silent on the matter, or claim these structures are made of cholesterol, salt, and sucrose—something that clearly is not the case, as I also discussed with Big Pharma insider, Sasha Latypova.[31]

Hopefully people will wake up and understand there is much more to these injections than the cover story of mRNA—that somehow in the fraudulent manufacturing process, cannot quite be produced at large scale, just like records of the isolation of a COVID 19 virus cannot quite be found anywhere on the planet by any agency. As Dr. Hughes likes to ask questions, one could wonder what black project are we dealing with here that two thirds of humanity have been injected with? And who owns those who control the narrative?

You either love Truth or you don't. Time is not on our side in saving people from the worldwide effects of these shots. Mortality rates are increasing everywhere. The longer denial persists about what is in these injections, and what it does to human blood, the more people will go without treatment. Additionally, they will continue to expose themselves to electromagnetic fields that enhance the growth of these structures and may tragically "die suddenly." I argue that urgent research and treatment recommendations are needed to save the human species.

What is in the COVID 19 "Vaccines"? Evidence of a Global Crime Against Humanity – Interview with Dr. David Hughes

NOVEMBER 08, 2022[32]

The full interview with Dr. Hughes can be found on my Substack. This interview gives detailed information about the worldwide research on the COVID 19 injections and the live blood analysis findings from healthcare practitioners and researchers around the world.[33]

Dr. Hughes wrote regarding his efforts: "This work was an attempt to synthesize and make publicly available all existing independent investigations into the COVID 19 'vaccine' contents beginning in July 2021. There is now sufficient evidence to demonstrate that the world has been lied to regarding the COVID 19 'vaccine' contents. No informed consent was given; hence this represents a violation of the Nuremberg Code. 5.4 billion people have been injected, which represents arguably the biggest crime in history."[34]

Dr. Hughes and I were part of an International Interdisciplinary Research Team that investigated the contents of COVID 19 injectables correlated with live blood analyses.[35] He is a senior lecturer in International Relations at the University of Lincoln in the UK. He holds undergraduate and master's degrees from the University of Oxford and a PhD from Duke University. Appalled by the COVID era of mass atrocity and the ruling class project to bring about a new dark age of technocratic enslavement, he is working to expose the Deep State mechanisms that have brought humanity to the edge of the abyss—but also to highlight the revolutionary potential that arises when the old order breaks down and the new one is not yet born.[36] His recent papers include: *COVID-19 "Vaccines" for Children in the UK: A Tale of Establishment Corruption* and *Wall Street, the Nazis, and the Crimes of the Deep State*.[37]

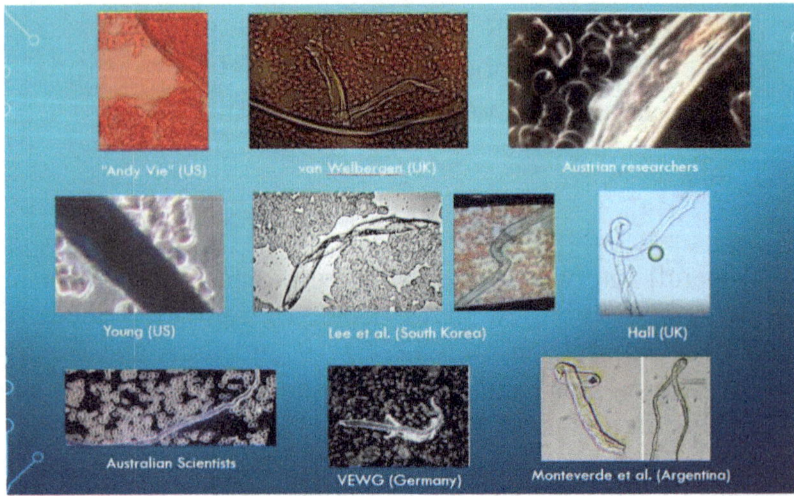

Figure 22. Multiple nanotechnological structures in COVID 19 injected blood found around the world. All contain similar filament structures and rouleaux formation. Dr. David Hughes.[38]

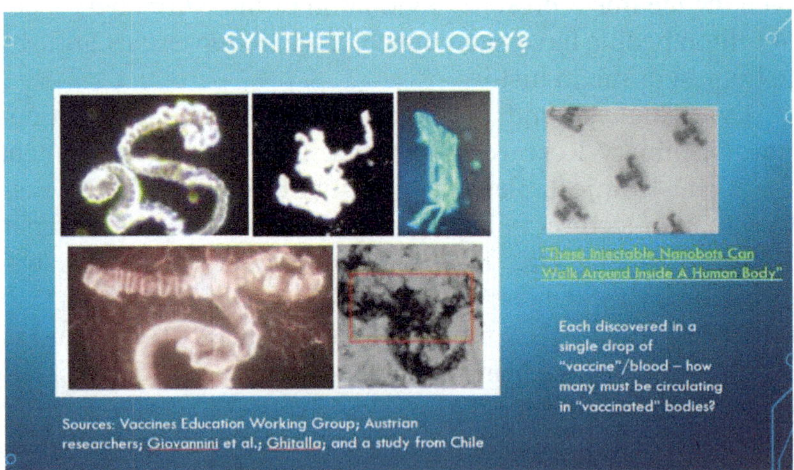

Figure 23. Multiple synthetic biological structures in COVID 19 injected blood from around the world. Dr. David Hughes.[39]

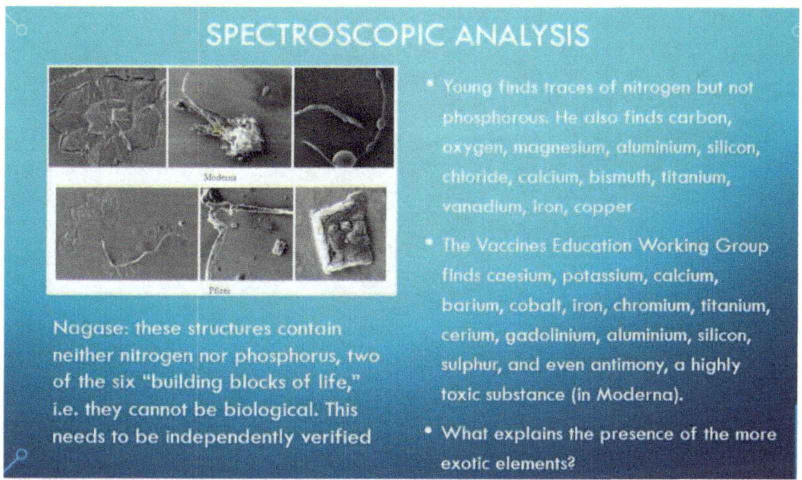

Figure 24. Spectroscopic analysis of Moderna and Pfizer vials from around the world show metals and unusual self-assembly nanotechnology structures. Dr. David Hughes.[40]

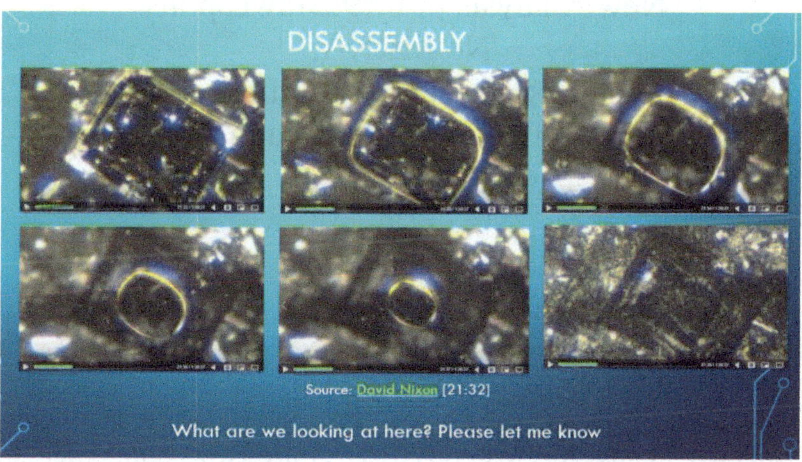

Figure 25. Dr. David Nixon finds assembly of microchip developed from Pfizer vial. Dr. David Hughes.[41]

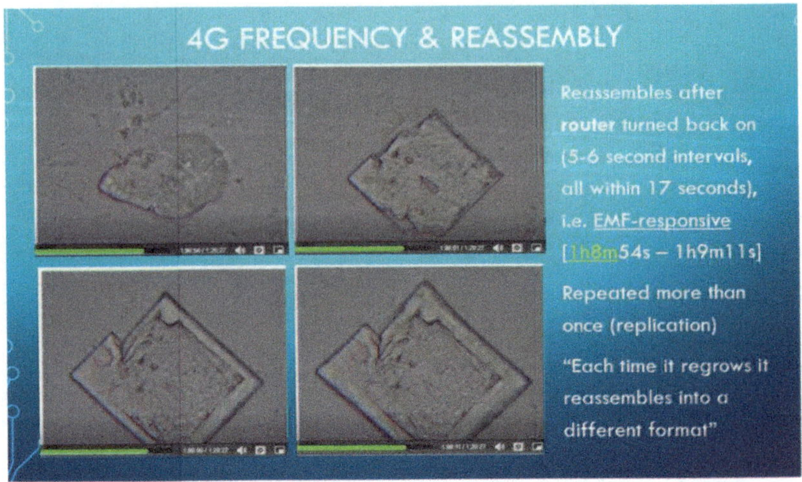

Figure 26. Disassembly of microchip developed from Pfizer vial found by Mat Taylor. Dr. David Hughes.[42]

New Analysis of C19 Bioweapons: No MRNA, but Toxic Metals and Silicone – Scientific Findings by Dr. Geanina Hagimă

NOVEMBER 25, 2023[43]

Electron microscopy investigations of COVID vaccines Comirnaty, Omicron, and Moderna via SEM and EDX, are presented in this segment.

Scanning electron microscopy (SEM) and energy-dispersive X-ray spectroscopy (EDX) are two complementary techniques often used together for materials characterization. These are the key differences between SEM and EDX analysis:

- SEM provides visual information about the surface features, morphology, and topography of a sample.
- EDX provides information about the elemental composition of the sample, indicating which chemical elements are present and in what quantities.[44]

In a 2023 interview with my colleague, Dr. Geanina Hagimă, she revealed her most recent research findings using electron microscopy on the Comirnaty COVID 19 shot which contains carbon, oxygen, silicon, titanium, yttrium, and magnesium. Once again, her research shows no element of life, no phosphorus or nitrogen. This means there is no mRNA or DNA in the "vaccine" vials.[45,46]

However, we are especially concerned about the undisclosed presence of silicone, titanium, and yttrium. Yttrium is used in biosensor and optoelectronics. Silicone is used in nanotechnology for nano- and microelectronics, optoelectronics, and biophotonics. Titanium has wide applications in nanotechnology biosensing. None of these elements are disclosed by the companies that produce these "vaccines." Dr. Hagimă's microscopy work on the Comirnaty COVID 19 shots also revealed self-assembling nanotechnology and quantum dot technology.[47]

In the graphs that follow, nickel is considered an artifact. That's because the measurement is taken in one spot and the entire solution or particle cannot be analyzed all at once. This is why many measurements are necessary. Although this gives some idea of what is in the vial, it does not completely, 100%, analyze all contents. These tests are very expensive which adds to the challenge of analysis.

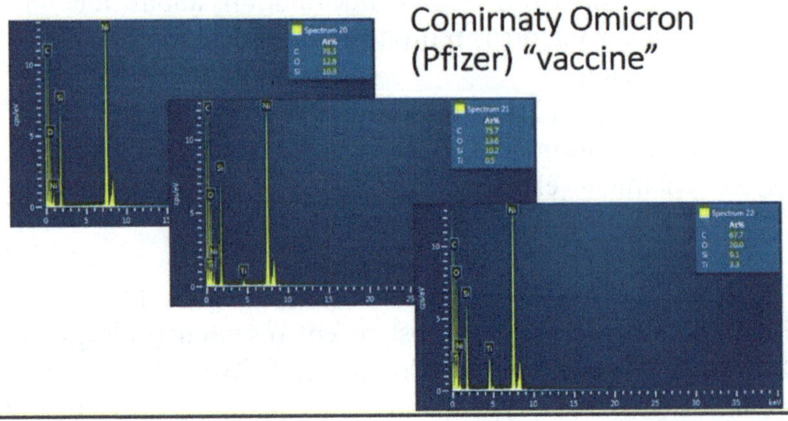

Figure 27. EDX SEM Pfizer Comirnaty Omicron "vaccine" shows carbon, oxygen, silicone, and titanium in multiple and different concentrations. Dr. Geanina Hagimă.[48]

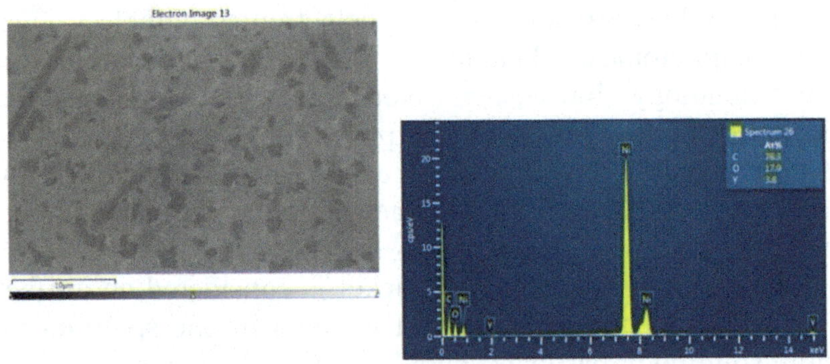

Figure 28. Electron microscopy of Pfizer Comirnaty Omicron "vaccine" shows nanoparticles on the left. EDX SEM on the right shows those particles to contain carbon 78.3%, oxygen 17.9%, and yttrium 3.8%. Dr. Geanina Hagimă.[49]

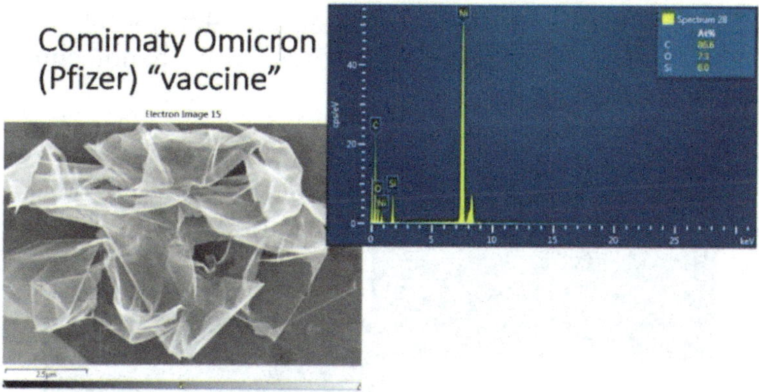

Figure 29. Electron microscopy of Pfizer Comirnaty Omicron "vaccine" shows nanoparticles on the left. EDX SEM on the right shows those particles to contain carbon, oxygen, and silicone. Dr. Geanina Hagimă.[50]

The Moderna COVID 19 injection contains substantial amounts of silicone, carbon, and oxygen. Carbon and oxygen could make up graphene oxide but could also be some other carbon-based material.

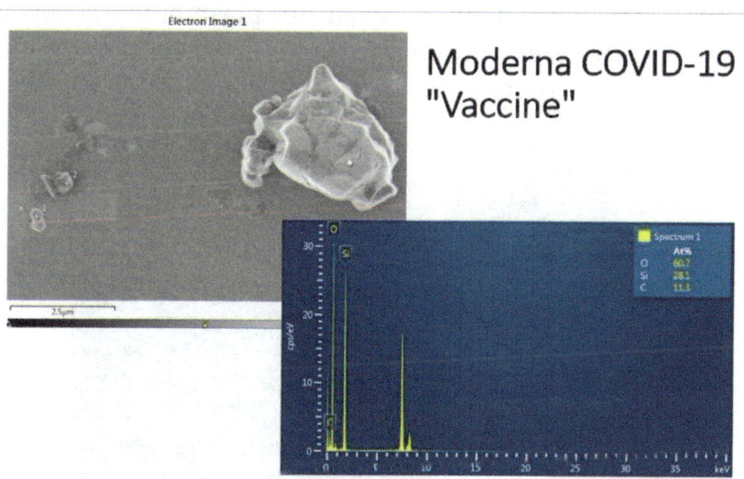

Figure 30. Electron microscopy of Moderna COVID 19 "vaccine" shows nanoparticles on the left. EDX SEM on the right shows those particles to contain carbon, oxygen, and silicone. Dr. Geanina Hagimă.[51]

Some measurements showed up to 43.2% undisclosed silicone which is a part of self-assembly nanotechnology biosensor manufacturing.

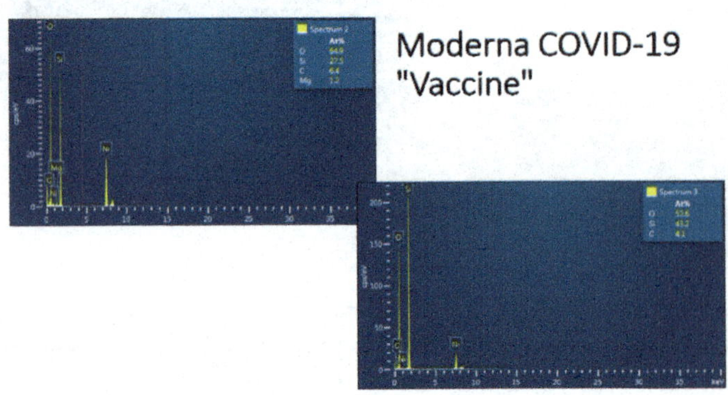

Figure 31. Moderna COVID 19 EDX SEM on the left shows particles contain oxygen 64.3%, silicone 27.3%, carbon 6.4, and magnesium 1.2%. On the right oxygen 52.6%, silicone 43.2%, and carbon 4.1%. Dr. Geanina Hagimă.[52]

Other undisclosed metals found in the Moderna COVID 19 "vaccine" are tin, which is used in plasmonic biosensing nanotechnology, and aluminum, which is used for building nanotechnology biosensors.[53]

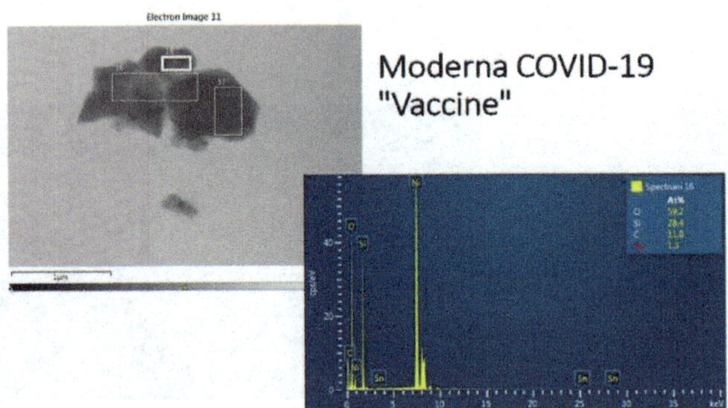

Figure 32. Electron microscopy of Moderna COVID 19 "vaccine" shows nanoparticles on the left. EDX SEM on the right shows particles contain oxygen 59.2%, silicone 28.4%, carbon 11.0%, and tin 1.3%. Dr. Geanina Hagimă.[54]

The lack of elements of life—indicating there is no mRNA in the COVID 19 vials—are consistent with Dr. Daniel Nagase and Steve Kirschs' findings.[55,56] Neither one of them found mRNA in the vials. The German Working Group for COVID Vaccine Analysis also found many metals used for nanotechnology applications.[57] In the UK, a forensic report showed graphene oxide in the vials.[58]

Electron microscopy of the pneumococcal "vaccine" also shows aluminum, silicone, sodium, phosphorus, chloride, carbon, and oxygen. Dr. Hagimă and I have separately performed microscopy on the Prevnar pneumococcal "vaccine" and found self-assembling nanotechnology in those "vaccines" as well.[59] Dr. Hagimă's results are presented below:

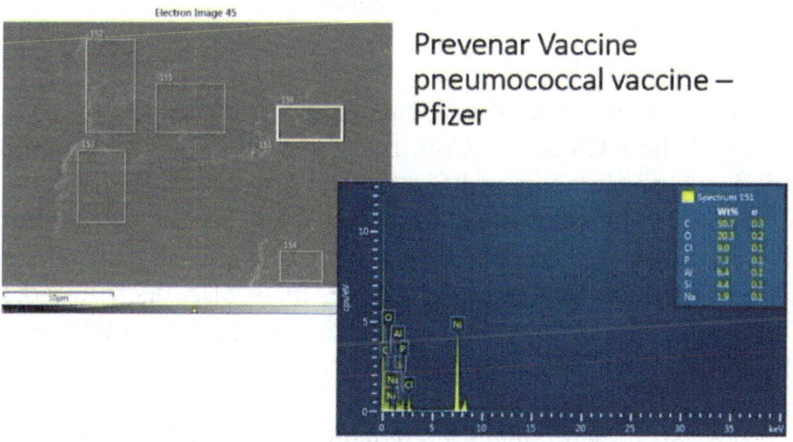

Figure 33. Electron microscopy of Prevenar "vaccine" shows nanoparticles on the left. EDX SEM on the right show the particles contain carbon 50.7%, oxygen 20.3%, chloride 9.0%, phosphorus 7.3%, aluminum 6.4%, silicone 4.4%, and sodium 1.9%. Dr. Geanina Hagimă.[60]

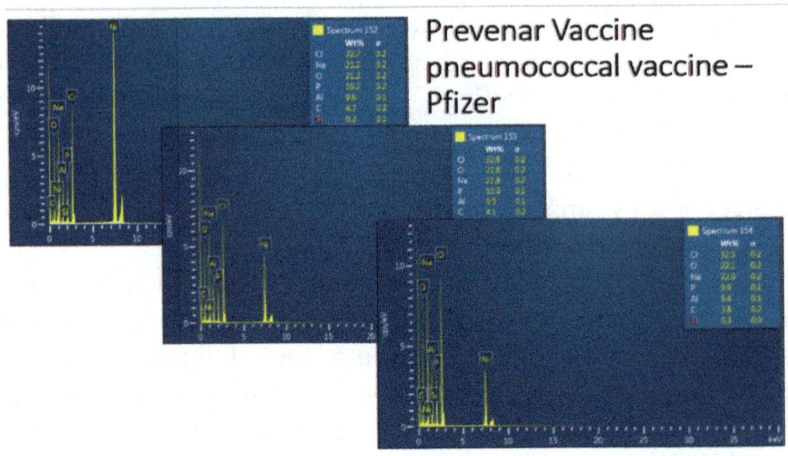

Figure 34. Prevenar "vaccine" EDX SEM shows three measurements: chloride, sodium, oxygen, phosphorus, aluminum, carbon, and silicone in different concentrations. Dr. Geanina Hagimă.[61]

We now have new evidence that confirms the previous testing of the COVID 19 Comirnaty and Moderna bioweapons containing no elements of life—phosphorus or nitrogen—hence no mRNA. Undisclosed elements like silicone, titanium, yttrium, and other metals used for nanotechnology biosensing applications, as demonstrated above, have also been found in Comirnaty, Moderna, Pneumovax, and even dental anesthetics. Therefore:

We call for an immediate worldwide halt of the COVID 19 vaccination program and an immediate investigation of ALL vaccines, including all childhood vaccines, for any undisclosed toxic heavy metals and metal building blocks used in nanotechnology.

We also call for the evaluation of all dental anesthetics worldwide that have been shown to contain self-assembly nanotechnology and biosensors.

And we also call for an investigation of these injectables via liquid gas chromatography, as well as investigations of all chemical polymer compositions, self-assembly hydrogel plastics, and polymer building blocks of nanotechnology with biosensing and photoelectronic capabilities, as seen currently in every human live blood analysis.

Dr. Ana Maria Mihalcea, MD, PhD, and
Dr. Geanina Hagimă, MD

Toxic Metal Nano Contaminants in Childhood Vaccinations and Adverse Effect Correlation

SEPTEMBER 11, 2022[62]

These metal nanostructures are most concerning to me as a physician. Such findings to me are reason enough to stop the shots.[63,64]

Even more worrisome is that it has long been known that these metals have been found in every childhood "vaccine" offered by every childhood "vaccine" company, and yet have remained undisclosed. No doctor has ever given informed consent regarding these toxic components anywhere in the world.

I include this next important analysis by world renown nanopathologist, Dr. Antoinetta Gatti, published in the *International Journal of Vaccines & Vaccination* in 2017:

> Electron-microscopy investigation method was applied to the study of vaccines, aimed at verifying the presence of solid contaminants by means of an Environmental Scanning Electron Microscope equipped with an X-ray microprobe. The results of this new investigation show the presence of micro- and nanosized particulate matter composed of inorganic elements in vaccines' samples which is not declared among the components and whose unduly presence is, for the time being, inexplicable. A considerable part of those

particulate contaminants has already been verified in other matrices and reported in literature as non-biodegradable and non-biocompatible. 44 types of vaccines coming from 2 countries (Italy and France) were analyzed.

The investigations verified the physical-chemical composition of the vaccines considered according to the inorganic component as declared by the Producer. In detail, we verified the presence of saline and aluminum salts, but further presence of micro-, sub-micro- and nanosized, inorganic, foreign bodies (ranging from 100 nm to about ten microns) was identified in all cases, whose presence was not declared in the leaflets delivered in the package of the product.

Sample metals found:

Aluminum
Chromium
Tungsten
Steel
Iron
Lead
Silicon
Copper
Bismuth
Platinum
Nickel
Silver
Gold
Zirconium
Hafnium
Strontium

Some metallic particles made of Tungsten or stainless steel were also identified. Other particles containing Zirconium, Hafnium, Strontium and Aluminum (Vivotif, Meningetec); Tungsten, Nickel, Iron (Priorix, Meningetec); Antimony (Menjugate kit); Chromium (Meningetec); Gold or Gold, Zinc (Infarix Hexa, Repevax), or Platinum, Silver, Bismuth, Iron, Chromium (MMRvaxPro) or Lead, Bismuth (Gardasil) or Cerium

(Agrippal S1) were also found. The only Tungsten appears in 8/44 vaccines, while Chromium (alone or in alloy with Iron and Nickel) in 25/44. The investigations revealed that some particles are embedded in a biological substrate, probably proteins, endotoxins and residues of bacteria. As soon as a particle comes in contact with proteic fluids, a nano-bio-interaction occurs and a 'protein corona' is formed. The nano-bio-interaction generates a bigger-sized compound that is not biodegradable and can induce adverse effects, since it is not recognized as self by the body.[65]

Table 2 List of the vaccines according to their manufacturers with the chemical composition of the debris identified in each sample. The elements most represented are reported

N	Company	Name	Alluminum	Elements Identified
1	Allergopharma - Germany	Allergoid	yes	Al
2	Aventis Pasteur MSD Lyon - Francie	Typhim Vi	no	BrKP, PbSi, FeCr, PbClSiTi
3	Baxter AG	Tetabulin	no	SiMg, Fe, SiTiAl, SBa, Zn
4	Berna Biotech	Vivotif Berna	no	FeAl, ZrAlHf, SrAl, BiAlCl
5	Berna Biotech	Inflexal V	no	CuSnPbZn, Fe, CaSiAl, SiAl, NaPZn, ZnP, AlSiTi
6	Chiron	Anatetall	Al(OH)3	FeAl, SZnBaAl
7	Chiron	Morupar	no	/
8	GlaxoSmithKline- Belgium	Mencevax ACWY	no	FeCrNi, ZrAl, FeCrNiZrAlSi
9	GlaxoSmithKline	Infanrix	Al(OH)3	Al, AlTi, AlSi
10	GlaxoSmithKline Biologicals	Infanrix hexa	Al(OH)3	SBa, FeCu, SiAl, FeSi, CaMgSi, AlCaSi, Ti, Au, SCa, SiAlFeSnCuCrZn, CaAlSi
11	GlaxoSmithKline Biologicals	Infanrix hexa	Al(OH)3 ,AlPO4. 2H2O	W, FeCrNi, Ti
12	GlaxoSmithKline	Typherix	no	Ti, TiW, AlSiTiWCr, SBa, W, SiAl, AlSiTi
13	GlaxoSmithKline	Priorix	no	WCa, WFeCu, SiAl, SiMg, PbFe, Ti, WNiFe
14	GlaxoSmithKline	Engerix-B	no	Al (precipitates)
15	GlaxoSmithKline	Varilrix	no	FeZn, FeSi, AlSiFe, SiAlTiFe, MgSi, Ti, Zr, Bi
16	GlaxoSmithKline	Fluarix	no	AlCu, Fe, AlBi, Si, SiZn, AlCuFe, SiMg, SBa, AlCuBi, FeCrNi, SPZn
17	GlaxoSmithKline Biologicals	Cervarix	Al(OH)3	AlSi, FeAl, SiMg, CaSiAl, CaZn, FeAlSi, FeCr, CuSnPb
18	Novartis Vaccines and Diagnostics	Anatetall	Al(OH)3	Al, FeCrNi, AlCr, AlFe, BaS, ZnAl
19	Novartis Vaccines and Diagnostics	Dif-Tet-All	Al(OH)3	Fe, SBa, SiSBa, AlZnCu, AlZnFeCr
20	Novartis Vaccines and Diagnostics	Menjugate kit	Al(OH)3	SiAl, Ti, FeZn, Fe, Sb, SiAlFeTi, W, Zr
21	Novartis Vaccines and Diagnostics	Focetria	no	Fe, FeCrNiCu, FeCrNi, SiFeCrNi, Cr, SiAlFe, AlSiTiFe, AlSi, SiMgFe, Si, FeZn
22	Novartis	Agrippal S1	no	Ca, Fe, SBa, SBaZn, Cr, Si, Pb, Bi, e FeSiAlCr, SiAlSBaFe, CaAlSi, Zn, CeFeTiNi, FeCrNi
23	Novartis Vaccines and Diagnostics	Agrippal S1	no	SiAlK, Si, SiMgFe, CaSiAl, SBaZn
24	Novartis vaccines	Agrippal	no	Cr, Ca, SiCaAl, ZrSi, SBa, CuZn, SCa
25	Novartis Vaccines and Diagnostics S	Fluad	no	CaSiAl, FeSiTi, SiMgAlFe, SBa
26	Novartis Vaccines and Diagnostics	Menveo	no	CaSiAl, SiAlFe, FeCrNi, Fe, Al, SBa
27	Pfizer	Prenevar 13	no	FeCr
28	Pfizer	Prevenar 13	no	W, CaAlSi, Al, CaSiAlFe, FeS, FeCr, FeCrNi, Fe, , CaP, FeTiMn, Ba, SiMgAlFe
29	Pfizer	Meningitec - ctrl	no	Cr, Si
30	Pfizer	Meningitec - ctrl	no	FeCrNi, W
31	Pfizer	Meningitec	no	CaSiAl, CaSi, SiAlFeTi, FeCrNi, W, Fe, Pb
32	Pfizer	Meningitec	no	Cr (precipitates), Ca, AlSi
33	Pfizer	Meningitec	no	W, SiCa, CaSi, Pb, FeCrNi, Cr
34	Wyeth Pharmaceutical - UK	Meningitec	no	SiAlFe, SiAlTi, SiMgFe, W, Fe, Zr, Pb, Ca, Zn, FeCrNi
35	Sanofi Pasteur MSD-France	Vaxigrip	no	Fe, FeCrNi, SiAlFe, AlSi, SiAlFeCr
36	Sanofi Pasteur MSD	Stamaril Pasteur	no	CaSiAl, AlSi, Fe, SiMgFe, SiMgAlFe, CrSiFeCr, CrSiCuFe
37	Sanofi Pasteur MSD	Gardasil	AlPO4. 2H2O	AlCuFe, PbBi, Pb, Bi, Fe
38	Sanifi Pasteur MSD	Gardasil	AlPO4. 2H2O	CaAlSi, AlSi, SiMgFe, Al, Fe, AlCuFe, FeSiAl, BiBaS, Ti, TiAlSi
39	Sanofi Pasteur	Vaxigrip	no	Ca, CrFe, FeCrNi, CaSZn, CaSiAlTiFe, Ag, Fe
40	Sanofi Pasteur	Vaxigrip	no	SiMgFe, CaSiAl, AlSiFe, AlSi, FeCr, FeZn, Fe
41	Sanofi Pasteur MSD	Repevax	AlPO4 .2H2O	Bi, Fe, AlSiFe, SiMg, SBa, Ca
42	Sanofi Pasteur MSD S	Repevax	AlPO4.2H2O	Ti, Br, AuCuZn, Ca, SiZn, SiAuAgCu, SiMgFe, FeCrNi, AlSiMgTiMnCrFe, SiFeCrNi, FeAl
43	Sanofi Pasteur MSD	M-M-R vaxPro	no	Si, SiFeCrNi, FeCrNi FeNi Fe, [illegible] CaAlSiFeV, SBa, Pt, PtAgBiFeCr
44	Virbac S.A. - Carros - France	Feligen CRP	no	Ca, SiAl

Citation: Gatti AM, Montanari S. New quality-control investigations on vaccines: micro- and nanocontamination. *Int J Vaccines Vaccin*. 2017;4(1):7–14. DOI: 10.15406/ijvv.2017.04.00072

Figure 35. List of 44 childhood "vaccines" and the metals found in each. Dr. Antoinetta Gatti.[66]

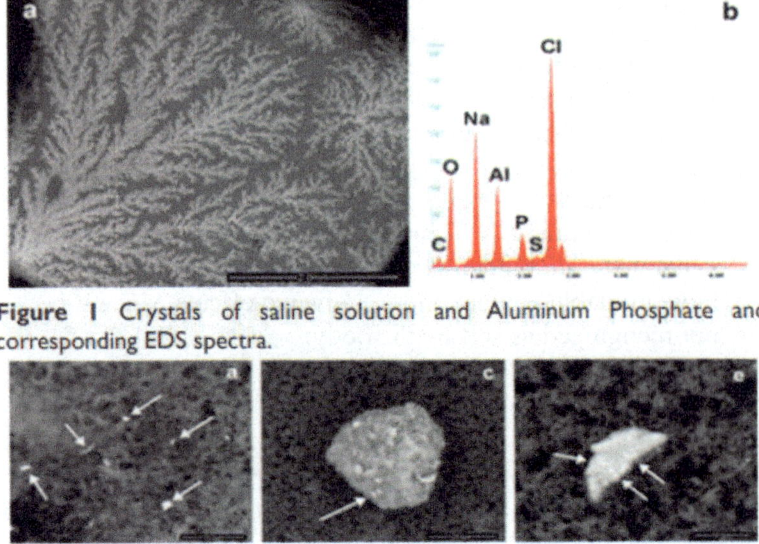

Figure 1 Crystals of saline solution and Aluminum Phosphate and corresponding EDS spectra.

Figure 2 Images of single particles, cluster of micro- and nanoparticles (<100nm) andaggregates with their EDS spectra. They are respectively composed of (a,b) Aluminum, Silicon, Magnesium, Titanium, Chromium, Manganese, Iron, (c,d) Iron, Silicon, Calcium Titanium, Chromium, (e,f) Aluminum, Copper. The arrows show the points where EDS spectra were taken.

Figure 36. Nanoparticles identified in childhood "vaccines." Dr. Antoinetta Gatti.[67]

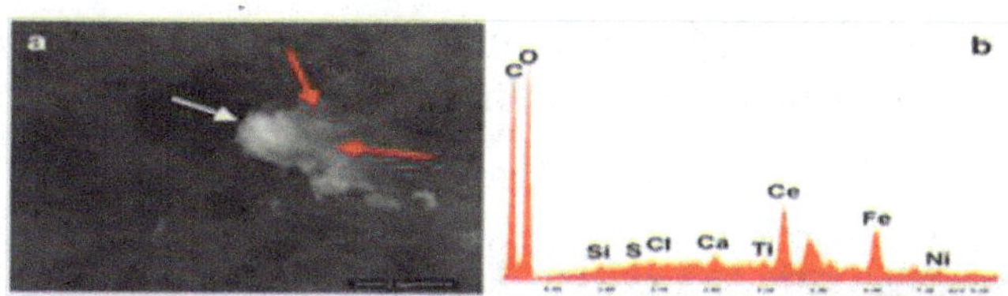

Figure 6 show an organic aggregate containing a debris made of Cerium, Iron, Nickel, Titanium. The red arrow indicates the organic layer (less atomically dense) that covers the Cerium particle.

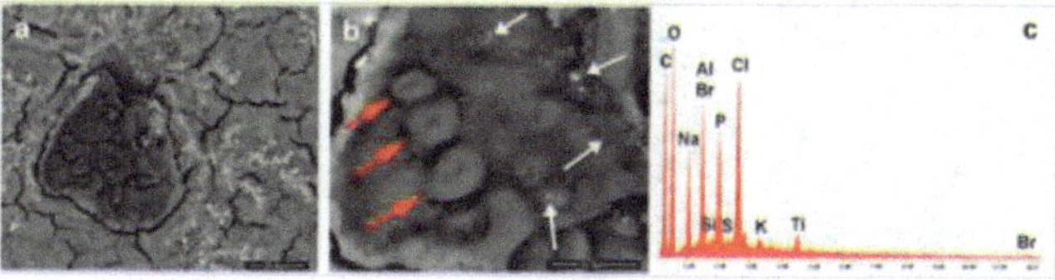

Figure 7 Image of an area in a Repevax drop where the morphology of red cells (red arrows) were identified. It is impossible to know whether they are human or animal origin. Among the debris of saline and Aluminum phosphate, there is the presence of debris (white arrows) composed of Aluminum, Bromine, Silicon, Potassium, Titanium.

Figure 37. Nanoparticles identified in childhood "vaccines." Dr. Antoinetta Gatti.[68]

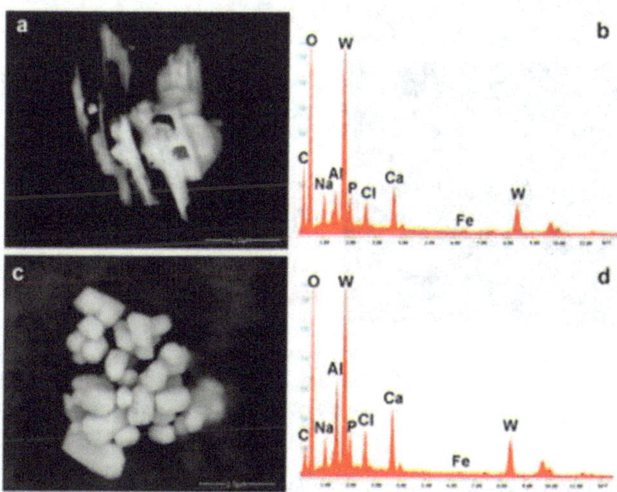

Figure 3 Images of Tungsten particles identified in drops of Prevenar and Infarix. They are composed respectively of Tungsten, Aluminum, Iron but in different concentrations. The arrows show the points where EDS spectra were taken.

Figure 38. Nanoparticles identified in childhood "vaccines." Dr. Antoinetta Gatti.[69]

This looks remarkably similar to the C19 nanoparticles found in the German Working Group analysis.[70]

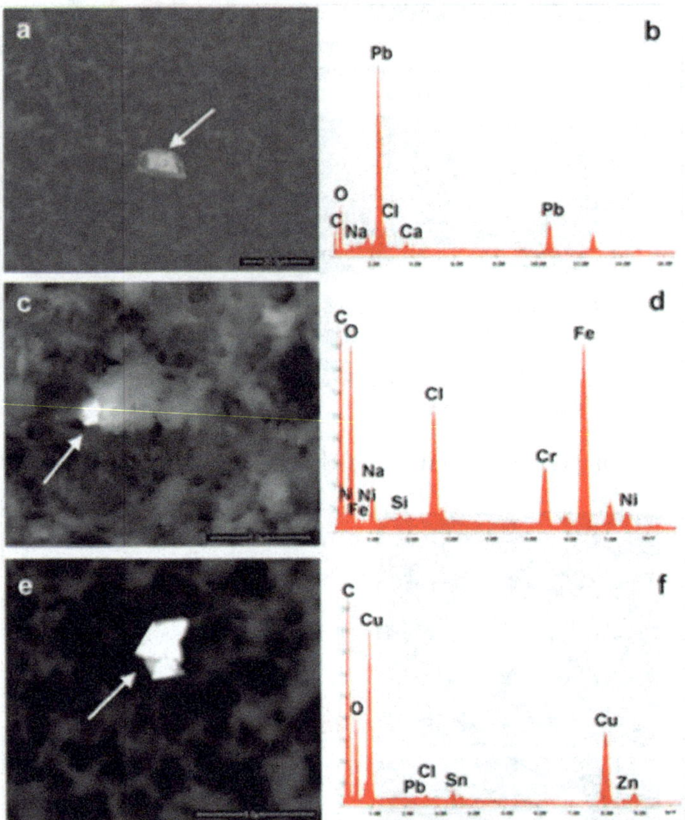

Figure 5 show particles surrounded by an organic compound. They are composed of Lead (a,b), Iron, Chromium, Nickel (stainless steel; c,d), Copper, Tin, Lead (e,f). The arrows show the points where EDS spectra were taken.

Figure 39. Nanoparticles identified in childhood "vaccines." Dr. Antoinetta Gatti.[71]

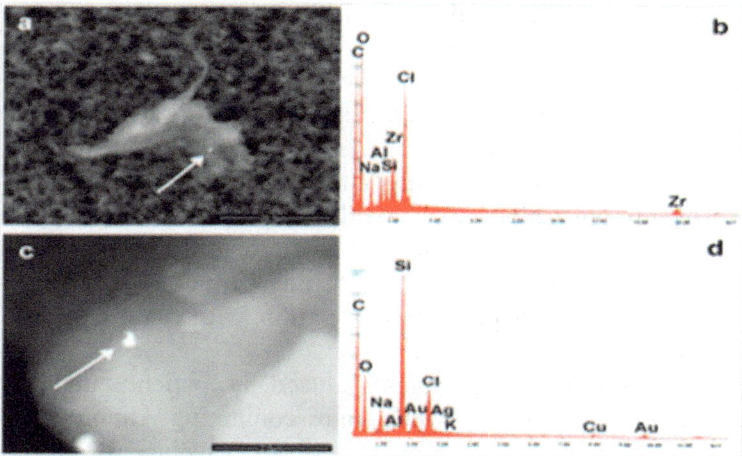

Figure 4 Images show examples of nano biointeraction. The aggregate (a,b) identified in Gardasil contains nanoparticles of Chlorine, Silicon, Aluminum, Zirconium, while the debris found in Repevax contains Silicon, Gold, Silver (c,d). The arrows show the points where EDS spectra were taken.

Figure 40. Nanoparticles identified in childhood "vaccines." Dr. Antoinetta Gatti.[72]

When looking at the side effect profile of many other so called "vaccines" we see quite similar adverse effects as we do with the COVID 19 platform. We know that the COVID 19 injections have higher adverse event rates than any other vaccine in prior history; however, the correlation of adverse effects is comparable. The importance of showing the childhood "vaccine" images above is that these same particles were also found in the COVID shots.

The 2017 study by Dr. Gatti tells us:

> The notice of Tripedia DTaP by Sanofi Pasteur reports 'Adverse events reported during post-approval use of Tripedia vaccine include idiopathic thrombocytopenic purpura, SIDS, anaphylactic reaction, cellulitis, autism, convulsion/grand mal convulsion,

encephalopathia, hypotonia, neuropathy, somnolence and apnea.' The epidemiological studies carried out did not show clear evidence of those associations, even if in 2011 the National Academy of Medicine (formerly, IOM) admitted: 'Vaccines are not free from side effects, or adverse effects.' Specific research on components of the vaccines like adjuvants (in most instances, Aluminum salts) are already indicated as possibly responsible for neurological symptoms and in some cases, in-vivo tests and epidemiological studies demonstrated a possible correlation with neurological diseases.

Neurological damages induced in patients under hemodialysis treated with water containing Aluminum are reported in worldwide-adopted vaccines against Human Papillomavirus (HPV), the debate was reawakened due to some adverse effects reported by some young subjects. Specific studies communicated the existence of symptoms related to never-described-before syndromes developed after the vaccine was administered. For instance, Complex Regional Pain Syndrome (CRPS), Postural Orthostatic Tachycardia Syndrome (POTS), and Chronic Fatigue Syndrome (CFS). The side-effects that can arise within a relatively short time can be local or systemic. Pain at the site of injection, swelling and uncontrollable movement of the hands (though this last symptom can also be considered systemic) are described. Among the systemic effects, fever, headache, irritability, epileptic seizures, temporary speech loss, lower limbs dysesthesia and paresis, hot flashes, sleep disorders, hypersensitivity reactions, muscle pain, recurrent syncope, constant hunger, significant gait impairment, incapacity to maintain the orthostatic posture are reported.[73]

Because of the dangerous labelling of people who question vaccines as "anti-vaxxers," public discussions, particularly in the medical field about "vaccine adverse effects," are rare. But if this is a toxic phenomenon that could be associated with a dose dependent response against toxic metals, why would we not discuss it? It has no correlation with the term "vaccine" against whatever infectious agent of concern, but rather a concern about the toxic poisoning effects from metals injected repeatedly into human beings. We know that heavy metals have synergistic toxic effects, and they are poisons. It is interesting that every "vaccine" adverse effect, like postural tachycardia syndrome (PoTS), chronic fatigue, neurological disorders, and many others mentioned above, can be direct symptoms of metal toxicity.[74]

Dr. Paul Thomas, an Oregon pediatrician who had his license revoked for voicing his concerns about childhood "vaccine" toxicity, has also been speaking about aluminum and mercury toxic adjuvants in the shots. He writes: "Long-term biodistribution of nanomaterials used in medicine is largely unknown. This is the case for alum, the most widely used 'vaccine' adjuvant, which is a nanocrystalline compound spontaneously forming micron/submicron-sized agglomerates. Although generally well tolerated, alum is occasionally detected within monocytelineage cells long after immunization in presumably susceptible individuals with systemic/neurologic manifestations or autoimmune (inflammatory) syndrome induced by adjuvants (ASIA)."[75]

We are witnessing unprecedented adverse effects from the COVID 19 "vaccines" which have been shown to contain toxic heavy metals. Studies like Dr. Gatti's reveal that all other "vaccines" tested have also been found to contain different combinations of toxic metals. Is the dose and composition of metal combinations affecting the phenomena of debilitating COVID 19 "vaccine" injuries that we are witnessing? Furthermore, does the fact that metals have been found in chemtrails and processed foods, including baby formula, add to the environmental bioaccumulation in a person's body and thereby cause adverse effects from different shots unique to that individual? Would therefore a high toxic body burden of heavy metals and low nutritional supplementation—without chelators like vitamin C, NAC, and glutathione—additionally affect the severity of symptoms?

Why do we allow injections that contain poisonous metals? To call someone an "anti-vaxxer" who asks this question is pure lunacy, for the question is about their poisonous effects, not supposed vaccination against a pathogen. Why exactly have physicians been suppressed and their license taken away who have spoken out against "vaccines" and their adjuvant toxicity? And why are mainstream physicians so silent about self-assembling metal nanostructures in COVID 19 injected people? Why is there such an overlap of COVID 19 vax injury and symptoms of heavy metal poisoning?

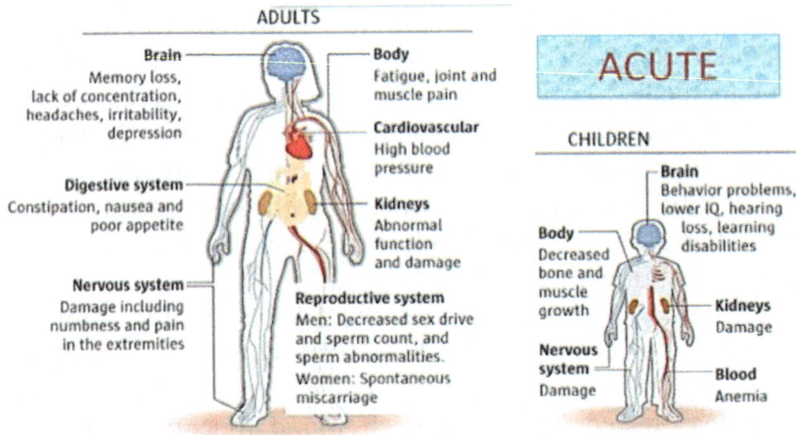

Figure 41. Signs and symptoms of heavy metal toxicity in the body. Top Natural Remedy.[76]

If it quacks like a duck, walks like a duck, and looks like a duck, could it be that there might be a scientific correlation with it being a duck? In other words, if it looks like metal poison and presents metal-like poison—we see metal poisons in the vials and we see metal poisons in the blood of the injected—could there be a scientific correlation to metal poisoning being a part of the picture? It seems it might be worthwhile adding metal detoxification into all vaccine injury protocols. So, shouldn't the detoxification of metals with EDTA Chelation be standard of care, as I have frequently discussed in multiple articles?

Chemical Analysis Comparison of Hydrogel Filaments from C19 Shots and Environmental Geoengineering Sources – What Happened to Humanity's Blood?

APRIL 07, 2023[77]

The filaments seen in live blood, COVID 19 "vaccine" contents, and studies of environmental poisoning via geoengineering can come from different sources; however, there are some remarkable similarities present in all that are worthy of further study. In my view, this assault of hydrogel-based, synthetic biology is the platform of the transhumanist agenda to modify and transform all life on earth, as I will state repeatedly.

My own and Clifford Carnicoms' ongoing working hypothesis is that the platform for all these synthetic filaments has one commonality: self-assembling polymers, aka hydrogel. We know that Clifford found chemical signatures in the CDB filaments (aka Morgellons or advanced nanotechnology) that strongly suggested the presence of polyvinyl alcohol, a hydrogel polymer. It is well known that the lipid nanoparticle, supposed mRNA, shot delivery system is a hydrogel-based polymer known as polyethylene glycol. We will investigate the chemical similarities of known compositions of COVID 19 vial contents and analysis of environmental filaments known as Morgellons or CDB.

In a report from the United Kingdom, *Qualitative Evaluation of Inclusions in Moderna, AstraZeneca and Pfizer Covid-19 Vaccines, Project CUNIT-2-112Y6580*, the microscopic growth of filaments was noted. The UK report suggests carbon species like graphene in the vaccines they studied using microscopy. Further identification in the chemical analysis of these filaments has not been done by this group, so we cannot rule out that other chemical compounds have also been involved in this filament growth. The same filament growth has been documented by many other COVID 19 vial content researchers and overlaps with what we have been seeing in live blood analysis, which includes the CDB filaments observed by Clifford Carnicom for the past 30 years.

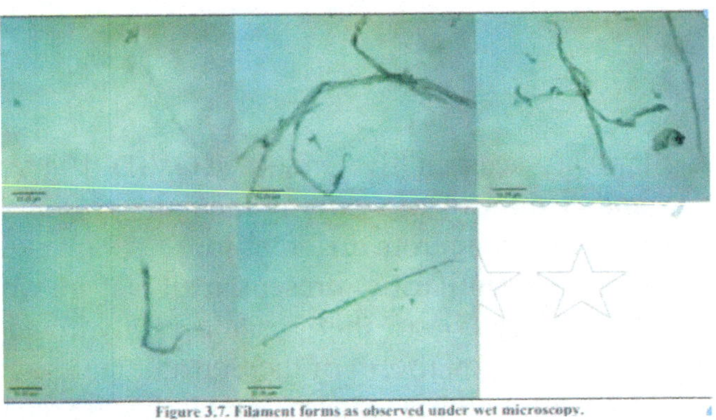

Figure 42. Moderna COVID 19 "vaccine" filament growth. Project CUNIT-2-112Y6580.[78]

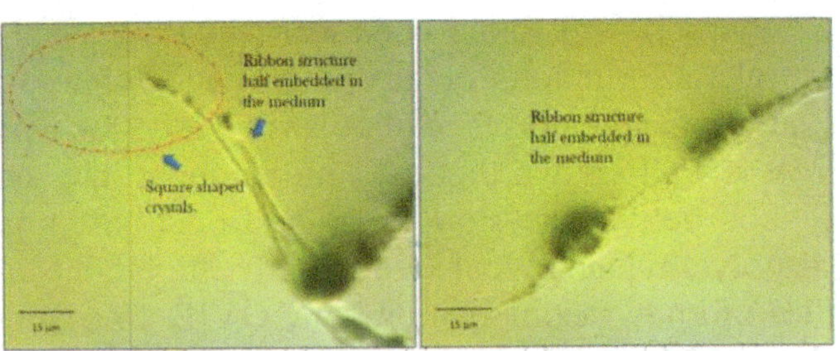

Figure 43. Moderna COVID 19 "vaccine" filament growth. Project CUNIT-2-112Y6580.[79]

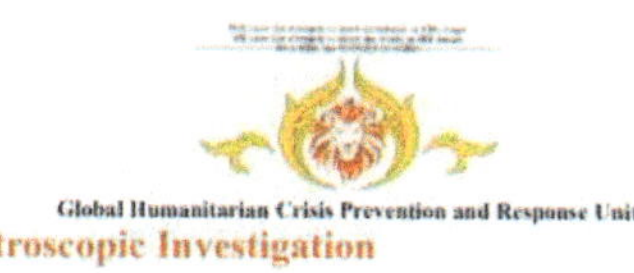

3.2.2. Raman Spectroscopic Investigation

Representative inclusions from Moderna 01 were examined by Raman spectroscopy. The investigation clearly showed that all the inclusions have a strong carbon signal with confirmed graphene compositions of some representative forms.

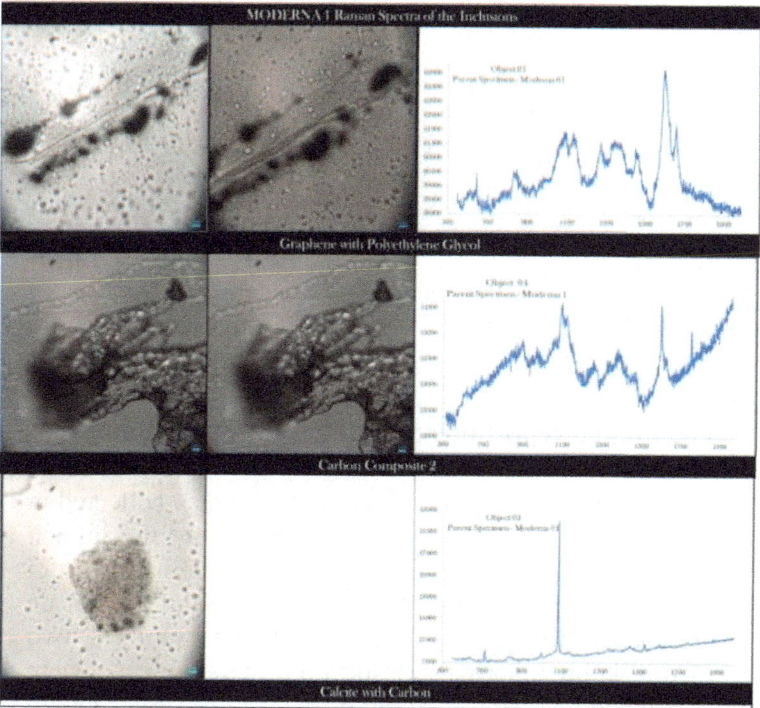

Figure 44. Moderna COVID 19 "vaccine" Raman spectroscopy analysis. Project CUNIT-2-112Y6580.[80]

In 2012, an environmental filament analysis was conducted in France at a series of collection points identified on a map. The image below shows filaments that were found in the environment, as a result of geoengineered spraying in the area.

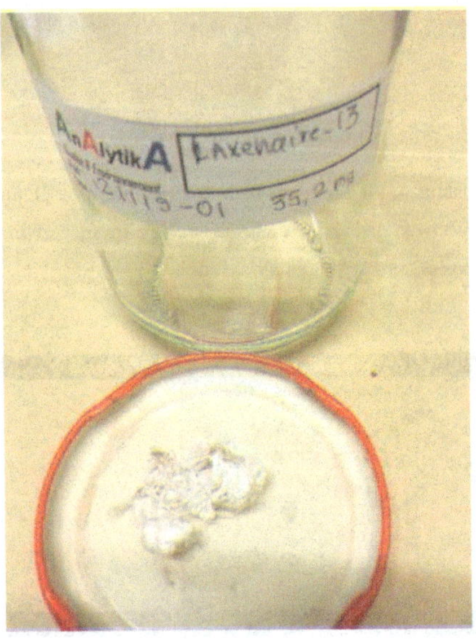

Figure 45. Environmental filament following geoengineering projects in France 2012. Bernard Tailliez.[81]

The French report provides the following summary:

> Several samples of «air borne filaments» collected in November and December 2012 throughout the French territory were sent to our laboratory (originating from Thénioux, Saint Clément des Levées, Saint Martin de Crau, and Malabat ... For each of these samples, two Curie-Point thermal desorption experiments were conducted at 445°C, directly as well as after in-situ methylation (a process allowing detection of polar compounds potentially present). The organic compounds generated in this series of eight experiments were each time-separated by gas chromatography and identified by mass spectrometry (GC/MS). The data obtained were interpreted and the detailed results are presented in this analytical report. It appears that these «air borne filaments» are complex organic polymers, containing

> many synthetic chemicals, as evidenced by GC/MS screening of their thermal decomposition products.
>
> Many organic molecules commonly encountered in the composition of jet fuels and jet reactor lubricants were evidenced in this investigation. The four samples studied contain several toxic synthetic compounds (phthalates) and three of them contain DEHP, a member of this family of particular concern due to its properties of endocrine disruptors. All organic molecules, particularly the heterocyclic compounds, present in the «air borne filaments» samples represent a strong concern, for public health as well as environmental protection.[82]

Phthalates are synthetic chemicals used to make plastics flexible and to make products smell good. They are found in car interiors, shower curtains, deodorant, cosmetics, medical devices, and children's products and toys.

Complex organic polymers are hydrogels. Hydrogel-forming natural polymers include proteins, such as collagen and gelatine, and polysaccharides, such as starch, alginate, and agarose. Synthetic polymers that form hydrogels are traditionally prepared using chemical polymerization methods.

I have been speaking about the fact that the hydrogel filaments seen in the blood are similar to plastics and are not parasites or worms.

The method of preparation leads to formations of some important classes of hydrogels. These can be exemplified by the following:

- Homopolymeric hydrogels are referred to polymer networks derived from a single species of monomer, which is a basic structural unit comprised of any polymer network. Homopolymers may have cross-linked skeletal structure depending on the nature of the monomer and polymerization technique.
- Copolymeric hydrogels are comprised of two or more different monomer species with at least one

hydrophilic component, arranged in a random, block or alternating configuration along the chain of the polymer network.

- Multipolymer interpenetrating polymeric hydrogel (IPN), an important class of hydrogels, is made of two independent cross-linked synthetic and/or natural polymer components, contained in a network form. In semi-IPN hydrogel, one component is a cross-linked polymer and the other component is a non-cross-linked polymer.[83]

This document reveals other synthetic chemicals identified in the French environmental filament analysis:

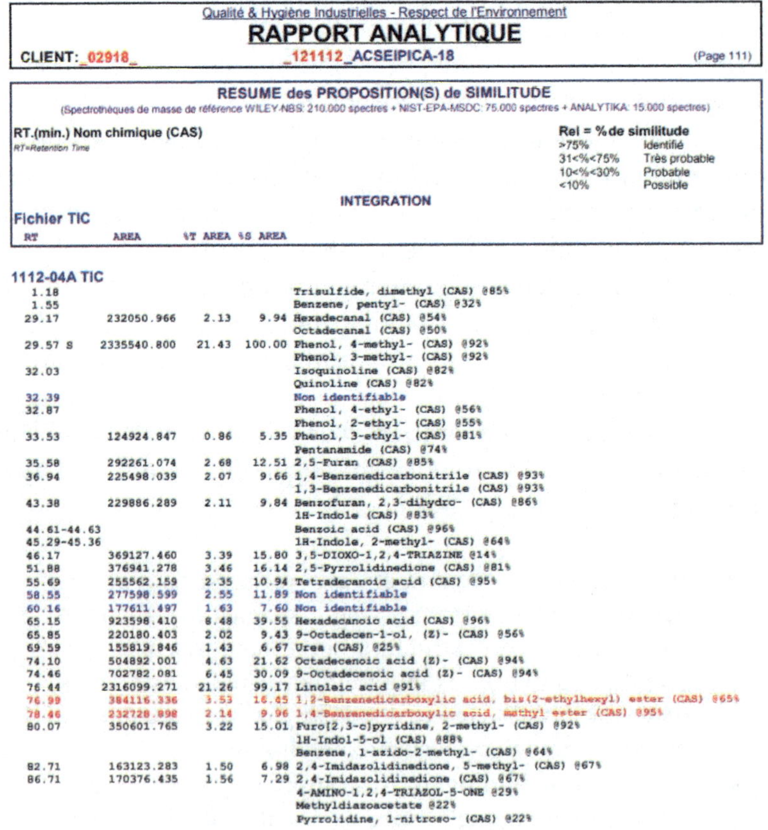

Qualité & Hygiène Industrielles - Respect de l'Environnement

RAPPORT ANALYTIQUE

CLIENT: _02918_ _121112_ACSEIPICA-18 (Page 111)

RESUME des PROPOSITION(S) de SIMILITUDE

(Spectrothèques de masse de référence WILEY-NBS: 210.000 spectres + NIST-EPA-MSDC: 75.000 spectres + ANALYTIKA: 15.000 spectres)

RT.(min.) Nom chimique (CAS)
RT=Retention Time

Rel = %de similitude	
>75%	Identifié
31<%<75%	Très probable
10<%<30%	Probable
<10%	Possible

INTEGRATION

Fichier TIC

1112-04A TIC

RT	AREA	%T AREA	%S AREA	
1.18				Trisulfide, dimethyl (CAS) @85%
1.55				Benzene, pentyl- (CAS) @32%
29.17	232050.966	2.13	9.94	Hexadecanal (CAS) @54%
				Octadecanal (CAS) @50%
29.57 S	2335540.800	21.43	100.00	Phenol, 4-methyl- (CAS) @92%
				Phenol, 3-methyl- (CAS) @92%
32.03				Isoquinoline (CAS) @82%
				Quinoline (CAS) @82%
32.39				Non identifiable
32.87				Phenol, 4-ethyl- (CAS) @56%
				Phenol, 2-ethyl- (CAS) @55%
33.53	124924.847	0.86	5.35	Phenol, 3-ethyl- (CAS) @81%
				Pentanamide (CAS) @74%
35.58	292261.074	2.68	12.51	2,5-Furan (CAS) @85%
36.94	225498.039	2.07	9.66	1,4-Benzenedicarbonitrile (CAS) @93%
				1,3-Benzenedicarbonitrile (CAS) @93%
43.38	229886.289	2.11	9.84	Benzofuran, 2,3-dihydro- (CAS) @86%
				1H-Indole (CAS) @83%
44.61-44.63				Benzoic acid (CAS) @96%
45.29-45.36				1H-Indole, 2-methyl- (CAS) @64%
46.17	369127.460	3.39	15.80	3,5-DIOXO-1,2,4-TRIAZINE @14%
51.88	376941.278	3.46	16.14	2,5-Pyrrolidinedione (CAS) @81%
55.69	255562.159	2.35	10.94	Tetradecanoic acid (CAS) @95%
58.55	277598.599	2.55	11.89	Non identifiable
60.16	177611.497	1.63	7.60	Non identifiable
65.15	923598.410	8.48	39.55	Hexadecanoic acid (CAS) @96%
65.85	220180.403	2.02	9.43	9-Octadecen-1-ol, (Z)- (CAS) @56%
69.59	155819.846	1.43	6.67	Urea (CAS) @25%
74.10	504892.001	4.63	21.62	Octadecenoic acid (Z)- (CAS) @94%
74.46	702782.081	6.45	30.09	9-Octadecenoic acid (Z)- (CAS) @94%
76.44	2316099.271	21.26	99.17	Linoleic acid @91%
76.99	384116.336	3.53	16.45	1,2-Benzenedicarboxylic acid, bis(2-ethylhexyl) ester (CAS) @65%
78.46	232728.898	2.14	9.96	1,4-Benzenedicarboxylic acid, methyl ester (CAS) @95%
80.07	350601.765	3.22	15.01	Furo[2,3-c]pyridine, 2-methyl- (CAS) @92%
				1H-Indol-5-ol (CAS) @88%
				Benzene, 1-azido-2-methyl- (CAS) @64%
82.71	163123.283	1.50	6.98	2,4-Imidazolidinedione, 5-methyl- (CAS) @67%
86.71	170376.435	1.56	7.29	2,4-Imidazolidinedione (CAS) @67%
				4-AMINO-1,2,4-TRIAZOL-5-ONE @29%
				Methyldiazoacetate @22%
				Pyrrolidine, 1-nitroso- (CAS) @22%

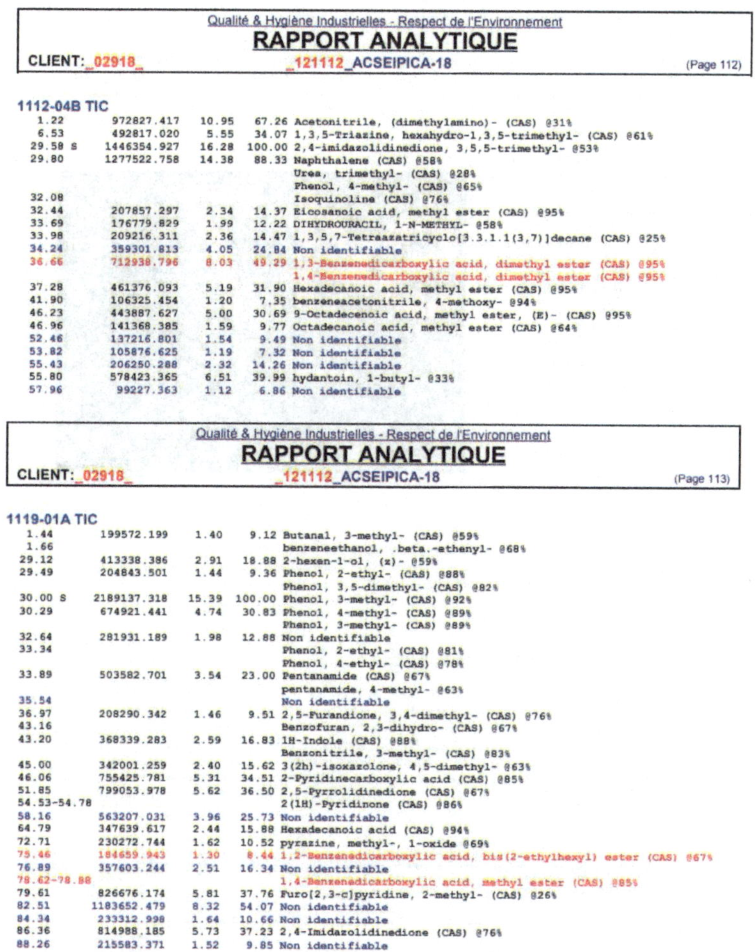

Qualité & Hygiène Industrielles - Respect de l'Environnement

RAPPORT ANALYTIQUE

CLIENT: _02918_ _121112_ACSEIPICA-18 (Page 112)

1112-04B TIC

1.22	972827.417	10.95	67.26	Acetonitrile, (dimethylamino)- (CAS) @31%
6.53	492817.020	5.55	34.07	1,3,5-Triazine, hexahydro-1,3,5-trimethyl- (CAS) @61%
29.58 s	1446354.927	16.28	100.00	2,4-imidazolidinedione, 3,5,5-trimethyl- @53%
29.80	1277522.758	14.38	88.33	Naphthalene (CAS) @58%
				Urea, trimethyl- (CAS) @28%
				Phenol, 4-methyl- (CAS) @65%
32.08				Isoquinoline (CAS) @76%
32.44	207857.297	2.34	14.37	Eicosanoic acid, methyl ester (CAS) @95%
33.69	176779.829	1.99	12.22	DIHYDROURACIL, 1-N-METHYL- @58%
33.98	209216.311	2.36	14.47	1,3,5,7-Tetraazatricyclo[3.3.1.1(3,7)]decane (CAS) @25%
34.24	359301.813	4.05	24.84	Non identifiable
36.66	712938.796	8.03	49.29	1,3-Benzenedicarboxylic acid, dimethyl ester (CAS) @95%
				1,4-Benzenedicarboxylic acid, dimethyl ester (CAS) @95%
37.28	461376.093	5.19	31.90	Hexadecanoic acid, methyl ester (CAS) @95%
41.90	106325.454	1.20	7.35	benzeneacetonitrile, 4-methoxy- @94%
46.23	443887.627	5.00	30.69	9-Octadecenoic acid, methyl ester, (E)- (CAS) @95%
46.96	141368.385	1.59	9.77	Octadecanoic acid, methyl ester (CAS) @64%
52.46	137216.801	1.54	9.49	Non identifiable
53.82	105876.625	1.19	7.32	Non identifiable
55.43	206250.288	2.32	14.26	Non identifiable
55.80	578423.365	6.51	39.99	hydantoin, 1-butyl- @33%
57.96	99227.363	1.12	6.86	Non identifiable

Qualité & Hygiène Industrielles - Respect de l'Environnement

RAPPORT ANALYTIQUE

CLIENT: _02918_ _121112_ACSEIPICA-18 (Page 113)

1119-01A TIC

1.44	199572.199	1.40	9.12	Butanal, 3-methyl- (CAS) @59%
1.66				benzeneethanol, .beta.-ethenyl- @68%
29.12	413338.386	2.91	18.88	2-hexen-1-ol, (z)- @59%
29.49	204843.501	1.44	9.36	Phenol, 2-ethyl- (CAS) @88%
				Phenol, 3,5-dimethyl- (CAS) @82%
30.00 S	2189137.318	15.39	100.00	Phenol, 3-methyl- (CAS) @92%
30.29	674921.441	4.74	30.83	Phenol, 4-methyl- (CAS) @89%
				Phenol, 3-methyl- (CAS) @89%
32.64	281931.189	1.98	12.88	Non identifiable
33.34				Phenol, 2-ethyl- (CAS) @81%
				Phenol, 4-ethyl- (CAS) @78%
33.89	503582.701	3.54	23.00	Pentanamide (CAS) @67%
				pentanamide, 4-methyl- @63%
35.54				Non identifiable
36.97	208290.342	1.46	9.51	2,5-Furandione, 3,4-dimethyl- (CAS) @76%
43.16				Benzofuran, 2,3-dihydro- (CAS) @67%
43.20	368339.283	2.59	16.83	1H-Indole (CAS) @88%
				Benzonitrile, 3-methyl- (CAS) @83%
45.00	342001.259	2.40	15.62	3(2h)-isoxazolone, 4,5-dimethyl- @63%
46.06	755425.781	5.31	34.51	2-Pyridinecarboxylic acid (CAS) @85%
51.85	799053.978	5.62	36.50	2,5-Pyrrolidinedione (CAS) @67%
54.53-54.78				2(1H)-Pyridinone (CAS) @86%
58.16	563207.031	3.96	25.73	Non identifiable
64.79	347639.617	2.44	15.88	Hexadecanoic acid (CAS) @94%
72.71	230272.744	1.62	10.52	pyrazine, methyl-, 1-oxide @69%
75.46	184659.943	1.30	8.44	1,2-Benzenedicarboxylic acid, bis(2-ethylhexyl) ester (CAS) @67%
76.89	357603.244	2.51	16.34	Non identifiable
78.62-78.88				1,4-Benzenedicarboxylic acid, methyl ester (CAS) @85%
79.61	826676.174	5.81	37.76	Furo[2,3-c]pyridine, 2-methyl- (CAS) @26%
82.51	1183652.479	8.32	54.07	Non identifiable
84.34	233312.998	1.64	10.66	Non identifiable
86.36	814988.185	5.73	37.23	2,4-Imidazolidinedione (CAS) @76%
88.26	215583.371	1.52	9.85	Non identifiable

Figure 46. Analytic report from France on environmental filament shows many different chemicals identified. Bernard Taillez.[84]

Let's now look at the chemical composition of the Pfizer lipid nanoparticles, as found in the following document obtained by a Freedom of Information Act (FOIA) request in Australia: *Nonclinical Evaluation Report BNT162b2 [mRNA] COVID-19 vaccine (COMIRNATYTM) Submission No: PM-2020-05461-1-2.* Sponsor: Pfizer Australia Pty Ltd January 2021.

1.3. PRODUCT FORMULATION

BNT162b2 vaccine is supplied as a preservative-free concentrated suspension formulation for intramuscular (IM) administration after dilution. The vaccine contains a nucleoside-modified messenger RNA, encoding the SARS-CoV-2 Spike-glycoprotein (S), produced by *in-vitro* transcription process and encapsulated into solid-lipid nanoparticles (LNP). The LNP is composed of four lipids: ALC-0315, ALC-0159, DSPC, and cholesterol. Quantities of mRNA, lipids and excipients are presented below in Table 1-1.

Table 1-1. Product formulation

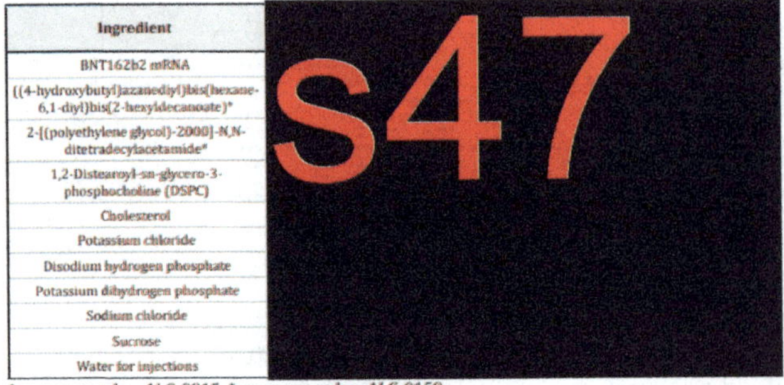

Ingredient
BNT162b2 mRNA
((4-hydroxybutyl)azanediyl)bis(hexane-6,1-diyl)bis(2-hexyldecanoate)*
2-[(polyethylene glycol)-2000]-N,N-ditetradecylacetamide[a]
1,2-Distearoyl-sn-glycero-3-phosphocholine (DSPC)
Cholesterol
Potassium chloride
Disodium hydrogen phosphate
Potassium dihydrogen phosphate
Sodium chloride
Sucrose
Water for injections

* company code = ALC-0315; [a] company code = ALC-0159

1.4. EXCIPIENTS

2-[(Polyethylene glycol)-2000]-N,N-ditetradecylacetamide (ALC-0159) and ((4-hydroxybutyl)azanediyl)bis(hexane-6,1-diyl)bis(2-hexyldecanoate)(ALC-0315) are novel excipients and are not listed on the TGA's ingredient database. These excipients will be referred to as ALC-0159 and ALC-0315 in this report, respectively. As per the Sponsor's statement, ALC-0315 has been

Document 6

Nonclinical Evaluation of BNT162b2 [mRNA] COVID-19 vaccine (COMIRNATY) Submission No. PM-2020-05461-1-2

optimised for RNA encapsulation and intracellular delivery, and ALC-0159 has been engineered to regulate LNP size (40 – 180 nm) and transfection potency. Batch data for multiple batches of proposed vaccine showed particle size (D50) in the range of 58 – 94 nm (Table 1-3). The lipids protect the mRNA from degradation, and facilitate cell uptake, hence they are a major determinant of potency (Jayaraman et al. 2012). The Sponsor indicated that these novel excipients, ALC-0159 and ALC-0315 are structurally and functionally similar to the lipid excipients PEG2000-C DMG and DLin-MC3-DMA, respectively, used in a siRNA-LNP drug product Onpattro™ (patisiran), which is approved in the US, Europe (by EMA) and Canada.

Details of these lipids are shown below.

Product	Novel lipid excipient (CAS no, Molecular formula and weight in Da)	Structure	Chemical name
BNT162b2 V9	**ALC-0159** (*CAS no.* 1849616-42-7, $(C_2H_4O)_nC_{31}H_{62}NO_2$, n=45-50 and 2400-2600 Da)		2-[(polyethylene glycol)-2000]-N,N-ditetradecylacetamide
	ALC-0315 (*CAS no* 2036272-55-4, $C_{48}H_{95}NO_5$ and 766 Da)		((4-hydroxybutyl)azanediyl)bis (hex ane-6,1-diyl)bis(2-hexyldecanoate)
Onpattro™ (patisiran)	PEG2000-C-DMG (NA, $(C_2H_4O)_nC_{34}H_{73}NO_5$, n=47 and 2650±300 Da)		(α-[3'-{[1,2-di(myristyloxy)proponoxyy] carbonylamino}propyl]-ω-methoxy, polyoxyethylene)
	DLin-MC3-DMA (NA, $C_{43}H_{79}NO_2$ and 642.09 Da)		(6Z,9Z,28Z,31Z)-heptatriaconta-6,9,28,31-tetraen-19-yl-4-(dimethylamino) butanoate

Figure 47. Product formulation of lipid nanoparticles in Pfizer C19 "vaccine" in Australia.[85]

I find it curious that the chemical structure between the environmental fibers analyzed in France, and the Pfizer COVID 19 lipid nanoparticles from Australia, have overlap. Note that butanal is a chemical component of the environmental filaments. In comparison, the COVID 19 Pfizer shot lipid nanoparticles contain (6Z,9Z,28Z,31Z)- hepatatriaconta-6,9,28,31- tetraene-19-yl-4- (dimethylamino) butanoate.

- Butyraldehyde, also known as butanal, is an organic compound with the formula CH 3 (CH 2) 2 CHO. This compound is the aldehyde derivative of butane. It is a colorless flammable liquid with an unpleasant smell. It is miscible with most organic solvents.

- Aldol condensation in the presence of a base forms 2-ethyl-2-hexenal, which is then hydrogenated to form 2-ethylhexanol, a precursor to the plasticizer bis(2-ethylhexyl) phthalate.

- Butanoate is a sodium salt of butyric acid, an oily, colorless liquid with an unpleasant odor. Butyraldehyde (Butanol) can be produced by the catalytic dehydrogenation of *n*-butanol. Butyric acid is manufactured by catalyzed air oxidation of butanal (butyraldehyde).[86]

Hence the chemical compounds found in the geoengineered filaments and those in the Pfizer vials are similar, and both can be building blocks of hydrogel polymers. This is another piece in the puzzle that Clifford Carnicom and I have been sounding the alarm about. We also found aromatic carbon hydrogen signatures in vaccinated and unvaccinated blood that can indicate the presence of hydrogel.

Alarming New Report from "Vaccine" Analysis in Germany and Other Countries

AUGUST 08, 2022[87]

In August of 2022, a group of scientists from Germany published their analysis of COVID 19 injections. Known as the German Working Group for COVID Vaccine Analysis, they made their initial findings publicly available in a wide-ranging report:

1. Toxic substances were found in all samples of COVID 19 vaccines – without exception.

2. The blood samples of all the people who had been vaccinated showed marked changes.

3. The greater the stability of the envelope of lipid nanoparticles, the more frequent are vaccine side effects.

4. In all samples of COVID 19 vaccines, without exception, components were found, using several methods of measurement, that: – are, in the quantities found, toxic according to medical guidelines, – had not been declared by the manufacturers as present in the vaccines, – are for the most part metallic, – are visible under the dark-field microscope as distinctive and complex structures of different sizes, – can only partially be explained as a result of crystallization or decomposition processes, – cannot be explained as contamination from the manufacturing process.

5. The comparison of blood samples from unvaccinated and vaccinated individuals by means of darkfield microscopy showed noticeable changes in the blood of each person who had been vaccinated with the

COVID 19 vaccines. This was evident even if those people hadn't at that point displayed any visible reaction to the vaccinations. Complex structures similar to those in the vaccines were found in the blood samples of the vaccinated. Using artificial intelligence (AI) image analysis, the difference between the blood of vaccinated and unvaccinated people was confirmed.

6. The stability of the lipid nanoparticle envelope is closely correlated with the incidence of vaccine side effects and injury. The more stable this envelope, the greater the amount of mRNA that penetrates cells, where the production of spike proteins then takes place. These results correspond with the findings of pathologists who have carried out autopsies on people who died due to vaccine injury. Spike proteins were detected in damaged tissue. Researchers suspect that the spike protein is, in itself, toxic.

The following predominantly metallic elements were unexpectedly detected in the doses from AstraZeneca, BioNTech/Pfizer and Moderna:

- Alkali metals: caesium (Cs), potassium (K),
- Alkaline earth metals: calcium (Ca), barium (Ba),
- Transition metals: cobalt (Co), iron (Fe), chromium (Cr), titanium (Ti),
- Rare earth metals: cerium (Ce), gadolinium (Gd),
- Mining group/metal: aluminium (Al),
- Carbon group: silicon (Si) (partly support material/slide),
- Oxygen group: sulphur (S).[88]

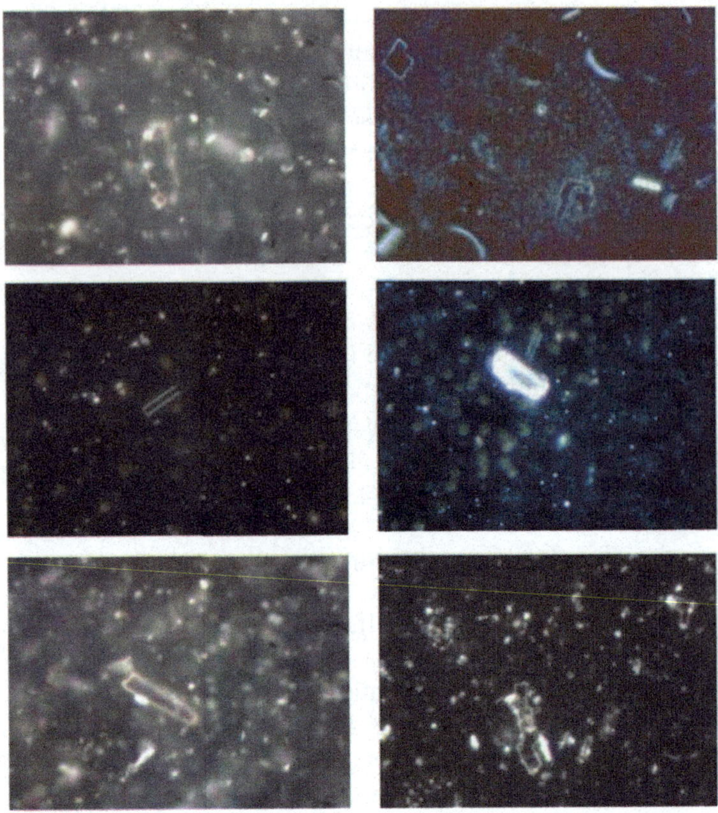

***Figure 7:** The Comirnaty vaccine from BioNTech/Pfizer exhibits a diversity and large number of unusual objects. The vast number of crystalline platelets and shapes can hardly be interpreted as impurities. They appear regularly and in large numbers in all samples.*

Figure 48. Comirnaty “vaccine” – unusual objects found in darkfield microscopy. German Working Group for COVID Vaccine Analysis.[89]

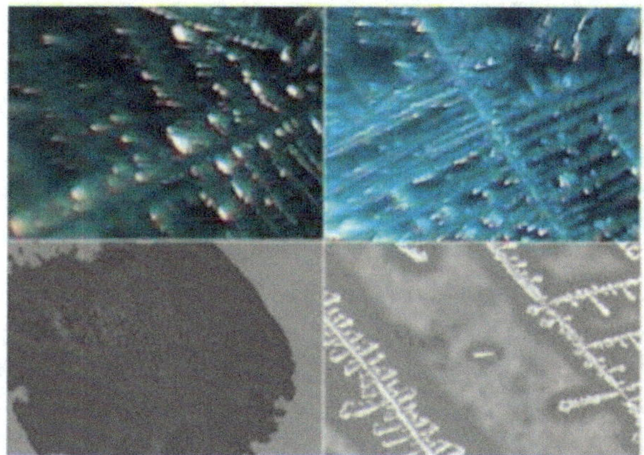

Figure 7: Crystal formation of mRNA-1273 (Moderna) in the reflected light microscope (top) and in the scanning electron microscope (bottom)

Figure 49. Comirnaty "vaccine" – unusual objects found in darkfield microscopy. German Working Group for COVID Vaccine Analysis.[90]

Dr. Sam Bailey, from New Zealand, also found nano-structures in the COVID 19 injections:[91]

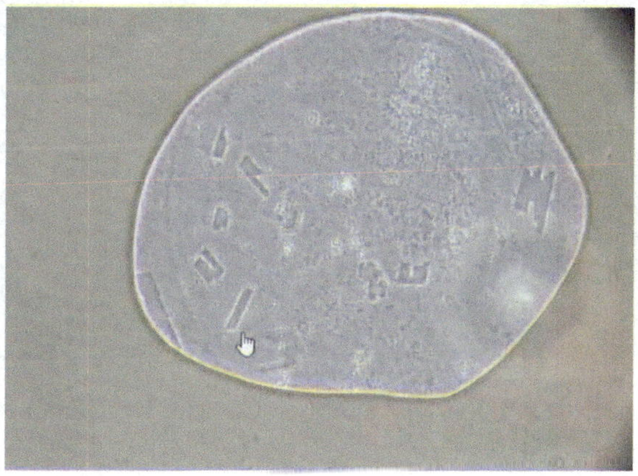

Figure 50. Pfizer COVID 19 vial analysis, New Zealand. Dr. Sam Bailey.[92]

Dr. Daniel Nagase from Canada conducted mass spectroscopy that did not identify any phosphorous or nitrogen in the COVID 19 injections sample. This means there were no elements related to life that constitute molecules like RNA, DNA, or proteins. He did, however, find self-assembling nanotechnology and metals:[93,94]

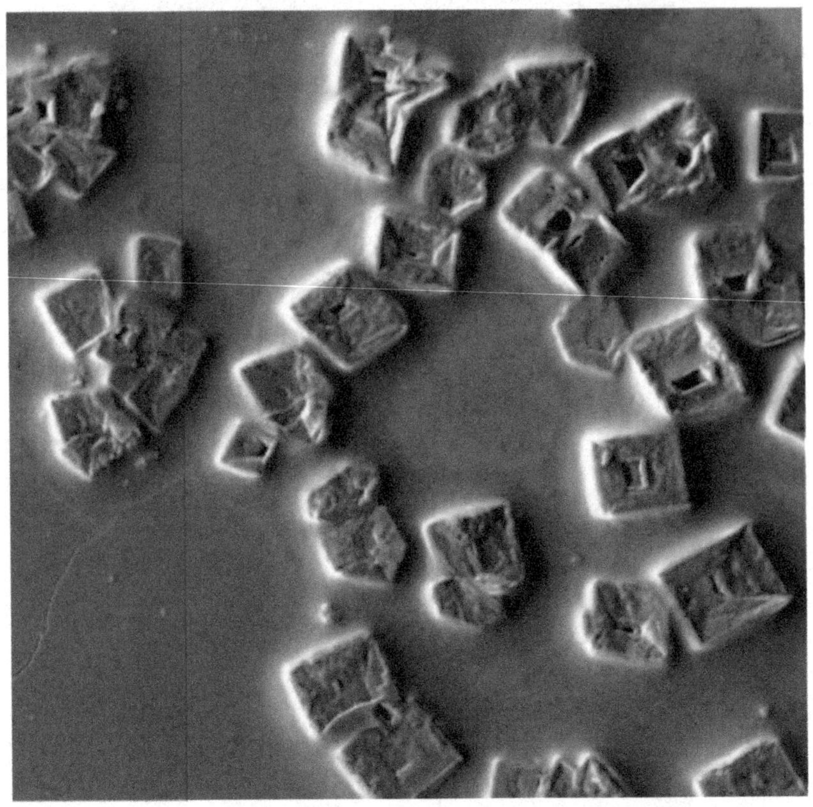

Figure 51. Pfizer COVID 19 vial analysis, Canada. Dr. Daniel Nagase.[95]

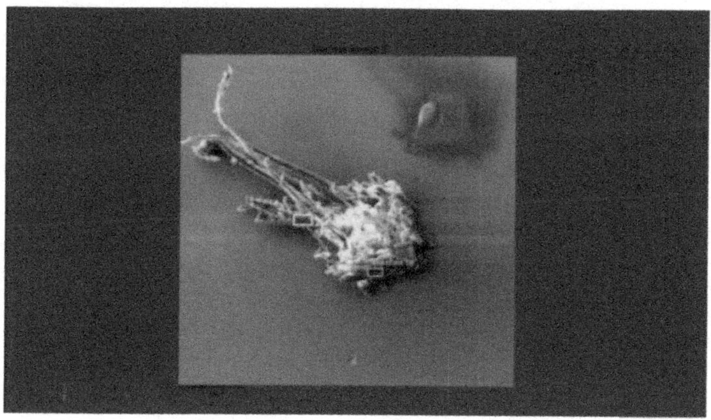

Figure 52. Pfizer COVID 19 vial analysis, Canada. Dr. Daniel Nagase.[96]

Extensive documentation of nanoparticles in the blood of vaccinated people from Italy is recorded in the study *Dark-Field Microscopic Analysis on the Blood of 1,006 Symptomatic Persons After Anti-COVID mRNA Injections from Pfizer/ BioNtech or Moderna.*[97]

The abstract states: "In conclusion, such abrupt changes as we have documented in the peripheral blood profile of 948 patients have never been observed after inoculation by any vaccines in the past according to our clinical experience.

"The sudden transition, usually at the time of a second mRNA injection, from a state of perfect normalcy to a pathological one, with accompanying hemolysis, visible packing and stacking of red blood cells in conjunction with the formation of gigantic conglomerate foreign structures, some of them appearing as graphene-family superstructures, is unprecedented.

"Such phenomena have never been seen before after any 'vaccination' of the past.

"In our collective experience, and in our shared professional opinion, the large quantity of particles in the blood of mRNA injection recipients is incompatible with normal blood flow especially at the level of the capillaries."[98]

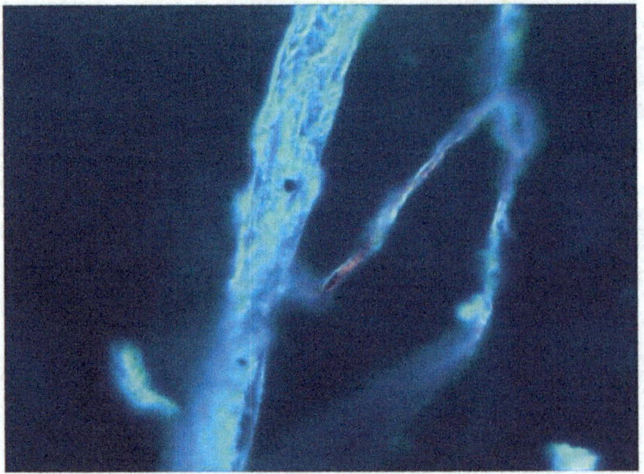

Figure 4. This image at 120x magnification (3x magnification digitally produced) highlights a typical self-aggregating structuring in fibro/tubular mode.

Figure 53. Self-assembly nanotechnology found in COVID 19 injected blood in Italy. *International Journal of Vaccine Theory, Practice, and Research,* Giovannini, *et al.*[99]

UK Forensic Report Finds Graphene: Qualitative Evaluation of Inclusions in Moderna, AstraZeneca, and Pfizer COVID 19 "Vaccines"

SEPTEMBER 14, 2022[100]

The Exposé reported on a Forensic Analysis of the C19 injection vials in the United Kingdom in 2022.[101] This report is of utmost significance as it has a meticulous chain of custody documentation, which is important to be able to submit as evidence in any court case. This forensic laboratory report has been presented in a police criminal case calling for immediate halt of the injections due to both corporate manslaughter and gross criminal manslaughter. The document names as defendants: AstraZeneca, Pfizer, Moderna, National Health Service (NHS), Medicines & Healthcare products Regulatory Agency (MHRA), Joint Committee on Vaccination and Immunization (JCVI), and Her Majesty's Government.[102]

EbMCsquared CIC commissioned independent analysis to investigate the contents of four injection vials (Moderna 01, Moderna 02, AstraZeneca, Pfizer) for any undeclared ingredients that may cause bodily harm. This is what the analysis found in all four vials:

Laboratory Report Summary

A summary of the findings detailed in the attached quality assured report is as follows:

RAMAN Spectroscopy discovered the following particles -

- Graphene
- SP3 Carbon
- Iron Oxide
- Carbon derivatives

Figure 54. UK forensic laboratory report summary. Project CUNIT-2-112Y6580. EbMCsquared CIC.[103]

And this is what the report says graphene can do to the body:

Toxicology Report Summary

A summary of the findings detailed in the attached toxicology report is as follows:

- Graphene nanomaterials (GFNs) can penetrate the body's natural barriers and damage the central nervous system
- Graphene oxide (GO):
    a. can damage internal organs
    b. damages the reproduction and development system
    c. destroys blood health
    d. damages and destroys cells
    e. can trigger cancer and accelerate ageing
    f. damages mitochondria and DNA
    g. triggers an inflammatory response and three different kinds of cell death
    h. causes changes in gene function

Figure 55. UK forensic toxicology report summary. Project CUNIT-2-112Y6580. EbMCsquared CIC.[104]

The identified toxic inclusions were stated in the report as:

1. Graphene nano ribbons coated with polyethylene glycol
2. Graphene composite form 1
3. Graphene composite form 2
4. Microcrystalline calcite with carbonaceous inclusions
5. Graphene nano forms with and without fluorescence
    a. Graphene nano objects
    b. Graphene nano scrolls

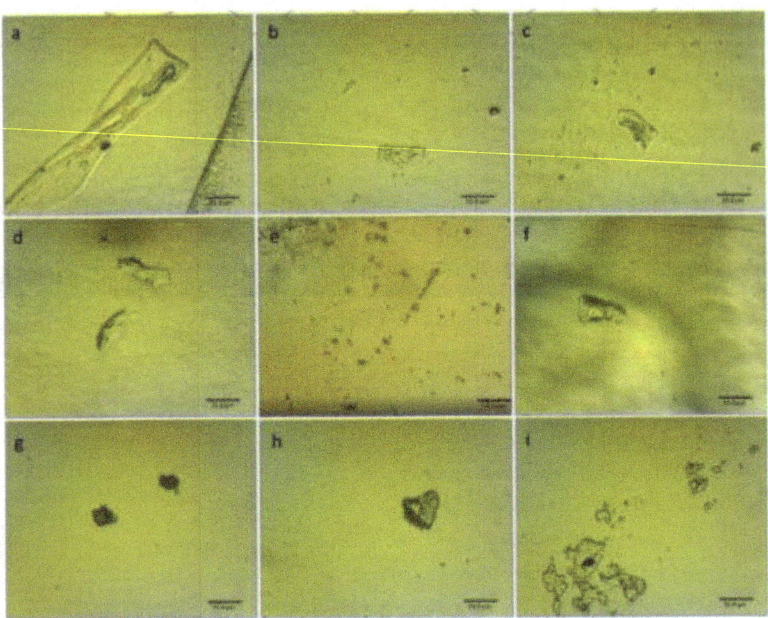
Figure 3.32. Representative inclusions found within Pfizer vaccine.

Figure 56. Microscopy of inclusions in Pfizer COVID 19 "vaccine." Project CUNIT-2-112Y6580. EbMCsquared CIC.[105]

3.1.1. Graphene Composites in the form of Nano Ribbons

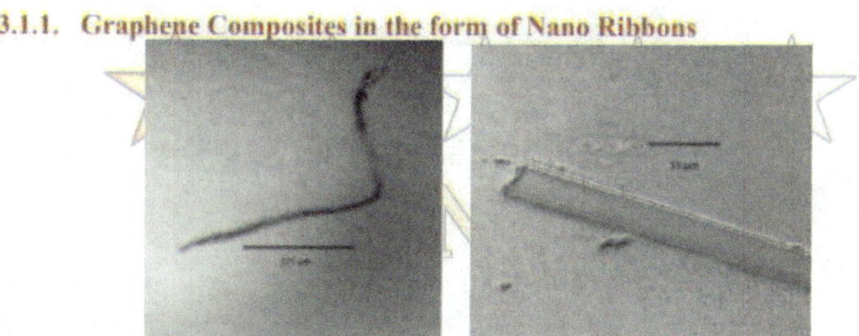

Figure. 3.1. Carbon Composite Ribbon Forms from a sample in Moderna 01. The first picture is of a wet sample and at a low magnification. The second picture is that of the same sample when it is dry and embedded in solution at a high magnification.

Figure 57. Microscopy of graphene composites in the form of nanoribbons – Moderna COVID 19 “vaccine.” CUNIT-2-112Y6580. EbMCsquared CIC.[106]

3.1.2. Graphene Composite form 1

GC1 appears in a translucent folded form of about 10-15microns across. The form is transparent to translucent in transmitted light and shows light structure within it.

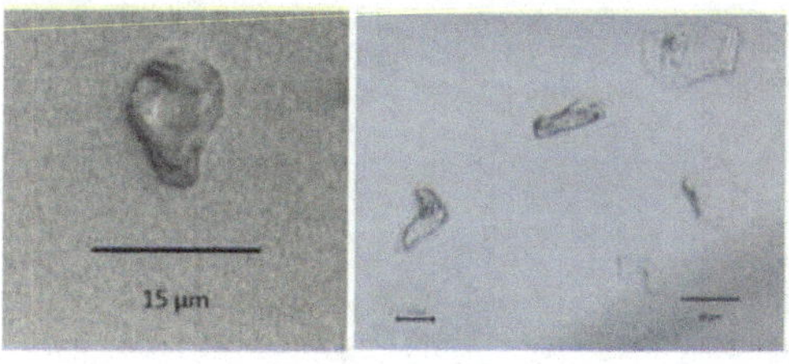

Figure 3.2. An assemblage of different forms with some embedded in the solution appearing translucent and those on the top show a good relief.

Figure 58. Microscopy of graphene composites – Moderna COVID 19 “vaccine.” Project CUNIT-2-112Y6580. EbMCsquared CIC.[107]

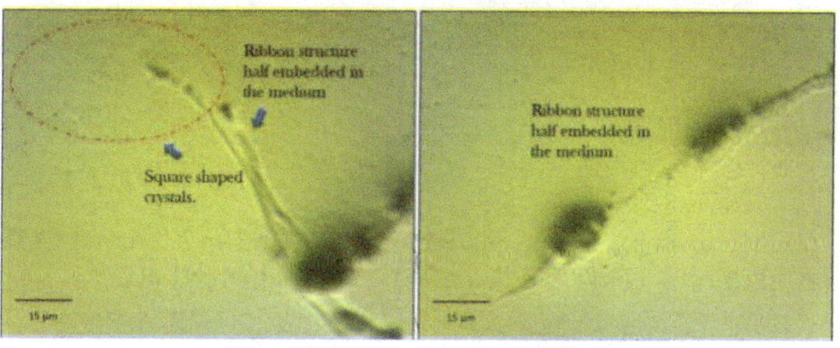

Figure 59. Microscopy of graphene ribbon structures – Moderna COVID 19 “vaccine.” Project CUNIT-2-112Y6580. EbMCsquared CIC.[108]

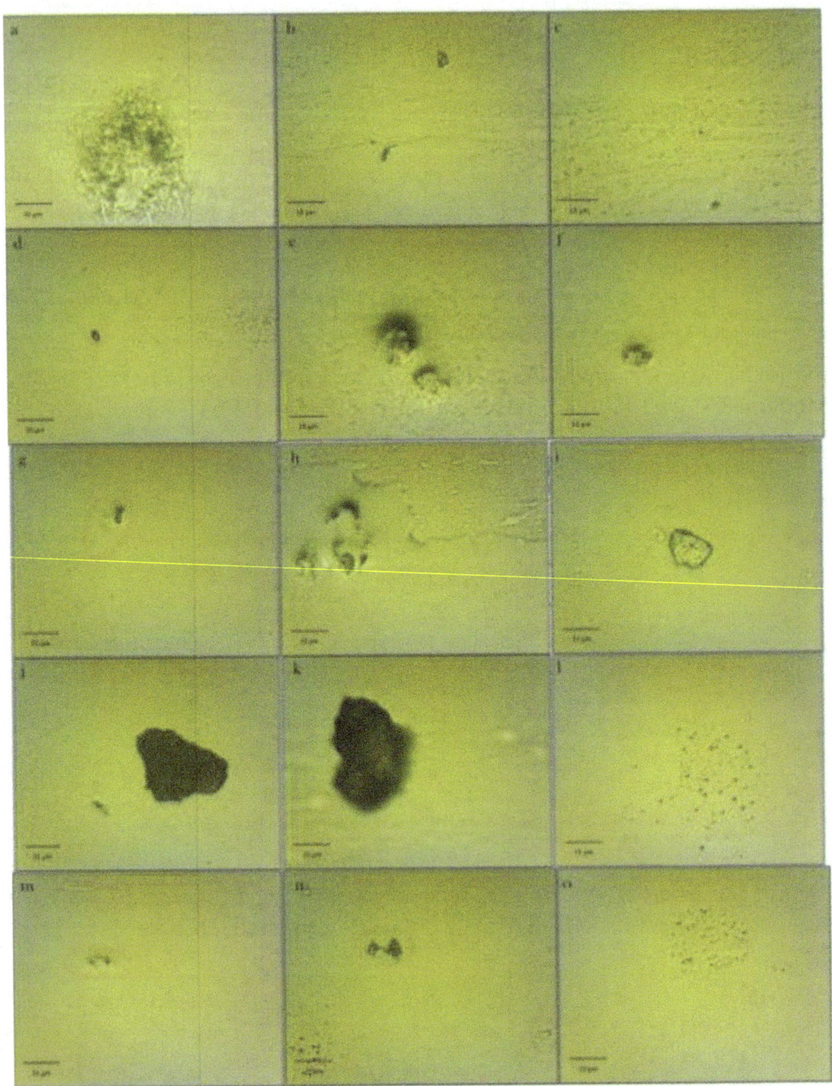

Figure 3.10. Various inclusions found within Moderna 01.

Figure 60. Microscopy of various inclusions found in Moderna COVID 19 "vaccine." Project CUNIT-2-112Y6580. EbMCsquared CIC.[109]

These particles were observed in ubiquity across the sample preparations and each of these structures began with the formation of a small, seed-like particle to which the surrounding particles aggregated, based on hydrophobic interactions. What seems to be obvious through observation, is that hydrophobic interactions appear to be the dominant driving force of the LNP growth, while electrostatic interactions guide the seed formation and stability of the final assembly.

The scientists used a motion detector to evaluate self-assembly of the nanostructures:

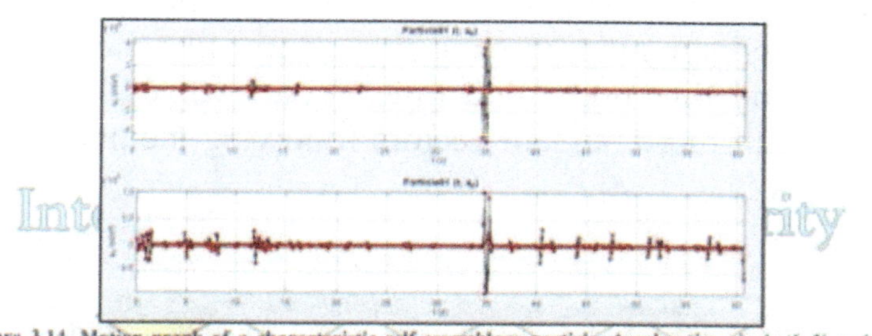

Figure 3.14. Motion graph of a characteristic self-assemblage particle. Accelerations in both X and Y directions show typical staggered forms that typify hydrophobic/philic jumps and movements.

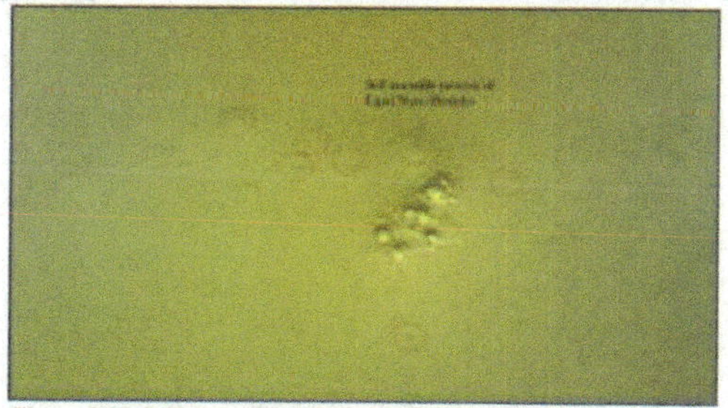

Figure 3.15. Self-Assembled Nano Particles with Payload of mRNA.

Figure 61. Self-assembly measured by motion – COVID 19 "vaccine." Project CUNIT-2-112Y6580. EbMCsquared CIC.[110]

The Astra Zeneca "vaccine" also showed nanoparticles with self-assembly observed.

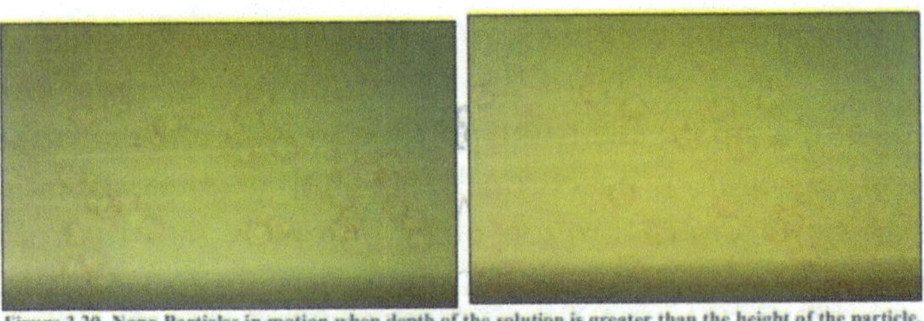

Figure 62. Self-assembly nanoparticles – AstraZeneca COVID 19 "vaccine." Project CUNIT-2-112Y6580. EbMCsquared CIC.[111]

These nanoscopic particles were quite noticeable as white specs in the beginning, moving in a swarm-like motion in the same general direction. With time, these evolved into bigger droplets with more random vectors following the principles of self-assembly.

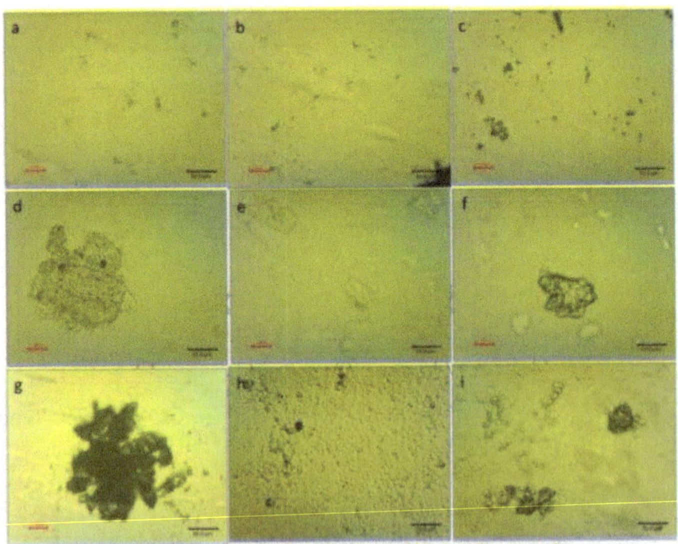

Figure 63. Self-assembly nanoparticles – AstraZeneca COVID 19 "vaccine." Project CUNIT-2-112Y6580. EbMCsquared CIC.[112]

We now have evidence from around the world that the COVID 19 injections all contain toxic, self-assembling nanoparticles. Based on this forensic evidence from the UK, a criminal case has been filed.

All over the world these evaluations must take place with the same meticulous rigor as shown by the examples presented here. Everyone responsible for these crimes against humanity needs to be investigated and criminally charged. From the CDC, NIH, FDA, Medical Boards, FSMB, Pfizer, Moderna, Astra Zeneca, Johnson & Johnson, and the government officials and military that developed and deployed this upon the population. That should include doctors who ordered the injections and did not stop, regardless of strong evidence for adverse effects. "I would have lost my job if I spoke up," will not fare well as a defense when you are charged criminally for manslaughter.

These many reports of toxic findings in the "vaccines" need to be looked at and discussed by EVERYONE. This is the injection of toxic POISON into 68% of the world's population. The motion detection of these elements as recorded and proving self-assembly, speaks for itself. The sinister intention behind this needs to be recognized.

This is what genocide by injection looks like. The shots need to be stopped immediately. We need justice. I fully support the notion of Nuremberg 2.0 for war criminals or domestic terrorists who have released this bioweapon on humanity.

New Images of Self-Assembly Structures in Pfizer Vials and Live Blood Analysis

OCTOBER 04, 2022[113]

Dr. David Nixon graduated from Otago University in 1992. He has spent 25 years in general practice, both in New Zealand and Australia. Dr. Nixon has worked in Brisbane for the last 12 years and is currently under supervision and restrictions from the Australian Health Practitioner Regulation Agency (AHPRA), due to his warnings of the serious public health risk posed by COVID 19, and for writing vaccination exemptions.

Dr. Nixon has been using darkfield microscopy live blood analysis to evaluate the effects of the COVID 19 injectables and is involved with an international team of doctors and researchers working in this area. He became aware of the dangers of the injectables and has looked at many Pfizer vials and experimented with them to determine what makes the structures grow. For a period of time, he and I closely collaborated. In one particular interview, we go through extensive images, as well as video footage, pointing out what the Pfizer ingredients look like coming right from the refrigerator.[114]

Dr. Nixon also examined the blood of vaccinated people, and the unvaccinated who were in contact with vaccinated individuals. Live blood analysis from shedding in the unvaccinated clearly showed the same abnormal features as seen in the vaccinated.[115] This has been replicated by many other doctors and scientists.[116]

These next images from Dr. Nixon were taken from a Pfizer vial sample and left overnight at room temperature—metallic rectangular structures developed:

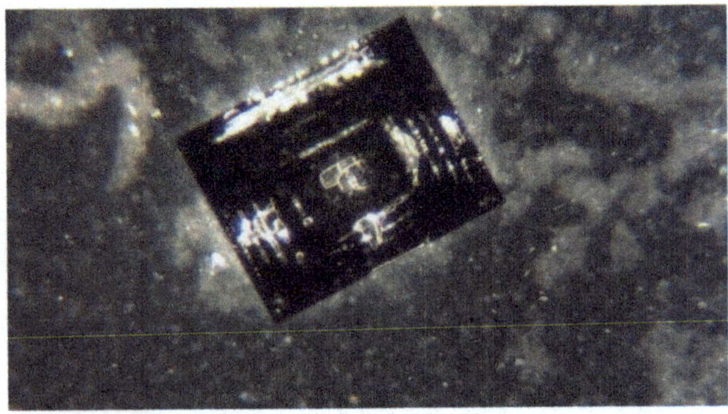

Figure 64. Self-assembled microchip developed from Pfizer COVID 19 injection. Dr. David Nixon.[117]

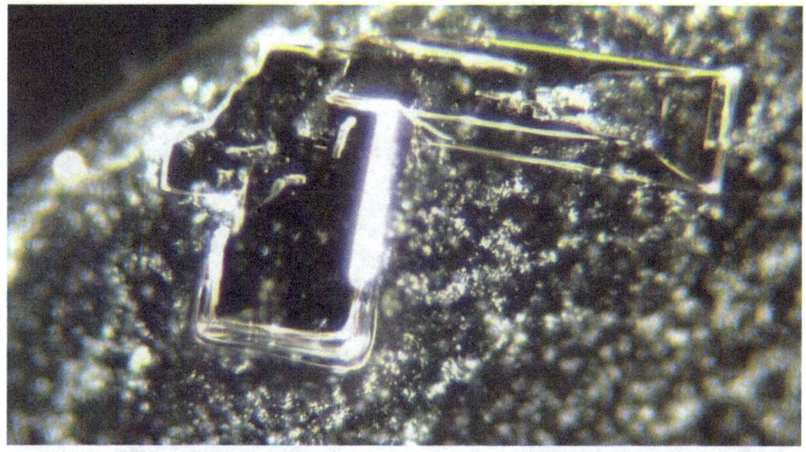

Figure 65. Self-assembled microchip developed from Pfizer COVID 19 injection. Dr. David Nixon.[118]

And under higher magnification:

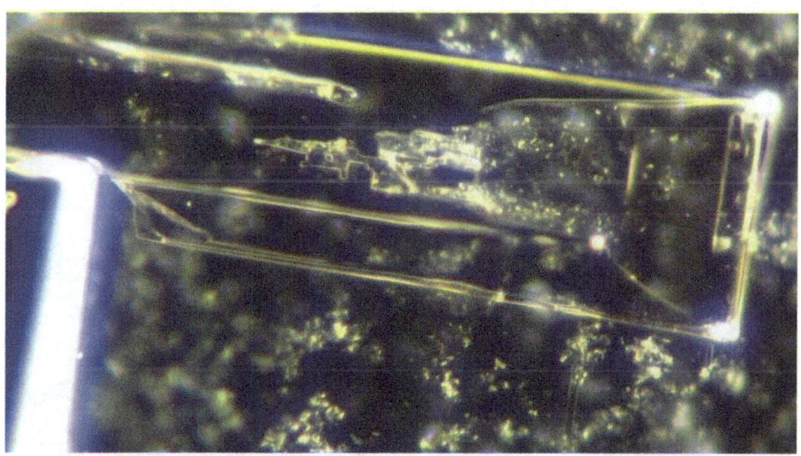

Figure 66. Self-assembled microchip developed from Pfizer COVID 19 injection. Dr. David Nixon.[119]

Below is a different complex structure that developed:

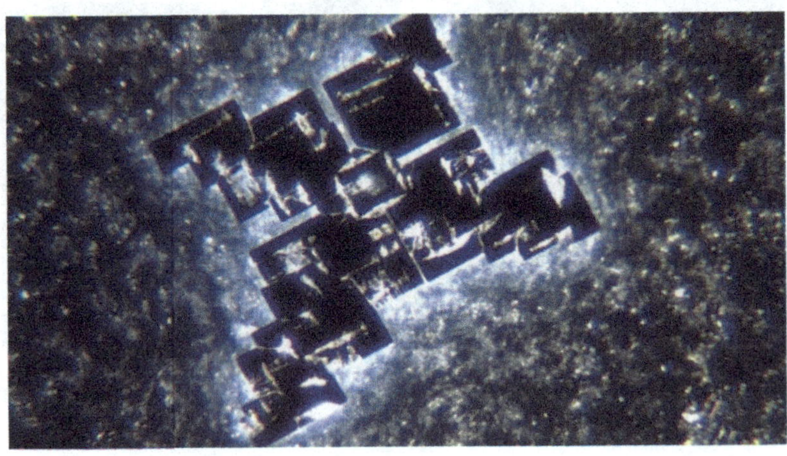

Figure 67. Self-assembled microchip developed from Pfizer COVID 19 injection. Dr. David Nixon.[120]

Higher magnification of a different structure:

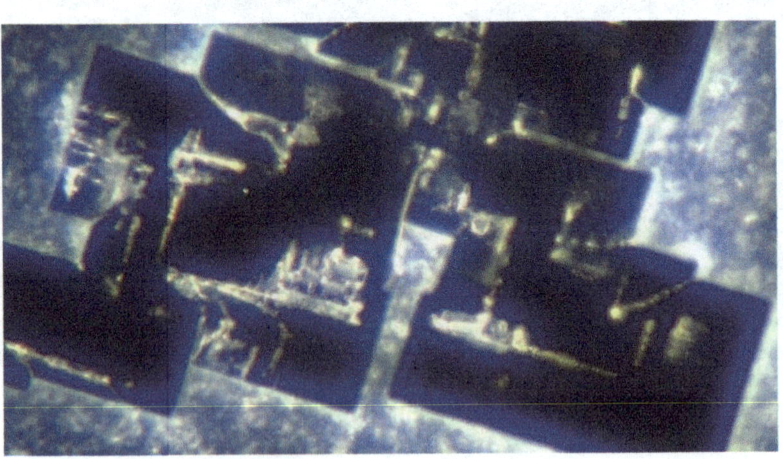

Figure 68. Self-assembled microchip developed from Pfizer COVID 19 injection. Dr. David Nixon.[121]

In Figure 69 we see a filament from a Pfizer COVID 19 sample left overnight. A Faraday cage was placed over it to shield from WiFi. Instead of crystalline structures, microtubes developed:

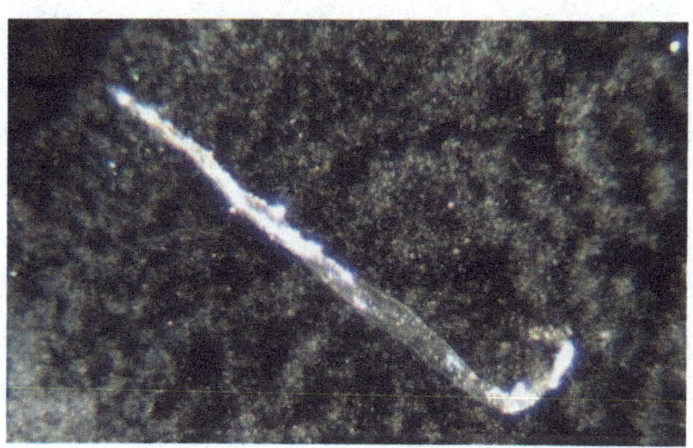

Figure 69. Self-assembled microchip developing into a filament from Pfizer COVID 19 injection. Dr. David Nixon.[122]

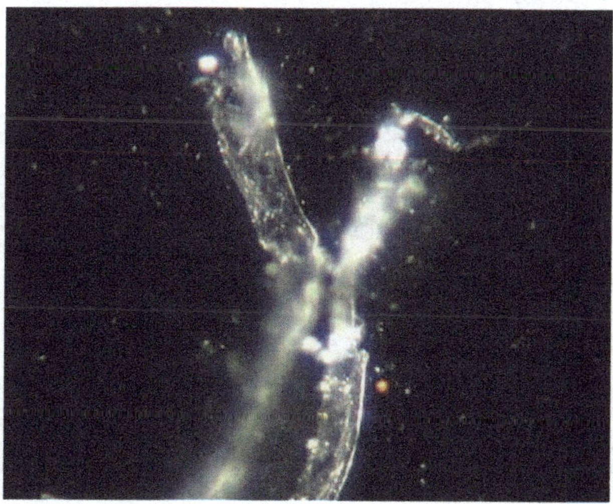

Figure 70. Self-assembled filament developed from Pfizer COVID 19 injection. Dr. David Nixon.[123]

Below is a similar carbon nanotube, possibly graphene, in a vaccinated person following two injections of Moderna. White blood cells are visible trying to degrade the structure:

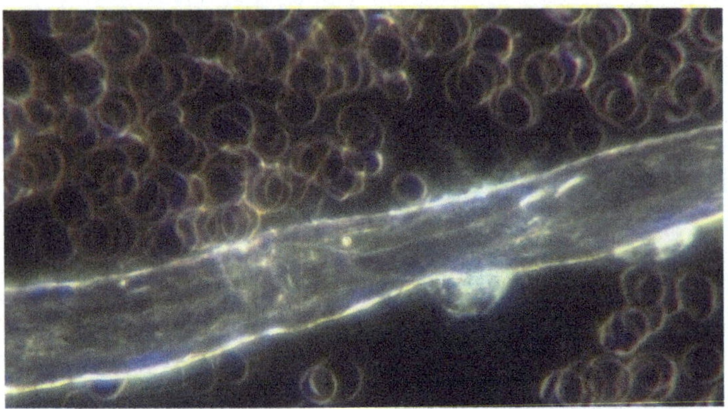

Figure 71. Self-assembled filament in COVID 19 injected blood. Magnification 400x. Dr. David Nixon.[124]

More complex carbon tubes in the blood of the same vaccinated person:

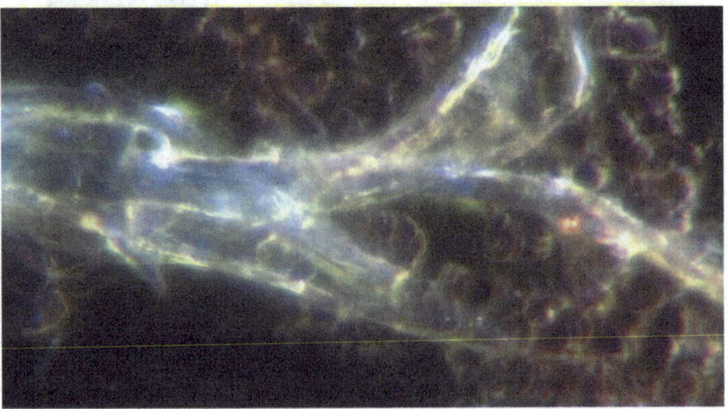

Figure 72. Self-assembled filament in COVID 19 injected blood. Magnification 2000x. Dr. David Nixon.[125]

Biomedical Clinics' Medical Director, Dr. Philippe van Welbergen, revealed that the graphene being injected into people is assembling and developing into larger fibers and structures, and acquiring magnetic properties or an electrical charge. The fibers also display indications of more complex structures with streaks.[126]

He also showed that "shards" of graphene are being transmitted from vaccinated to unvaccinated people, and it is destroying the red blood cells and causing blood clots in the unvaccinated.[127]

What are these structures? Why are these microscopic structures self-assembling from the vials? Why are vaccinated people emitting a MAC address? How do we dissolve these structures that are found in the blood of the vaccinated and the unvaccinated through shedding? We must address these observations with scientific rigor in order to find solutions.

The COVID 19 "Vaccine" Research of Dr. Shimon Yanowitz

SEPTEMBER 20, 2022[128]

Dr. Shimon Yanowitz is an independent scientist and researcher from Israel, with a background in electrical engineering and computer science. Dr. Yanowitz analyzed Pfizer BioNTech, Moderna, J&J, and Astra Zeneca vials and, after incubating them at body temperature, found extensive self-assembly nanostructures. In our interview, he showed the self-assembly of nanotechnology from previously frozen COVID 19 vials.[130] We closely collaborated for a period in 2022 and 2023. I consider his documentation of self-assembly nanotechnology of immense historic importance.

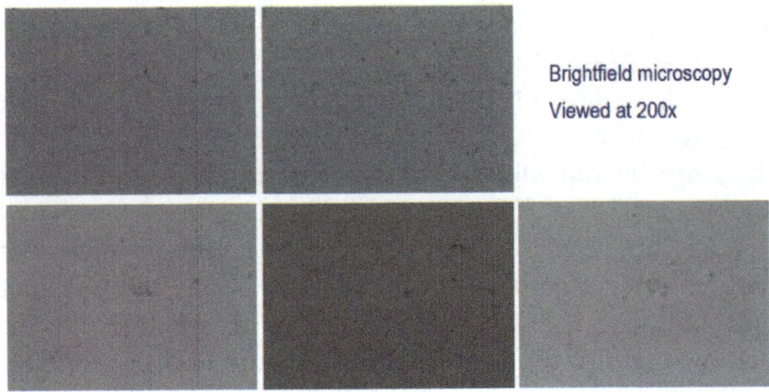

Figure 73. Analysis of Pfizer and Moderna COVID 19 "vaccines" after thawing. Dr. Shimon Yanowitz.[130]

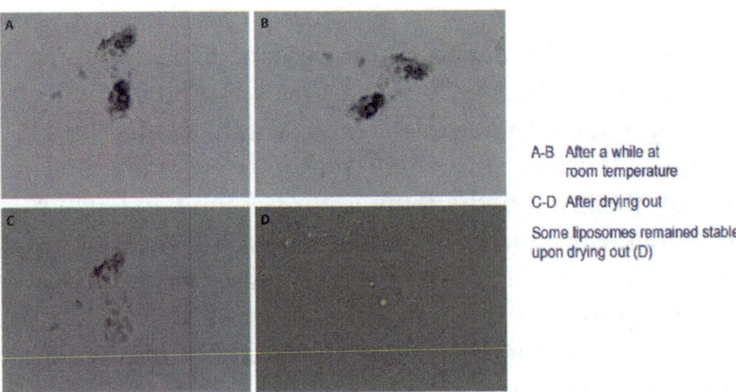

Figure 74. Liposomes from Moderna sample. Dr. Shimon Yanowitz.[131]

3. Moderna samples in Neubauer Improved Chamber, at room temperature

A-B Upon insertion to the chamber. Viewed in Brightfield.

C-F After 20-30 minutes in the chamber. Viewed in Phase Contrast. Filaments and structures started to form.

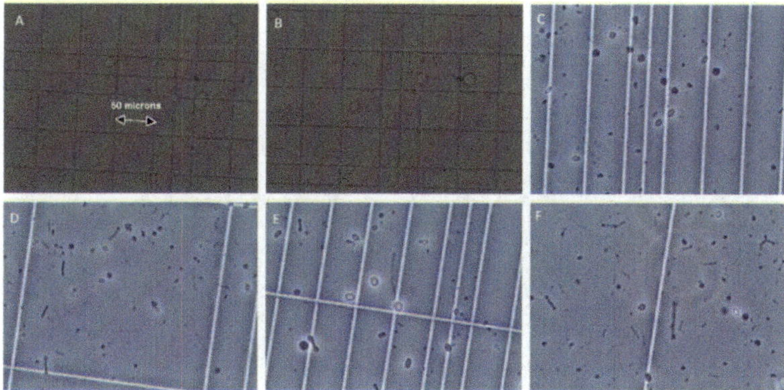

Figure 75. Moderna samples in Neubauer improved chamber. Dr. Shimon Yanowitz.[132]

4. Pfizer-Biontech samples in Neubauer Improved Chamber, at room temperature

A-C Upon insertion to the chamber. Viewed in Brightfield.

D-F After 20-30 minutes in the chamber. Viewed in Phase Contrast. Filaments and structures started to form.

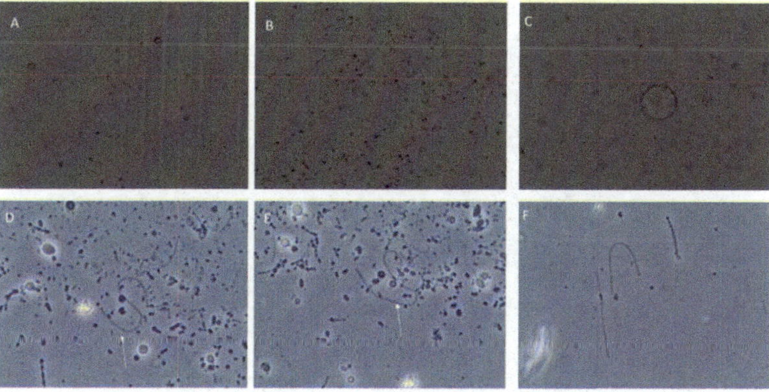

Figure 76. Pfizer vials show self-assembly nanotechnology. Dr. Shimon Yanowitz.[133]

Multicompartment liposomes in Pfizer (right) and Moderna (Left)

These liposomes are transparent

Their size in Pfizer is as much as 50 microns in diameter, twice the size of Moderna

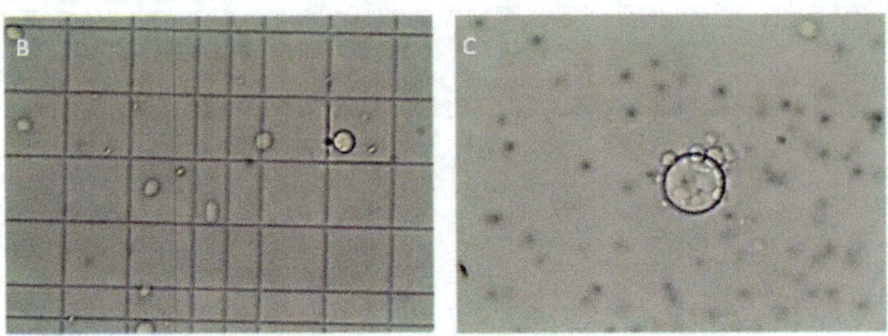

Figure 77. Self-assembly of liposomes. Dr. Shimon Yanowitz.[134]

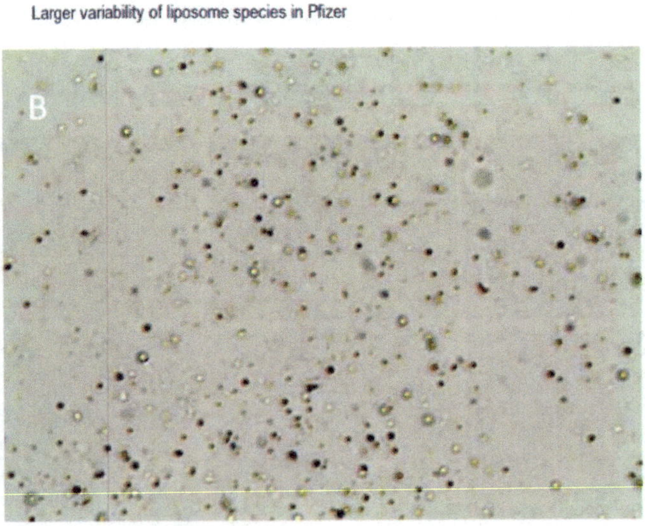

Larger variability of liposome species in Pfizer

Figure 78. Multiple liposome species. Pfizer COVID 19 injection. Dr. Shimon Yanowitz.[135]

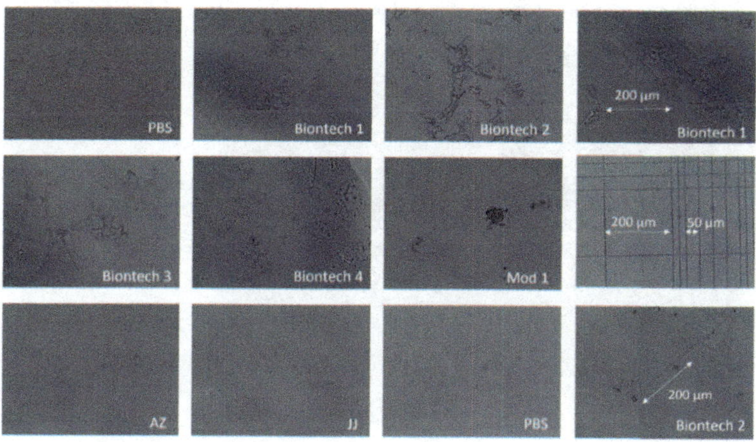

Figure 79. Self-assembly documented in incubated COVID 19 injectable samples. Dr. Shimon Yanowitz.[136]

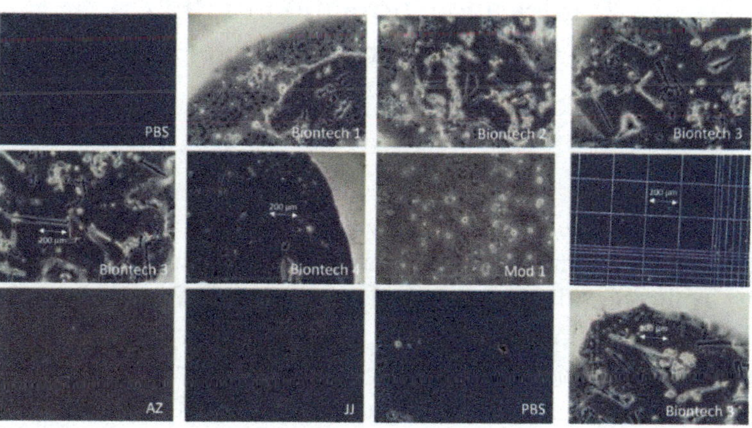

Figure 80. Self-assembly documented in incubated COVID 19 injectable samples. Dr. Shimon Yanowitz.[137]

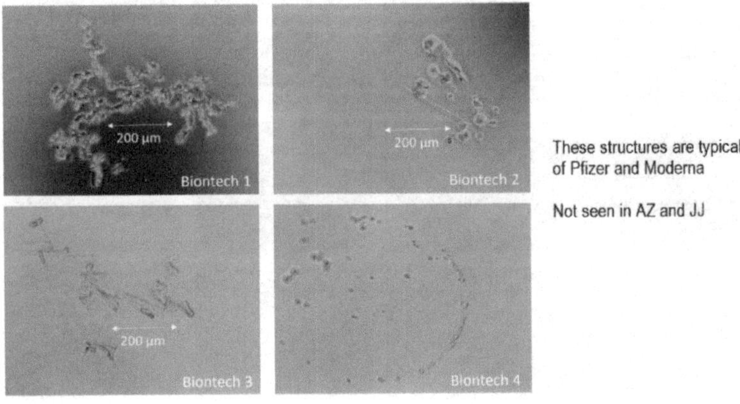

Figure 81. Self-assembly documented in incubated COVID 19 injectable samples. Dr. Shimon Yanowitz.[138]

Self-Assembling Microtechnology in Pfizer Vials – Ribbons, Microchips, Optical Communications Cables and Correlation to PEG, Graphene, and Hydrogel

DECEMBER 17, 2022[139]

In a later interview, Dr. David Nixon presented new images evaluating the nanorobots that are constructing the microchips now in the blood of everyone I have tested. We discussed the light transmission of certain microcircuitry and possible explanations regarding their optical communication, with input from Shimon Yanowitz and Matt Taylor. And we talked about the hydrogel construction base that appears to carry the software imprint on the self-assembly process. New images of live blood analyses from vaccinated people were presented by Dr. Nixon, and from unvaccinated who have visited my clinic, and all showed similar self-assembly and artificial technology structures. Dr. Yanowitz demonstrated self-assembling ribbons from COVID 19 vials and how they are the same as what we see in the live blood from shedding and environmental exposure to these toxins.[140]

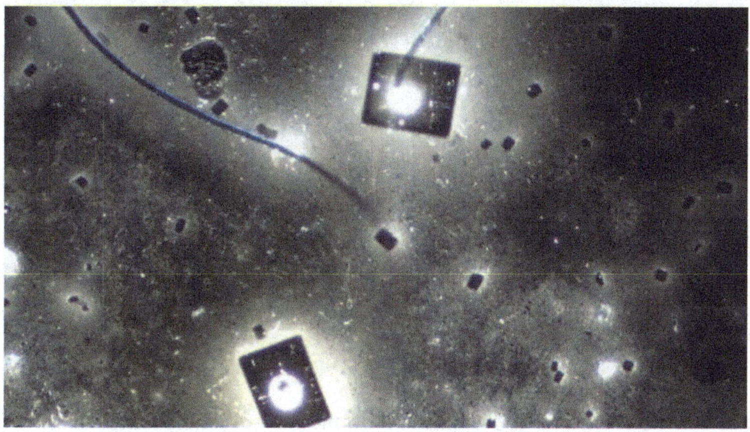

Figure 82. Self-assembled microchips from Pfizer vials with communication cables. Dr. David Nixon.[141]

Dr. Nixon, engineer Matt Taylor, and Dr. Shimon Yanowitz discussed the development of optical communication highways between crystalline microchips. My greatest concern in these findings is the rate of speed in the development of the ribbons, which I am convinced is the same as we are identifying through live blood analysis. Dr. Nixon showed that the ribbons develop within 2 days from invisible to a very large size.[142] If this same phenomenon is happening in people's bodies, that becomes a very grave concern in regard to the risk of developing blood clots.

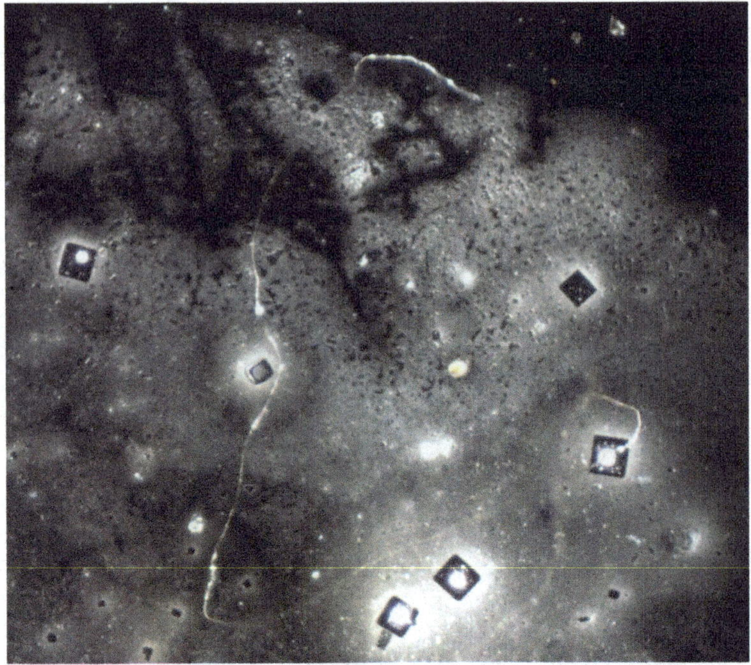

Figure 83. Self-assembling filaments connecting to microchips from Pfizer "vaccine" vial. Dr. David Nixon.[143]

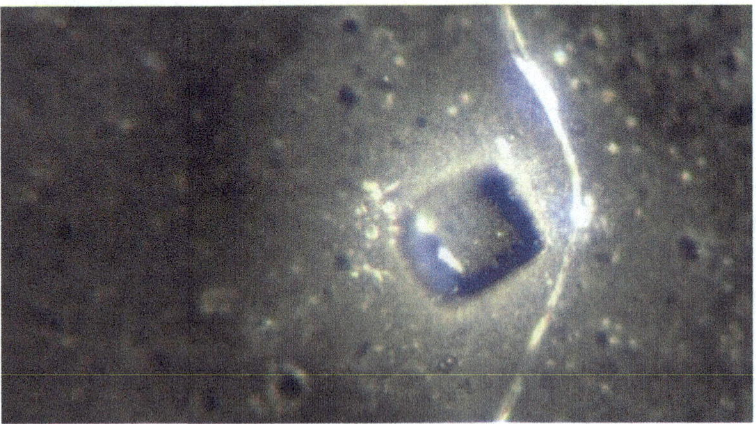

Figure 84. Self-assembled filament connecting to microchips from Pfizer "vaccine" vial. Dr. David Nixon.[144]

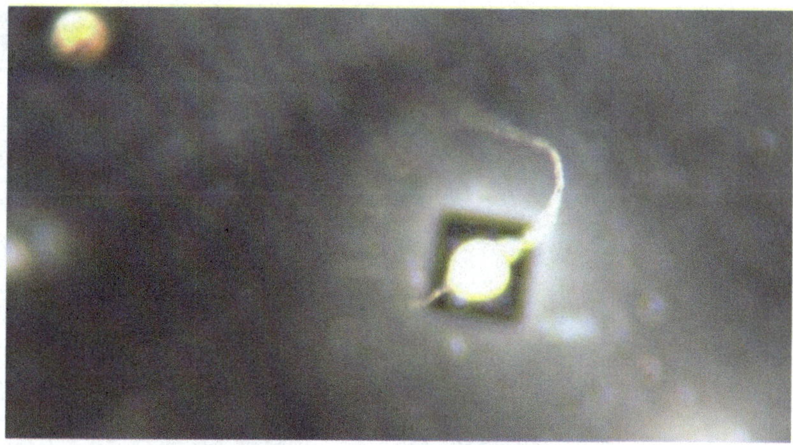

Figure 85. Self-assembled filament connecting to microchips from Pfizer "vaccine" vial. Dr. David Nixon.[145]

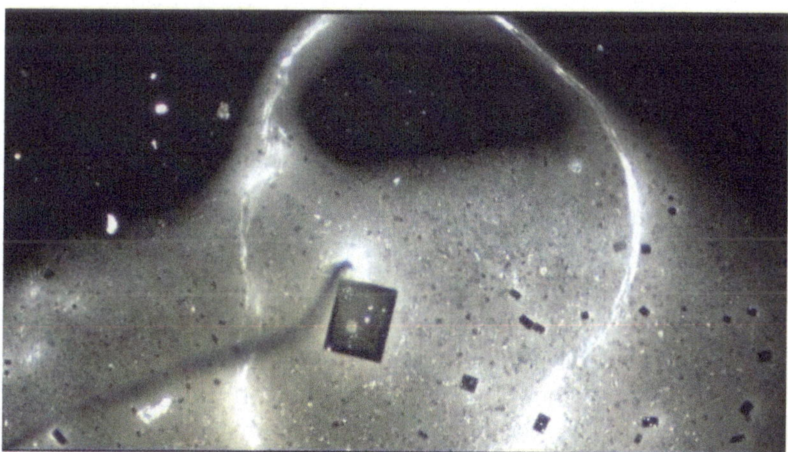

Figure 86. Self-assembled filament connecting to microchips from Pfizer "vaccine" vial. Dr. David Nixon.[146]

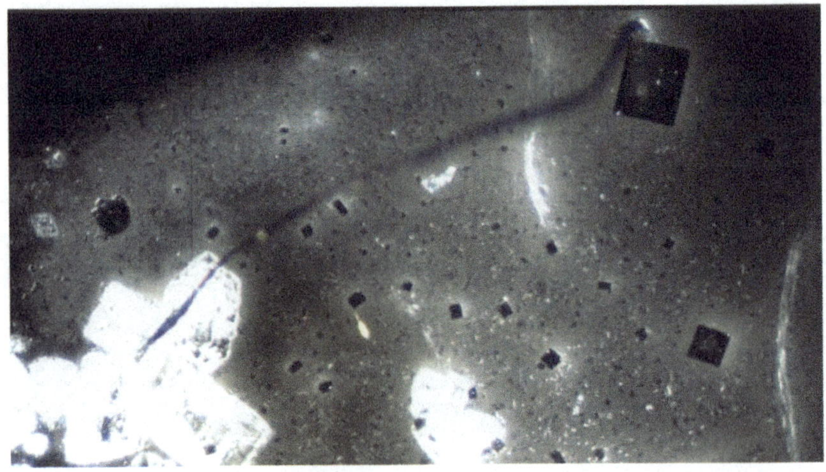

Figure 87. Self-assembled filament connecting to microchips from Pfizer "vaccine" vial. Dr. David Nixon.[147]

COVID 19 Injection Analysis Shows Dozens of Toxic Phthalates Associated with Endocrine Disruption and Heart Disease

JANUARY 20, 2024[148]

A while back, international attorney Todd Callendar showed me the chemical analysis of a COVID 19 injection that was taken from the vial of a vaccine injured person. It is challenging to get such analysis done and rather expensive. Those involved do not want to be public, so only limited information can be shared. When I first saw the results, I knew that this was confirmation that we have been right all along, and that there is a direct correlation between the chemistry of the contents of the COVID 19 injections and the geoengineered, environmental filaments that people know as Morgellons.

I want to acknowledge Clifford Carnicom and Elana Freeland. When I first met them, their work convinced me that the COVID 19 bioweapons are a continuation of the surveillance technology some call Morgellons but should rather be called "advanced self-assembly nanomaterials," which are plasmonic nanoantennas that transmit the resonant frequency of human DNA. German Researchers, Harald Kautz-Vella and Kristin Hauksdottir, wrote an excellent research article about this topic stating there may be multiple different technologies involved.[149] I believe what I have been seeing under the microscope is self-assembling nanotechnology, polymer plastics, and quantum dots—and that is what Clifford calls "Cross Domain Bacteria."

"The first possible mechanism when fibers are observed could be a reaction of Ca (NO3)2 and fluoride-tensides to Ca2F-nanocrystals, which, similar to piezoelectric crystals, develop magnetic properties when exposed to external fields. In a dry environment, these nanocrystals would theoretically form unstable, spiderweb-like structures. When triggered to become magnetic in a humid environment, they theoretically would be able to form droplets on command, by fusing smaller droplets by magnetic attraction to rain-size droplets.

"The second form of fibers observed, are the aluminum coated nylon fibers, as indicated by the manuscript from the U.S. Air Force Academy, Department of Chemistry. [Nylon belongs to the chemical family of polyamides, which Clifford Carnicom and I have found as chemical signatures via near infrared spectroscopy in human blood samples.] The fibers have been reported to hide planes from radar detection, as well as being used to deflect sunlight in the context of combating global warming. The Air Force calls them spoofer sprays.

"More complex medical applications consist of self-assembling nano-machines, like for example optical fibers, that by capillarity take in an up-concentrate of nano-dyes and other nanoparticles with special characteristics, like gold-nanoparticles. These fibers are able to collect light patterns coming in from the DNA, turning them into electromagnetic signals that are sent by the fiber-based so called plasmonic antennas out as a readable electromagnetic signal."[150]

I include below an analysis, conducted at Harvard, showing phthalates in environmental filaments, together with graphene carbon nanotubes, dyes, metals, and other chemicals:

Samples #2 & #3 Analysis Results

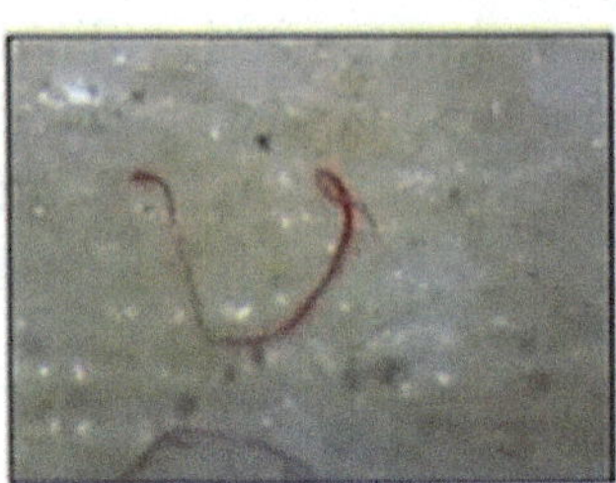

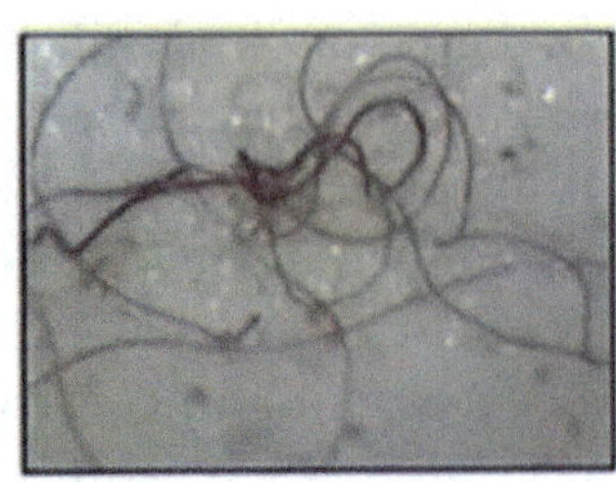

- Polycrystalline Sr, Mg-doped $LaGaO_3$(LSGM) nanowire
- P19 Protein
- Methotrexate

Black:

- TiO2/Polymer/Au/Al blend nanowire
- Terephthalic acid
- Dimethyl Terephthalate

Purple:

- Carbon Nanotube
- Radioactive sodium Iodide
- N-acetylglucosamine

Figure 88. Morgellons filament analysis. C. Hill.[151]

Sample Analysis Conditions: S-TEM EELS

S-TEM – Tecnai TF30

- *Beam energy: 200 keV*
- *FEG extraction: 4000 V*
- *Gun lens: 6*
- *C1 aperture: 30 µm*
- *C2 aperture: 100 µm*
- *Convergence: 9 mrad*
- *Spot size: 6*
- *Probe current: 0.5 nA*
- *Camera length: 80 mm*
- *Probe FWHM: 0.9 nm*

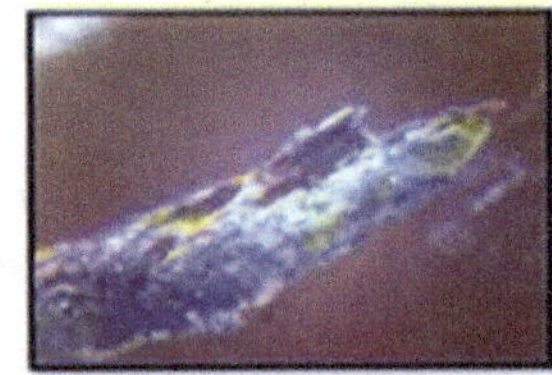

Sample #1 Analysis Results

- High resolution TEM revealed crystalline lattice spacings of metallic Palladium and Aluminum microtubule particle arrays bound to Amino Acids.
- Pd is bound to the N and S atoms in the side chains of Cysteine (Red), Methionine (Blue), and Hystidine (Green/Yellow). Hystidine is a metal binding residue in peptides due to the disprotenated N3 atom in the imadazole ring.

Sample also contains the following:

- Ni and Co magnetic nanowires with an outer diameter of 50-60 nm.
- Stacked Pyridine Ligand molecular wires containing Zn with Porphyrin cores.
- Ladder oligomers of Quinoxaline and Benzoanthracene.

Figure 89. s-TEM EELS analysis of Morgellons filaments. C. Hill.[152]

During a lecture by Dr. Ian Akyldiz, professor at Georgia Institute of Technology and senior engineer with the IEEE, he said about the supposed mRNA injections: "COVID MRNAS ARE NOTHING MORE THAN SMALL SCALE BIO-NANO MACHINES."[153] This development was thought to have also been connected to Arizona State through the DARPA MOLDICE program from 2001. All articles pertaining to this research are now no longer available on the internet.

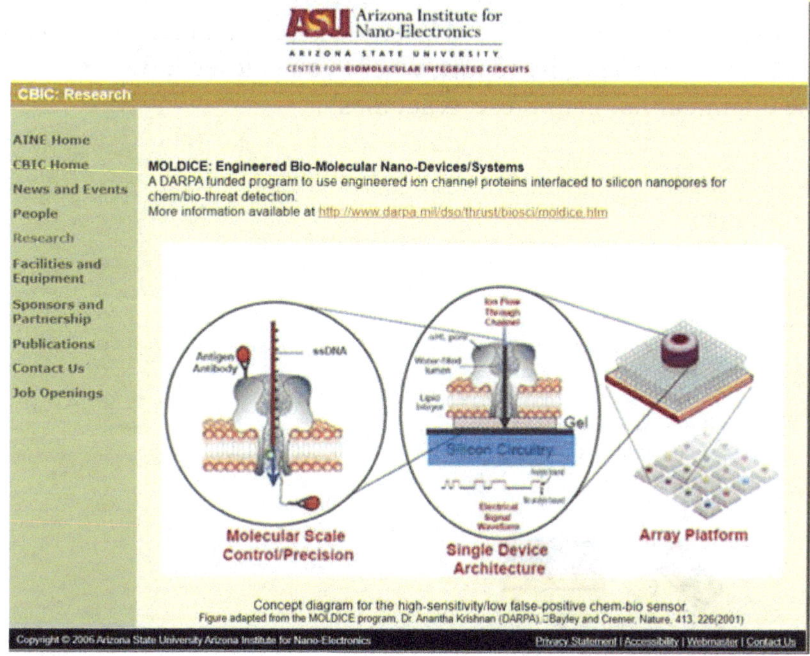

Figure 90. Engineered nanodevices used in chemical/biological threat detection. ASU, Arizona Institute for Nano-Electronics.[154]

I have repeatedly said that liquid gas chromatography needs to be done on all "vaccine" vials to look for these toxic chemicals. The plastics in the COVID 19 injections are extensive and most importantly, they are toxic endocrine disruptors, cancer causing, teratogenic, and more. A horrifying total of 146 chemicals have been found.

Similar phthalate derivatives were also found in another environmental filament analysis from 2012, and I have compared this to FOIA requests concerning the Pfizer COVID 19 "vaccine."[155] The same chemicals we discovered in the blood (polyamides and metals), were found in microchips implanted in targeted individuals back in 2011.[156]

Dr. Hildegarde Staninger wrote a 99-page report titled: *GLOBAL BRAIN CHIP AND MESOGENS – Nano Machines for Ultimate Control of False Memories.* Below are a few pages taken from this lengthy report, where you can see how extensive the chemical list is in these "vaccines":

Contents

Figure 91. Excerpt of chemical report of Pfizer COVID 19 "vaccine" analysis show many phthalates. Todd Callender.[157]

The findings of PLASTIC polymers correlate with the Moderna patent that discusses "stealth nanoparticles" made from these plastic materials. I have wanted the world to know that what we have been warning of is correct, and that once the bioweapons are seized and forensic analysis is done at a large scale, testing for these polymers must also be conducted.

(12) **United States Patent** (10) **Patent No.: US 11,622,972 B2**

Packer et al. (45) **Date of Patent: *Apr. 11, 2023**

(54) LIPID NANOPARTICLE COMPOSITIONS AND METHODS OF FORMULATING THE SAME

(71) Applicant: **ModernaTX, Inc.**, Cambridge, MA (US)

8,450,298	B2	5/2013	Mahon et al.
8,460,696	B2	6/2013	Slobodkin et al.
8,460,709	B2	6/2013	Ausborn et al.
8,568,784	B2	10/2013	Lillard et al.
8,569,256	B2	10/2013	Heyes
8,580,297	B2	11/2013	Essler et al.
8,642,076	B2	2/2014	Manoharan et al.

In some embodiments, the lipid nanoparticles described herein are stealth nanoparticles or target-specific stealth nanoparticles such as, but not limited to, those described in U.S. Pub. No. US20130172406, herein incorporated by reference in its entirety. The stealth or target-specific stealth nanoparticles can comprise a polymeric matrix, which can comprise two or more polymers such as, but not limited to, polyethylenes, polycarbonates, polyanhydrides, polyhydroxyacids, polypropylfumerates, polycaprolactones, polyamides, polyacetals, polyethers, polyesters, poly(orthoesters), polycyanoacrylates, polyvinyl alcohols, polyurethanes, polyphosphazenes, polyacrylates, polymethacrylates, polycyanoacrylates, polyureas, polystyrenes, polyamines, polyesters, polyanhydrides, polyethers, polyurethanes, polymethacrylates, polyacrylates, polycyanoacrylates, or combinations thereof.

Figure 92. Moderna lipid nanoparticle composition. United States Patent No.: US 11,622,972 B2.[158]

For a broader understanding, below are some toxicology explanations for the phthalates found in the C19 injections. Note they are used to create polymer fibers and have significant toxicity:

Benzyl butyl phthalate

Description - Benzyl butyl phthalate belongs to the class of organic compounds known as benzoic acid esters. These are ester derivatives of benzoic acid. Based on a literature review, a significant number of articles have been published on Benzyl butyl phthalate. This compound has been identified in human blood as reported by (PMID: 31557052). Benzyl butyl phthalate is not a naturally occurring metabolite and is only found in those individuals exposed to this compound or its derivatives. Technically Benzyl butyl phthalate is part of the human exposome. The exposome can be defined as the collection of all the exposures of an individual in a lifetime and how those exposures relate to health. An individual's exposure begins before birth and includes insults from environmental and occupational sources.

Bis(2-ethylhexyl) phthalate

Description - Di(2-ethylhexyl)phthalate, also known as DEHP or di-iso-octyl phthalate, belongs to the class of organic compounds known as benzoic acid esters. These are ester derivatives of benzoic acid. Di(2-ethylhexyl)phthalate is a primary metabolite. Primary metabolites are metabolically or physiologically essential metabolites. They are directly involved in an organism's growth, development, or reproduction. Di(2-ethylhexyl) phthalate is formally rated as a possible carcinogen (by IARC 2B) and is also a potentially toxic compound.

Dibutyl phthalate

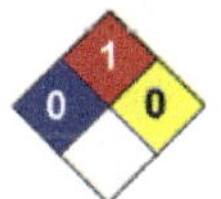

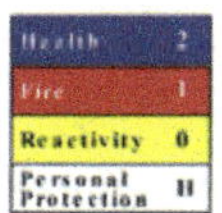

Dibutyl phthalate

Description - Dibutyl phthalate is found in cloves. DBP was added to the California Proposition 65 (1986) list of suspected teratogens in November 2006. It is a suspected endocrine disruptor. It was used in some nail polishes; all major producers began eliminating this chemical from nail polishes in the Fall of 2006. Dibutyl phthalate (DBP) is a commonly used plasticizer. It is also used as an additive to adhesives or printing inks. It is soluble in various organic solvents, e.g. in alcohol, ether, and benzene. DBP is also used as an ectoparasitic ide. Belongs to the class of organic compounds known as benzoic acid esters. These are ester derivatives of benzoic acid.

Di isobutyl phthalate

Diisobutyl phthalate (DIBP) is prepared by esterification process of isobutanol and phthalic anhydride. Its structural formula is C6H4(COOCH2CH(CH3)2)2. DIBP is an odorless plasticizer and has excellent heat and light stability. It is the lowest cost plasticizer for cellulose nitrate. DIBP has lower density and freezing point than the related compound dibutyl phthalate (DBP). Otherwise, it has similar properties DBP and can often be used as a substitute for it. Its refractive index is 1.488–1.492 (at 20 °C, D).

Biological Role(s):

1. teratogenic agent

2. A role played by a chemical compound in biological systems with adverse consequences in embryo developments, leading to birth defects, embryo death or altered development, growth retardation and functional defect.

3. PPAR modulator

Isophthalic acid

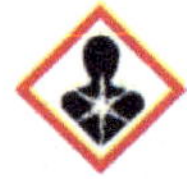

Isophthalic acid (PIA) is a non-toxic organic compound with the formula C6H4(CO2H)2. This colorless solid is an isomer of phthalic acid and terephthalic acid. These aromatic dicarboxylic acids are used as precursors (in the form of acylchlorides) to commercially important polymers. The high-performance polymer polybenzimidazole is produced from isophthalic acid.

Applications

Isophthalic acid (PIA) has three major uses:

1. PET (Polyethylene Terephthalate) copolymer, which is used in bottle resins and to a much lesser extent, for fibers. PIA (Purified Isophthalic Acid) reduces the crystallinity of PET, which serves to improve clarity and increase the productivity of bottle-making.
2. Unsaturated polyester resins, where the addition of PIA improves thermal resistance and mechanical performance, as well as resistance to chemicals and water.
3. Polyester/alkyd surface coating resins, where PIA increases resistance to water, overall durability and weatherability

Figure 93. Toxicology explanation from Pfizer COVID 19 injection analysis.[159]

One can see that not only are these chemicals endocrine disruptors, cancer causing, and teratogenic, but they are also used as precursors for polymers.

According to a study in the journal *Environmental Pollution*, phthalates are known causes of death from heart disease: "Daily exposure to phthalates, a group of chemicals used in everything from plastic containers to makeup, may lead to approximately 100,000 deaths in older Americans annually. The chemicals, which can be found in hundreds of products such as toys, clothing, and shampoo, have been known for decades to be 'hormone disruptors,' affecting a person's endocrine system. The toxins can enter the body through such items and are linked to obesity, diabetes, and heart disease… The research, which was carried out by New York University's Grossman School of Medicine and includes some 5,000 adults aged 55 to 64, shows that those with higher concentrations of phthalates in their urine were more likely to die of heart disease. However, higher concentrations did not appear to increase the risk of death by cancer. 'Our findings reveal that increased phthalate exposure is linked to early death, particularly due to heart disease.'"[160]

The epigenetic modification that occurs also causes harm to the next generation: "Phthalates are esters of phthalic acid which are used in cosmetics and other daily personal care products. They are also used in polyvinyl chloride (PVC) plastics to increase durability and plasticity. Phthalates are not present in plastics by covalent bonds and thus can easily leach into the environment and enter the human body by dermal absorption, ingestion, or inhalation. Several *in vitro* and *in vivo* studies suggest that phthalates can act as endocrine disruptors and cause moderate reproductive and developmental toxicities. Furthermore, phthalates can pass through the placental barrier and affect the developing fetus. Thus, phthalates have ubiquitous presence in food and environment with potential adverse health effects in humans. This review focusses on studies conducted in the field of toxicogenomics of phthalates and discusses possible transgenerational and multigenerational effects caused by phthalate exposure during any point of the life cycle."[161]

These next two quotes are from articles explaining that the leaching potential of phthalates of different plastics vary; however, polyamides, polypropylene, polyethylene terephthalate, and polyvinyl alcohol all leak phthalates that can then negatively affect the human body.

"The leaching potentials were plastic type-specific, where the pencil case (polyvinyl chloride, PVC) represented the highest migrations with total $\sum_{15}$ PAEs concentration of 6660 ± 513 ng/g, followed by the cleaning brush-1 (polyamide, PA, ~1830 ng/g) and rubber glove (1390 ± 57.5 ng/g). Conversely, the straw (polypropylene, PP), cleaning brush-2 (polyethylene terephthalate, PET) and shampoo bottle (PET) released the lowest amounts of PAEs, with 50.3 ± 8.21, 93.9 ± 91.8 and 104.35 ng/g, respectively. The release patterns of PAE congeners were polymer type-related, where di-*n*-butyl phthalate (DBP) dominated the leaching from PA, PP and PET microplastics (47–84%), diethyl phthalate leached the most from PVC and rubber microplastics (45–92%), while diisobutyl phthalate and DBP dominated the leaching from PE microplastics."[162]

"Phthalates are not chemically bound to the polymer so they can easily release into the environment, and finally enter the human body from various potential sources. Phthalates can be rapidly metabolized to their respective primary monoesters and further to oxidized metabolites in the human body."[163,164,165]

Further liquid gas chromatography and in-depth chemical analysis must be done on the COVID 19 bioweapons. We are in possession of extensive reports that show many toxic plastic chemicals in the COVID 19 bioweapons. I call upon brave scientists, toxicologists, and laboratories who are willing to save humanity and repeat this analysis for further confirmation and evidence for legal action.

Residual DNA Fragments Analysis Detected in Monovalent and Bivalent Pfizer/BioNTech and Moderna modRNA COVID 19 Shots Confirms Spider Silk Genes Encoded in the Spike Open Reading Frame

APRIL 03, 2024[166]

Dr. David Speicher has a PhD in the fields of clinical microbiology and virology. He has more than 20 years expertise in diagnostics of infectious diseases, has authored over 30 peer-reviewed publications, and has secured more than $1M in scientific funding.

Dr. Speicher investigated the DNA fragments in the COVID 19 injections and found spidroin gene sequences. These encode for dragline silk, the strongest form of spider silk. I have also investigated spider silk environmental filaments from California which were found after geoengineered chemtrails sprayed the area.[167]

As mentioned, Clifford Carnicom and I found the chemical signatures of polyamide proteins in the blood of both COVID 19 vaccinated and unvaccinated individuals. In analysis of the rubbery clots given to me by embalmer Richard Hirschman—clots from a deceased individual, a living COVID 19 vaccine injured individual, and an unvaccinated individual—similar polyamide materials were observed. All had polyamide signatures. Polyamides can be silk, wool or nylon. Dr. Speicher found that spidroins were encoded in the open reading frame of the spike gene. This explains why Clifford and I were unable to dissolve the clots with the most caustic agents—because one of the components could have been spider silk.

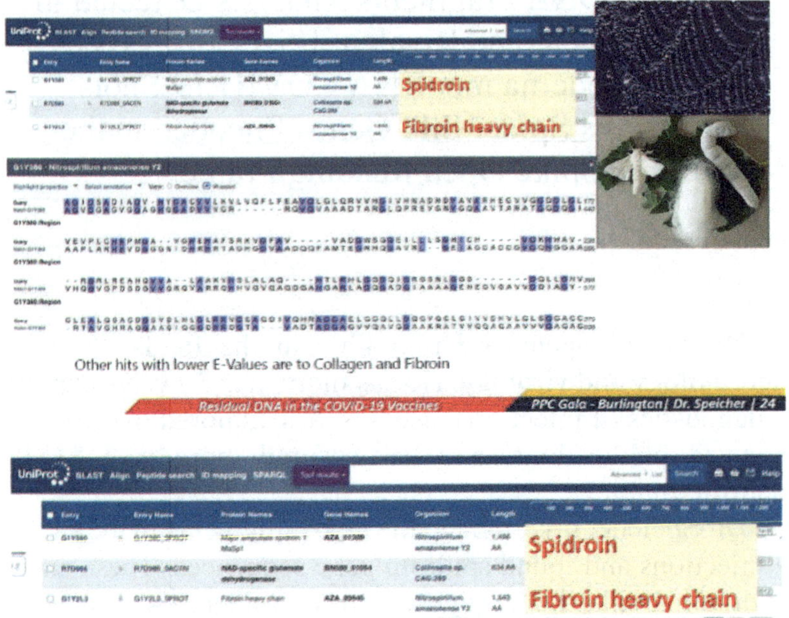

Figure 94. Analysis of DNA in COVID 19 injections shows spidroin sequences. Dr. David Speicher.[168]

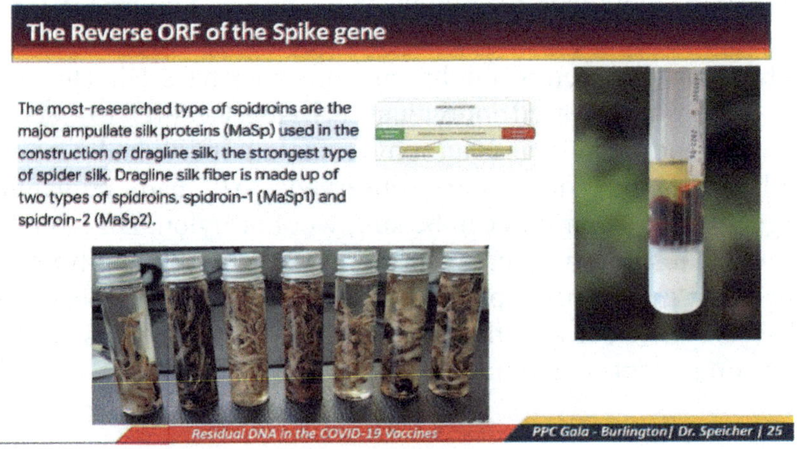

Figure 95. Analysis of DNA in COVID injections shows spidroin sequences. Dr. David Speicher.[169]

Dr. Speicher's work is huge confirmation of my research on the polyamide polymer presence in the residual DNA fragments he identified as dragon spider silk genes. This is devastating for humanity, as this material is stronger than steel. "Despite its mythical name, dragon silk is actually the work of genetic engineers. It's widely known, at least in the materials industry, that spider silk has exceptional strength, resilience and flexibility... Spider silk is five to 10 times stronger than conventional silkworm silk... It's also, in some cases, as much as twice as elastic. It's even tougher than Kevlar."[170]

Discussion of Argentinian COVID 19 Bioweapon Analysis Finding Building Blocks of Self-Assembling Nanotechnology

JUNE 06, 2024[171]

Dr. Marcela Sangorrin and Lorena Diblasis' research group from the National Scientific and Technical Research Council – National University of Comahue, Neuquén, Argentina, analyzed multiple brands of COVID 19 vials. The results are a big step forward for the world to understand what is in these so-called "vaccines." The team performed fluorescent microscopy, energy dispersive X-ray analysis with scanning electron microscopy, and inductive coupling mass spectroscopy. My interview with Lorena explains the findings in depth. I provide here a few key points from that interview in relation to this self-assembling nanotechnology.[172]

The Argentinian team compared the fluorescent microscopy of a graphene sample with the COVID 19 injections and found matches in the lambda bands of excitation filters, as well as the presence of similar nanoparticles.

This group's research found lanthanides in all COVID injections. There are multiple chemical components that have fluorescent attributes; however, lanthanides are rare earth metals with strong magnetic effects, which is significant because of their application in nanotechnology and use in the manufacturing of quantum dots, due to their unique fluorescence. Whistleblower Melissa McAtee, a former employee of Pfizer, reported that in the manufacturing process, she would see a fluorescent glow emanating from the COVID 19 vials.[173] In Chapter 3, I discussed the fluorescence of nano- and microrobots, filaments, and an orange glow that the COVID 19 injected, and now the uninjected due to shedding, are exhibiting.[174]

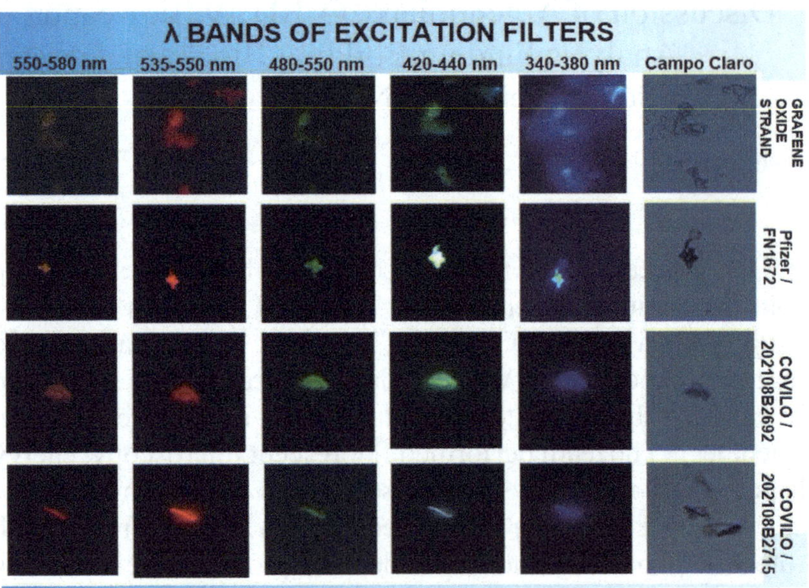

Figure 96. Fluorescent microscopy of COVID 19 injections compared to graphene. Dr. Marcela Sangorrin, *et al.*[175]

The lanthanide chemical group consists of lanthanum, cerium, praseodymium, neodymium, promethium, samarium, europium, gadolinium, terbium, dysprosium, holmium, erbium, thulium, and ytterbium.[176]

Below is the list of chemicals that the researchers in Argentina found in different COVID 19 "vaccine" bioweapons:

ANALYSIS BY ICP-MS, DATED 15-11-2023, THE SAMPLES WERE DIGESTED FOR 72 HOURS WITH 10% DOUBLE DISTILLED NITRIC ACID SOLUTION.

Simbolo	Isótopo	Nombre	AZTRAZ Nn0195	COVILO 202108 b2715	SPUTNIK 11 840621	MODERNA 045C22A	COMIRNATY SELY8	LIMITE DE DETECCION	LIMITE DE CUANTIFI
			C (µg/L)	C (µg/L)	C (µg/L)	C (µg/L)	C (µg/L)	LDM (µg/L)	LCM (µg/L)
Cd	111	Cadmio			10.43			0,9779	3,2272
Sn	118	Estaño		1.1910	88.12	17.37	0.2853	0,0172	0,0567
Te	125	Telurio		0.4000				0,3229	1,0655
Ba	137	Bario		20.5760	17.5860		68.5460	7,2082	23,7872
La	139	Lantano				0.3782	0.5615	0,2554	0,8428
Ce	140	Cerio	0.2166	1.2041	62.2631	0.1667	5.0681	0,1565	0,5165
Eu	153	Europio		0.0189			0.0215	0,0136	0,0448
Gd	157	Gadolinio			0.2658			0,0402	0,1326
Tb	159	Terbio	0.0037	0.0060	0.0060	0.0109	0.0002	0,0001	0,0005
Dy	163	Disprosio		0.0259		0.0190		0,0116	0,0382
Ho	165	Holmio		0.0056	0.0054	0.0045		0,0045	0,0147
Er	166	Erbio		0.0389			0.0617	0,0088	0,0291
Yb	172	Iterbio		0.0151	0.0057	0.0082		0,0024	0,0078
Pt	195	Platino		0.2850			0.4175	0,2628	0,8673
Pb	208	Plomo			23.7000		45.3000	6,3640	21,0011
U	238	Uranio	0.0218	0.1115		0.0233	0.2492	0,0006	0,0020

LANTHANIDES – QUANTUM DOTS?

Figure 97. ICP-MS of COVID 19 injections shows multiple undisclosed metals and lanthanides. Dr. Marcela Sangorrin, *et al.*[177]

ASTRAZENECA. Lote: NN0195			
Símbolo	Elemento	Isótopo/A	CC (ug/g)
B	Boro	11	0,1353
Na	Sodio	23	0,4095
Mg	Magnesio	24	0,238865
Al	Aluminio	27	0,069731
Si	Silicio	29	0,4045
P	Fósforo	31	0,259
K	Potasio	39	0,98
Ca	Calcio	43	9,978
Sc	Escandio	45	0,00235
Ti	Titanio	47	0,02495
V	Vanadio	51	0,002325
Cr	Cromo	53	0,03575
Mn	Manganeso	55	0,03235
Fe	Hierro	57	0,835
Co	Cobalto	59	0,00599
Ni	Níquel	60	0,09522
Cu	Cobre	63	0,086165
Zn	Zinc	66	0,9989
Ga	Galio	71	0,00006
Ge	Germanio	72	0,0018
Br	Bromo	79	0,3615
Rb	Rubidio	85	0,013765
Sr	Estroncio	88	0,034845
Y	Itrio	89	0,00098
Zr	Circonio	90	0,149325
Nb	Niobio	93	0,005535
Mo	Molibdeno	95	0,002655
Rh	Rodio	103	0,00035
Pd	Paladio	105	0,008525

ASTRAZENECA. Lote: NN0195			
Símbolo	Elemento	Isótopo/A	CC (ug/g)
Ag	Plata	107	0,00078
Cd	Cadmio	111	0,0003
Ba	Bario	137	0,03328
La	Lantano	139	0,002521
Ce	Cerio	140	0,002815
Pr	Praseodimio	141	0,000088
Nd	Neodimio	146	0,00056
Hf	Hafnio	178	0,17928
Ta	Tántalo	181	0,000895
W	Wolframio	182	0,00534
Re	Renio	185	0,00075
Ir	Iridio	193	0,014675
Pt	Platino	195	0,00444
Au	Oro	197	0,01175
Hg	Mercurio	201	0,3785
Tl	Talio	205	0,00646
Pb	Plomo	208	0,02384
Bi	Bismuto	209	0,03987
Th	Torio	232	0,00161
U	Uranio	238	0,000257

54 UNDECLARED CHEMICAL ELEMENTS

Símbolo	Elemento	Isótopo/A
F	Flúor	18,99
Tc	Tecnecio	98,9
Po	Polonio	209

Figure 98. ICP-MS of COVID 19 injections shows a total of 54 undisclosed chemical elements. Dr. Marcela Sangorrin, *et al.*[178]

Please note that uranium, a highly radioactive element that causes cancer, was also found. This is of special interest to me, as I have been finding uranium now in almost everyone I see in my office. I wonder if it too was being sprayed via geoengineering. Four years ago, I almost never saw uranium in metals testing.

As all lanthanides are chelated by EDTA, I have been advocating for the therapeutic use of EDTA to get these nanotechnology building blocks out of the body.[179] EDTA binds to lanthanides. The metals test below does not show all of them; however, gadolinium is a lanthanide and represents that chemical group. You can see the results of a 6-hour urine metals test from a C19 uninjected individual after 1500 mg of EDTA IV infusion:

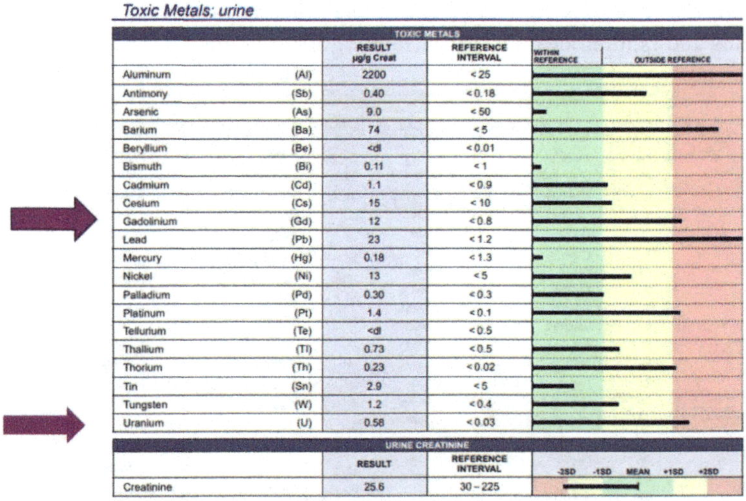

Toxic Metals; urine

TOXIC METALS		RESULT µg/g Creat	REFERENCE INTERVAL
Aluminum	(Al)	2200	<25
Antimony	(Sb)	0.40	<0.18
Arsenic	(As)	9.0	<50
Barium	(Ba)	74	<5
Beryllium	(Be)	<dl	<0.01
Bismuth	(Bi)	0.11	<1
Cadmium	(Cd)	1.1	<0.9
Cesium	(Cs)	15	<10
Gadolinium	(Gd)	12	<0.8
Lead	(Pb)	23	<1.2
Mercury	(Hg)	0.18	<1.3
Nickel	(Ni)	13	<5
Palladium	(Pd)	0.30	<0.3
Platinum	(Pt)	1.4	<0.1
Tellurium	(Te)	<dl	<0.5
Thallium	(Tl)	0.73	<0.5
Thorium	(Th)	0.23	<0.02
Tin	(Sn)	2.9	<5
Tungsten	(W)	1.2	<0.4
Uranium	(U)	0.58	<0.03

URINE CREATININE	RESULT	REFERENCE INTERVAL
Creatinine	25.6	30 – 225

Figure 99. Urine metals test after 1500 mg EDTA Chelation IV showing the elimination of many toxic metals and reduction of gadolinium and uranium. AM Medical.[180]

Also remember that Dr. Geanina Hagimă, in her analysis, found yttrium in the COVID 19 shots, which is also a lanthanide.[181]

In the Moderna patent, *Methods of Preparing Lipid Nanoparticles*, yttrium is included in the metals incorporated.[182] On page 80 is stated that radioactive ions are included, with yttrium also mentioned. That means uranium could also be knowingly used. The patent lists praseodymium and samarium, which are lanthanides with strong electrical conductivity. In the Argentinian analysis, the Astra Zeneca shot also has neodymium, a strong magnetic substance. Cerium is a lanthanide that was found in all C19 shots, including the Moderna, Sputnik, Astra Zeneca, Covelo, and Comirnaty. Europium, another lanthanide, was found in Covelo and Comirnaty.

[0402] In some embodiments, a therapeutic and/or prophylactic is a cytotoxin, a radioactive ion, a chemotherapeutic, a vaccine, a compound that elicits an immune response, and/or another therapeutic and/or prophylactic. A cytotoxin or cytotoxic agent includes any agent that may be detrimental to cells. Examples include, but are not limited to, taxol, cytochalasin B, gramicidin D, ethidium bromide, emetine, mitomycin, etoposide, teniposide, vincristine, vinblastine, colchicine, doxorubicin, daunorubicin, dihydroxyanthracinedione, mitoxantrone, mithramycin, actinomycin D, 1-dehydrotestosterone, glucocorticoids, procaine, teracaine, lidocaine, propranolol, puromycin, maytansinoids, *e.g.*, maytansinol, rachelmycin (CC-1065), and analogs or homologs thereof. Radioactive ions include, but are not limited to iodine (*e.g.*, iodine 125 or iodine 131), strontium 89, phosphorous, palladium, cesium, iridium, phosphate, cobalt, yttrium 90, samarium 153, and praseodymium. Vaccines include

Figure 100. Moderna patent excerpt showing metal nanoparticles were used in the formular. ModernaTX, Inc.[183]

In their fluorescent microscopy, the team from Argentina also found spherical, light-emitting technology that looks like quantum dots or what I call microrobots, as well as the filament structures we have become familiar with.

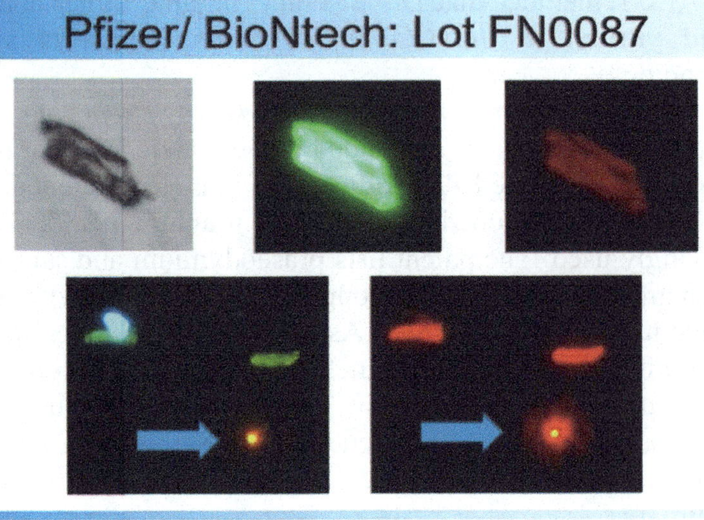

Figure 101. Structures in COVID 19 vials similar to what is now seen in live blood. Spherical, quantum dot microrobots were also found. Dr. Marcela Sangorrin, *et al.*[184]

In their analysis, the fluorescence was correlated to graphene, and it matched. As mentioned, lanthanides also have significant fluorescent capabilities and are used for quantum dot biosensing technology:

> Lanthanide (Ln) ions and quantum dots (QD) provide us with exceptional photophysical properties that cannot be found in any other luminescent material. Long luminescence lifetimes of supramolecular Ln complexes, combination of near infrared excitation and visible luminescence of Ln-doped upconversion nanoparticles, and color-tunability and high brightness of QDs have therefore been widely exploited for bioanalytical applications. One of the most frequently used techniques for analyzing biomolecular interactions is FRET (Förster resonance energy transfer), and the Ln-QD donor-acceptor FRET pair is one of the most versatile tools for

> FRET biosensing. Progress of technology development in biology, chemistry, and physics has significantly advanced Ln-to-QD FRET over the last five years, and current biosensing approaches include multiplexed detection of microRNAs, homogeneous clinical immunoassays, analysis of QD-bioconjugate morphology, and intra- and extracellular biosensing.
>
> Lanthanide (Ln) ions and semiconductor quantum dots (QDs) are inorganic luminescent compounds that are unlike all other fluorophores. Ln ions can emit photoluminescence (PL) with decay times up to milliseconds and can be excited in the near infrared (NIR) by using photon upconversion. QDs have narrow and size-tunable PL bands and a very strong and spectrally broad absorption. These particular photophysical properties (among many others) make the combination of Ln donors and QD acceptors in Förster resonance energy transfer (FRET) an exceptional tool for multiplexed, selective, and sensitive analysis of biomolecular interactions.[185]

In light of so many people who became magnetic after the COVID 19 bioweapon injections, the lanthanide discovery is very interesting. It may not just be graphene that is making people magnetic—after all, everyone nowadays is familiar with neodymium magnets!

> Another property of the lanthanides is their magnetic characteristics. The major magnetic properties of any chemical species are a result of the fact that each moving electron is a micromagnet. The species are either diamagnetic, meaning they have no unpaired electrons, or paramagnetic, meaning that they do have some unpaired electrons. The diamagnetic ions are: La^{3+}, Lu^{3+}, Yb^{2+} and Ce^{4+}. The rest of the elements are paramagnetic.[186]

Lanthanides have had huge applications in nanotechnology biosensing and bioimaging applications as well as in drug delivery:

> Upconverting luminescent nanoparticles (UCNPs) are 'new generation fluorophores' with an evolving landscape of applications in diverse industries, especially life sciences and healthcare. The anti-Stokes emission accompanied by long luminescence lifetimes, multiple absorptions, emission bands, and good photostability, enables background-free and multiplexed detection in deep tissues for enhanced imaging contrast. Their properties such as high color purity, high resistance to photobleaching, less photodamage to biological samples, attractive physical and chemical stability, and low toxicity are affected by the chemical composition; nanoparticle crystal structure, size, shape and the route; reagents; and procedure used in their synthesis. A wide range of hosts and lanthanide ion (Ln^{3+}) types have been used to control the luminescent properties of nanosystems. By modification of these properties, the performance of UCNPs can be designed for anticipated end-use applications such as photodynamic therapy (PDT), high-resolution displays, bioimaging, biosensors, and drug delivery.[187]

By no means does the finding of lanthanides exclude the presence of graphene. These two have been combined for their unique properties in many nanotechnology applications:

> The graphene 'gold rush' has resulted in the development of countless applications including electrochemical energy storage, sensors, and catalysts, using graphene (G) and graphene oxide (GO)-based materials. Surface functionalization with different metal species – single ions, neutral atoms or nanoparticles – is a frequently explored approach to the development of metal-graphene composites. Among the most attractive metals are lanthanides, whose electronic configuration

> consists of filled [Xe]6*s* levels and 4f orbitals that are gradually filled as the atomic number increases. These 4f orbitals are strongly shielded from the external environment by the 5*s*5*p*6*s* orbitals, and therefore the ligands of lanthanide complexes cause only small perturbations in the 4f electron structure, and the lanthanides retain their properties. Lanthanide ions are preferred dopants for diverse nanoparticles due to their outstanding properties such as stable luminescence, high fluorescence quantum efficiency and long luminescence lifetimes along with low toxicity. The combination of the unique characteristics of carbon nanomaterials, in particular graphene, with those of lanthanides, opens a way to the preparation of novel materials with unusual magnetic, luminescent, catalytic, biological and other properties useful for a broad spectrum of applications in different areas of science, technology, and medicine.[188]

The analysis performed by Dr. Sangorrin's research team cannot determine polymers. That's because polymers, such as polyethylene, are made from carbon and hydrogen.

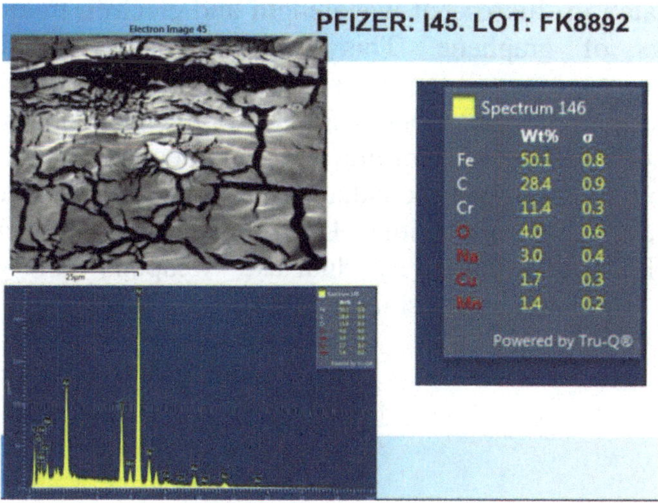

Figure 102. Mass spectroscopy shows undisclosed elements and metals. Dr. Marcela Sangorrin, *et al.*[189]

The 54 undisclosed elements discovered in Argentina are another huge find and step towards understanding the fact that all COVID 19 "vaccines" contain building blocks of nanotechnology.

The fact that semiconductive, paramagnetic, and fluorescent metals have been found as building blocks for self-assembling nanotechnology, biosensing, and bioimaging platforms is further confirmation that what we have been finding in the blood is being used for biosurveillance technology and human machine interface. Remember, in the center of the WEF fourth industrial revolution strategic intelligence is vaccination. If there was not self-assembling nanotechnology in these injections, how could vaccines be at the center of digital identity? Digital economy? Global governance? Cybersecurity? Digital communication? Unless they have injected the world's population via the COVID "vaccine" with self-assembling microchips to make all this possible.

This extraordinary analysis from Argentina found fluorescent building blocks of self-assembly nanotechnology, biosensors, and quantum dots in all analyzed vials, in addition to a match in fluorescent wavelength and electron microscopy findings of graphene. This certainly helps explain the fluorescent properties of the self-assembling nanotechnology now seen in human blood, and the orange facial glow and fluorescent filaments coming out of people's skin. Such elements are used in semiconductor nanoelectronics, biosensors, and bioimaging applications. Unfortunately, these electronics can also be utilized as dual-use weapons for genetic manipulation and nanotechnological warfare.[190]

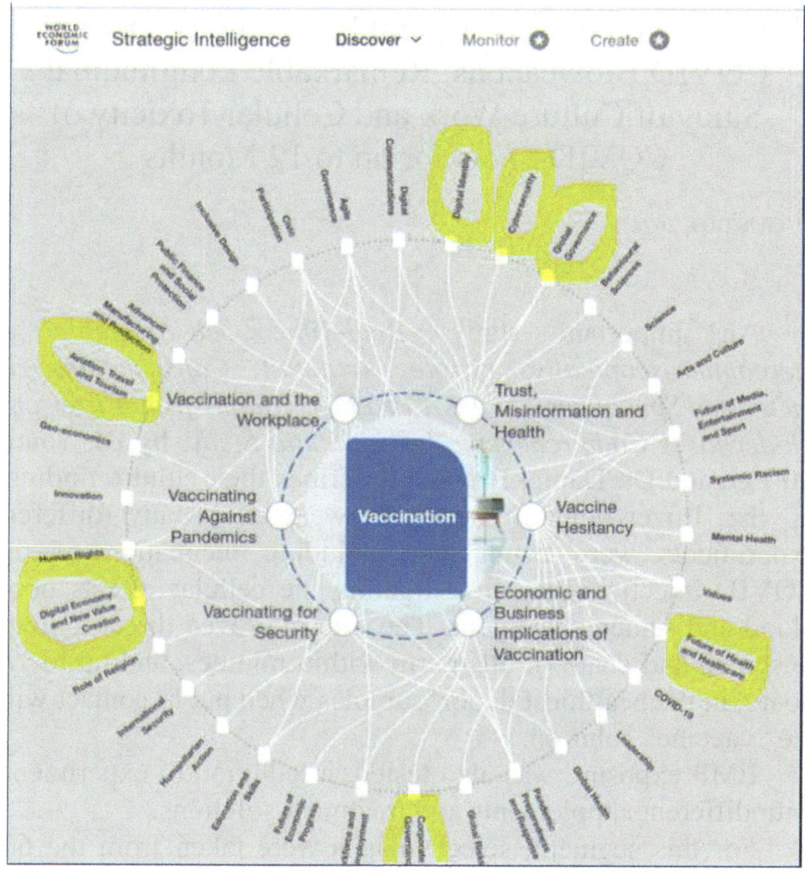

Figure 103. World Economic Forum Strategic Intelligence.[191]

Confirmation, yet again, of graphene in these horrendous shots should also be taken in the context of IEEE engineer, Dr. Ian Akyldiz' statements, since he helped develop the WBAN nanotechnology for human upload to the cloud and the AI controlled digital twin. As mentioned, Dr. Akyldiz famously stated: "COVID MRNAS ARE NOTHING MORE THAN SMALL SCALE BIO-NANO MACHINES."[192]

Confirmation of Self-Assembling Nanotechnology in COVID Bioweapons: Remarkable Longitudinal Study of Culture Work and Cellular Toxicity of COVID Shots for up to 12 Months

AUGUST 09, 2024[193]

An important study, *Real-Time Self-Assembly of Stereomicroscopically Visible Artificial Constructions in Incubated Specimens of mRNA Products Mainly from Pfizer and Moderna: A Comprehensive Longitudinal Study*, by Dr. Young Mi Lee and Dr. Daniel Broudy, describes their culture findings of the Pfizer and Moderna bioweapons. Many different experiments were conducted, including incubation of the COVID injections and investigating the cellular effects upon blood and semen specimens. These tests proved direct toxicity to semen and death of all sperm within minutes, and up to 1.5 hours, in the healthiest donor' samples when put in contact with the "vaccine" solution.

EMF exposure was also tested, in addition to experiments with different supplements and treatment solutions.

For this segment, select images were taken from the 66-page article. Please download the entire paper—this is one of the most comprehensive and long-term studies of COVID injections and their cellular effects to date. The conclusions are entirely consistent with all prior research findings of self-assembly nanotechnology in injectables.

I was part of an international team of scientists, together with Dr. Lee and Dr. Broudy, who were investigating the COVID injections and am exceedingly glad that their comprehensive research work was published in a peer-reviewed journal. Dr. Lee is a specialist in *in vitro* fertilization with her own laboratory and has been investigating the effects of the injections since 2021 in Korea under great danger for her career and life. She is a hero to humanity for her work. You can find my interview with Dr. Lee and Dr. Broudy, which reveals additional new findings, on my Substack—fifty-four COVID 19 "vaccine" vials (45 Pfizer, 7 Moderna, 1 AstraZeneca, 1 Novavax) were analyzed; 3-4 million nanoparticles per milliliter of COVID injection were found.[194]

> Observable real-time injuries at the cellular level in recipients of the 'safe and effective' COVID-19 injectables are documented here for the first time with the presentation of a comprehensive description and analysis of observed phenomena. The global administration of these often-mandated products from late 2020 triggered a plethora of independent research studies of the modified RNA injectable gene therapies, most notably those manufactured by Pfizer and Moderna. Analyses reported here consist of precise laboratory 'bench science' aiming to understand why serious debilitating, prolonged injuries (and many deaths) occurred increasingly without any measurable protective effect from the aggressively, marketed products. The contents of COVID-19 injectables were examined under a stereomicroscope at up to 400X magnification. Carefully preserved specimens were cultured in a range of distinct media to observe immediate and long-term cause-and-effect relationships between the injectables and living cells under carefully controlled conditions. From such research, reasonable inferences can be drawn about observed injuries worldwide that have occurred since the injectables were pressed upon billions of individuals. In addition to cellular toxicity, our findings reveal numerous—on the order of $3 \sim 4 \times 10^6$ per milliliter of the injectable—visible artificial self-assembling entities ranging from about 1 to 100 μm, or greater, of many different shapes. There were animated worm-like entities, discs, chains, spirals, tubes, right-angle structures containing other artificial entities within them, and so forth. All these are exceedingly beyond any expected and acceptable levels of contamination of the COVID-19 injectables, and incubation studies revealed

the progressive self-assembly of many artifactual structures. As time progressed during incubation, simple one- and two-dimensional structures over two or three weeks became more complex in shape and size developing into stereoscopically visible entities in three-dimensions. They resembled carbon nanotube filaments, ribbons, and tapes, some appearing as transparent, thin, flat membranes, and others as three-dimensional spirals, and beaded chains. Some of these seemed to appear and then disappear over time. Our observations suggest the presence of some kind of nanotechnology in the COVID-19 injectables.[195]

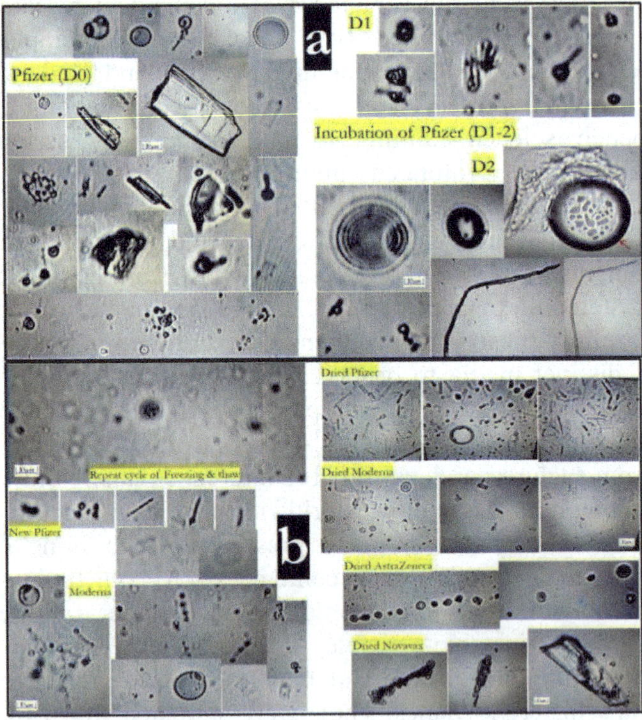

Figure 104. Direct microscopic findings observed in two dimensions magnified 400X: (a) Remnants and new Pfizer injectables, directly observed as well as after incubation for 1 -2 days. (b) Moderna and 4 dried COVID-19 injectables (Pfizer, Moderna, AstraZeneca, and Novavax). Lee, *et al.*, 2024.[196]

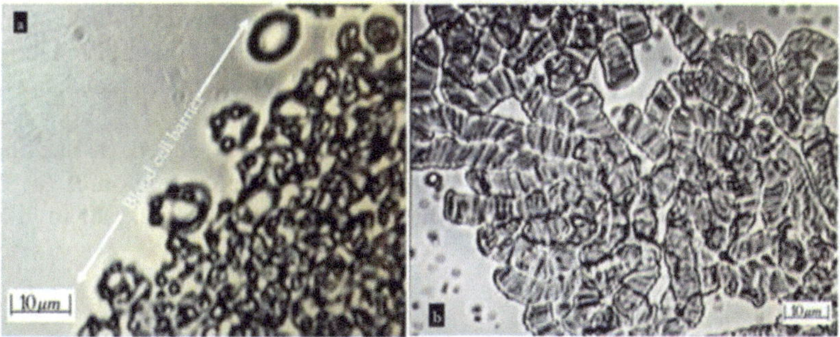

Figure 105. Interactions observed for whole blood(a)/plasma(b) with Novavax at 400X magnification: (a) Within 1 hour, blood cells formed a prominent barrier against “vaccine” contents. (b) After 30 minutes, severe aggregates of red blood cells in rouleaux appeared in the plasma specimen. Lee, *et al.*, 2024.[197]

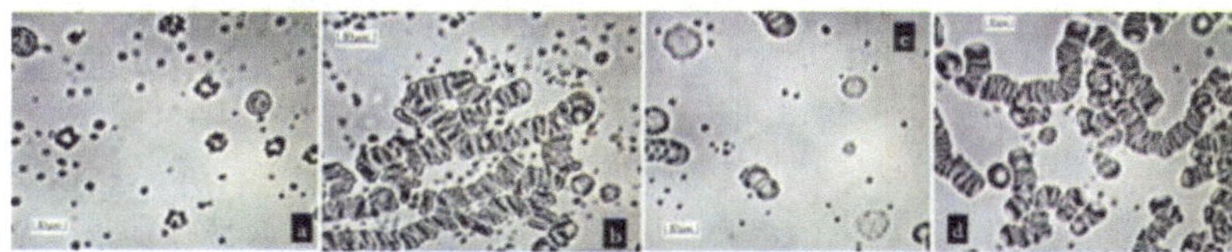

Figure 106. Plasma reactions after two hours with four COVID-19 injectables – Pfizer, Moderna, Novavax, and AstraZeneca: (a) Pfizer showing cellular collapse (pyknosis) of white blood cells and damaged platelets; (b) Moderna with stacks of red blood cells (rouleaux); (c) Novavax with the nucleus of white blood cells disintegrating (karyorrhexis), abnormal platelet aggregations, and some rouleaux of red blood cells; and (d) AstraZeneca with prominent Rouleau of red blood cells. Lee, *et al.*, 2024.[198]

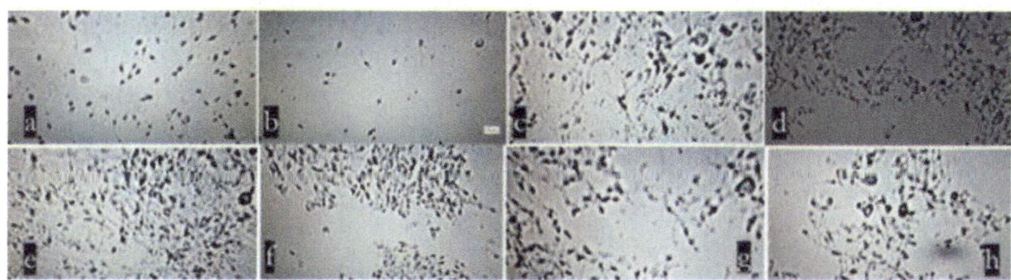

Figure 107. Reaction of semen to COVID-19 injectables at 200X magnification: (a) semen with normal saline as a control added after two

hours; (b) with flu vaccine added as a control after 1.5 hours showed sperm cells with intact morphology and with typical progressive natural reduction in sperm motility; (c) 30 minutes after Pfizer-1 injectable was added, sperm motility showed rapid reduction; (d) Pfizer-1 after one hour, all sperm motility ceased; (e) 30 minutes after Moderna. injectable added; (f) one hour after Moderna was added sperm cells were completely immotile; (g) 30 minutes after Novavax was added; (h) one hour after Novavax, all motility ceased. Lee, *et al.*, 2024.[199]

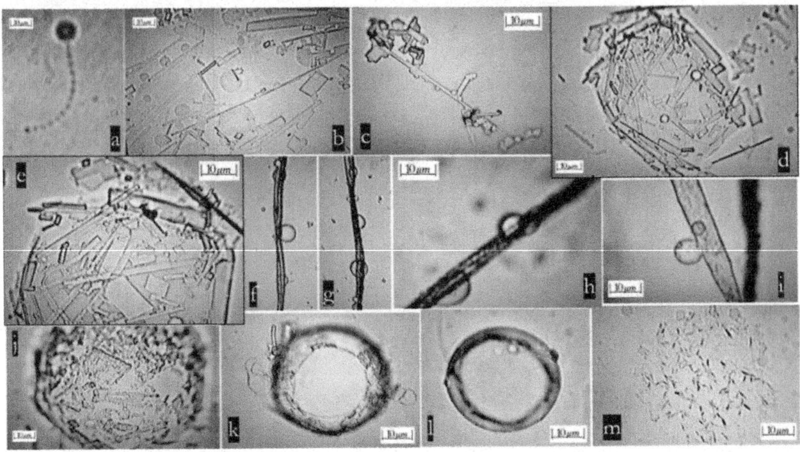

Figure 108. Findings for Pfizer incubation study for 372 days; (a) Day 22, this is what we describe as a beaded chain (at 400X magnification); (b) Day 24, 2- dimensional geometric self-assembly at the bottom (at 200X magnification) in normal saline; (c) Day 60, floating 3-dimensional detailed chip-like structures (at 400X magnification) in distilled water; (d) and (e) day 60, accumulated 3-dimensional chip-like structures within an oval shaped boundary (200X/400X) in distilled water; (f), (g), (h), (i) Floating filaments shedding bubbles inside and outside in normal solution at day 95 (100x/100x/200x/200x); (j), (k), (l), (m) Progressive degenerative changes in distilled water 200X (day 82/day 256/day 306/day 372). Lee, *et al.*, 2024.[200]

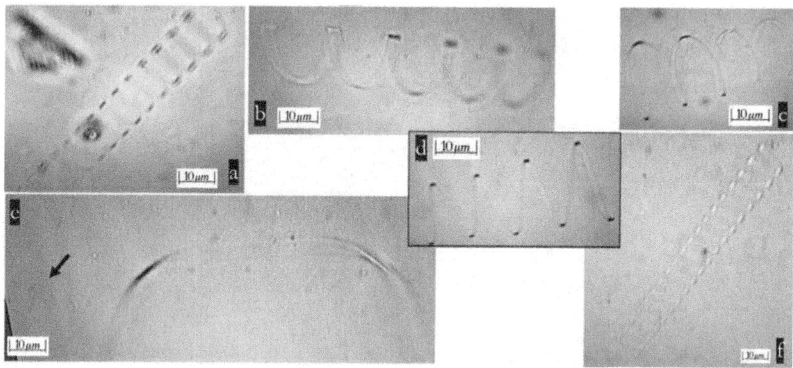

Figure 109. Various coils, ribbons, and spirals in Pfizer, distilled water: (a) Day 60 (at 200X magnification); (b) ~ (e) Day 74 (at 200X magnification); (f) Day 176 (at 100X magnification). Lee, *et al.*, 2024.[201]

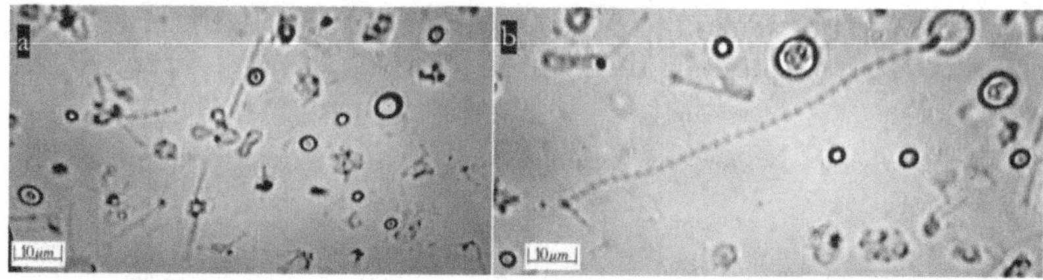

Figure 110. Beaded chains and assorted structures in Pfizer distilled water (Day 176, 400x): (a) Various artificial satellite-like structures, (b) Long beaded chains gathered on the central surface of the medium. Lee, *et al.*, 2024.[202]

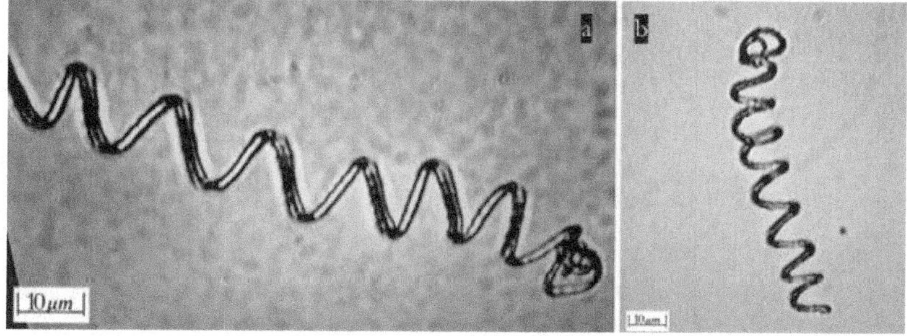

Figure 111. Typical algae-typed magnetic nanobot-like spirals in Pfizer in distilled water: (a) Day 176 (400x); (b) Day 337 (200x). Lee, *et al.*, 2024.[203]

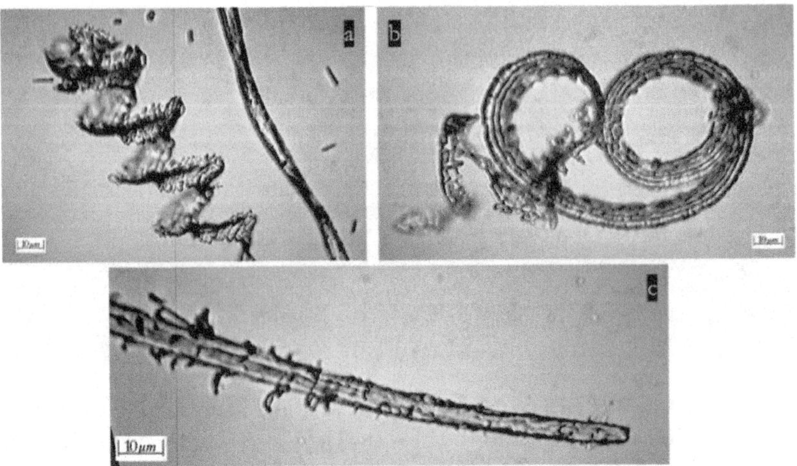

Figure 112. Various filaments — striated ribbons, sprouting in the late stage (Day 316) of incubation of Pfizer in distilled water: (a) and (b) curled striated ribbons (100x); (c) sprouting filaments in Pfizer (200x). Lee, *et al.*, 2024.[204]

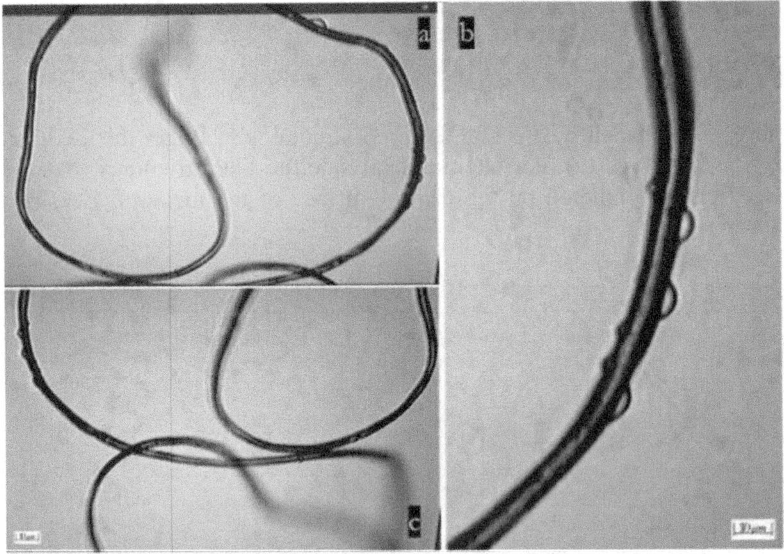

Figure 113. Bundle of transparent thin wire-like tubes with shedding bubbles in Pfizer incubation in distilled water (Day 331); floating in the uppermost layer (a- 40x/b-100x/c-40x). Lee, *et al.*, 2024.[205]

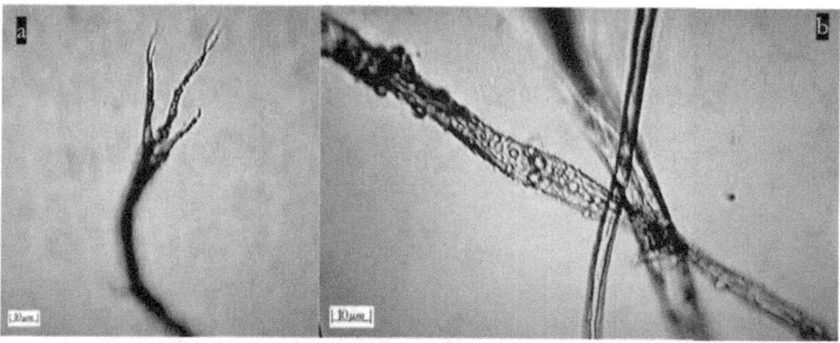

Figure 114. Tripod-like, striated filaments in Pfizer incubation in normal saline (Day 346, 200x): (a) More developed tripod-like structures or (b) Striated patterns on filaments. Lee, *et al.*, 2024.[206]

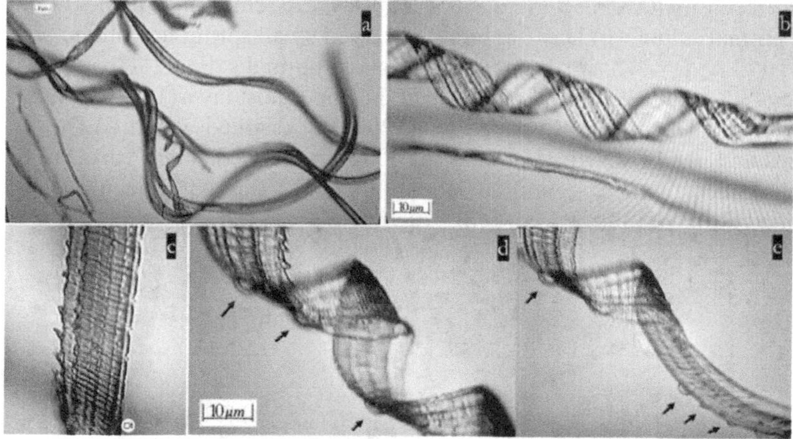

Figure115. Curled striated ribbons and bubbles in Pfizer incubation in distilled water (Day 406 and 499); (a), (b), and (c) uniquely striated curled ribbons in Pfizer in DW at 406 days of incubation (40X/100X/200X); (d), and (e); bubbles (arrows) appeared on the surface of the curled ribbons at 499 days incubation (200X). Lee, *et al.*, 2024.[207]

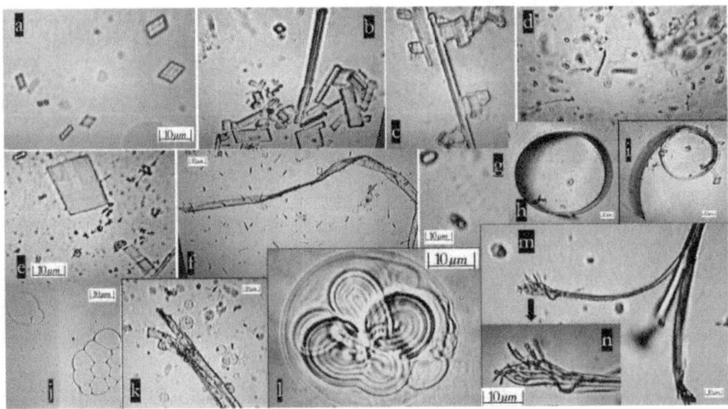

Figure 116. Geometric chip-like assembly, filaments, spirals, ribbons, and encapsulated wire bundles in the Moderna incubation study throughout Day 630 (100~400X): (a) Day 16; (b) Day 40; (c) Day 42; (d) Day 125; and (e) Day 126 (all 400x) in normal saline. (f) Day 126, chips and filament (100x) in normal saline; (g) Day 36, rarely observed small spring in distilled water; (h) and (i) Day 42, small circular ribbons in normal saline, (400x/200x); (j) Day 295, lobulated bubbles floating at the uppermost layer(100x) in distilled water; (k) Day 313, split-ended tape (200x) in distilled water; (l) Day 313, capsuled, well-packed wire bundles (400x) in distilled water; (m) Day 630, split-ended filament in normal saline (100x); (n) Day 630, magnified split-ended filament (400x). Lee, *et al.*, 2024.[208]

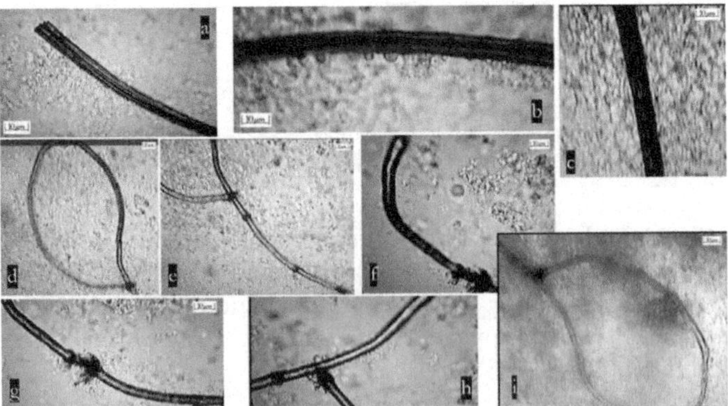

Figure 117. Findings of Moderna incubation study in plasma 2: (a) Day 133, dark pipe-like structure developed (100x); (b) with shedding bubbles (200x); (c) disappeared bubbles at Day 282(100x); (d) and (e) Day 133, snare-like lasso tubes (100x); (f), (g), and (h) Day 133, broken, disconnected points in

the lasso-like tube (200x); (i) Day 282, still the same figure maintained (100x). Lee, *et al.*, 2024.[209]

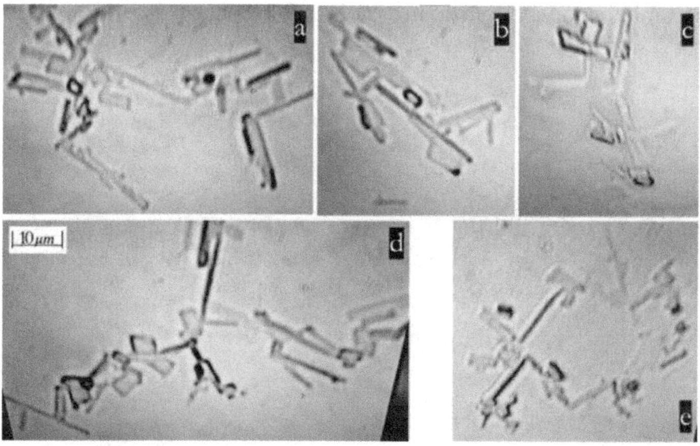

Figure 118. Heat (warming) study of Pfizer – after 48 hours of warming at BT in normal saline: (a), (b), (c), (d), and (e): Floating well-assembled 3-dimensional geometric structures on the surface of the media after 48 hours of warming (36.5°C) on the heat template. Accelerated development was similarly matched to the findings in the 2nd~ 3rd week of the unexposed incubation study (400x). Lee, *et al.*, 2024.[210]

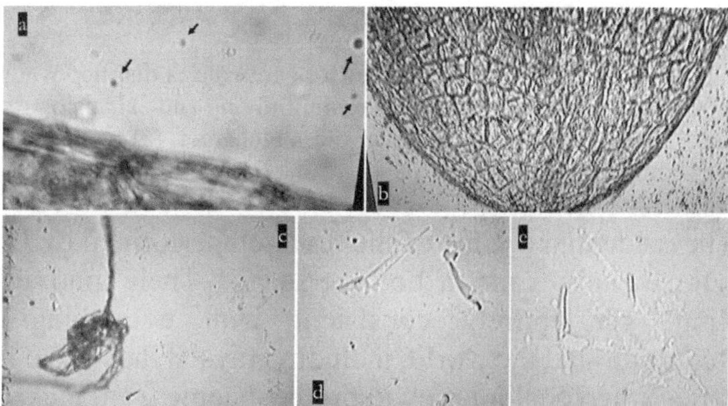

Figure 119. Recycling Pattern Study — Presumptive recycling pattern from the Moderna vaccine's skin extract (E1) in normal saline: (a) seed-like tiny dark particles (arrows) floating around the skin extract 1(E1) in the normal saline media (400x); (b) tiny particles scattered around the vaccinee's skin

extract, dark large material-crocodile skin-like structure (100x); (c) E1 seeds culture in normal saline – trace of the self-assembly at the bottom and floating filaments together after Day 366 incubation (100x); (d) and (e) Trace of the self-assembled geometric structures at Day 366 incubation (400x). Lee, *et al.*, 2024.[211]

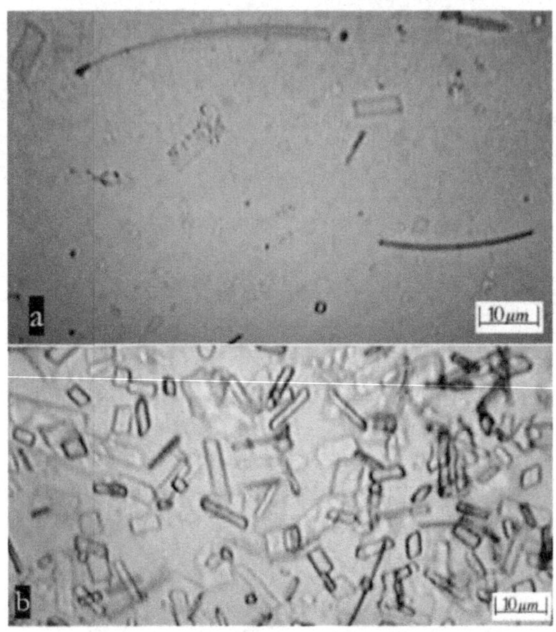

Figure 120. Study of wireless recharger for Moderna in distilled water (Day 36, 200X): Moderna showed immediate multiplying and expansion response just after 1 hour of exposure to the wireless recharger, (a) before exposure; (b) after 1 hour exposure.[212]

The evidentiary value of the research performed by Dr. Lee and Dr. Broudy cannot be overstated. Their findings are shocking, yet entirely consistent with everything other researchers around the world, including myself, have also found. In Dr. Lee's personal journey to protect people from the dangers of the COVID 19 bioweapon, she filed a lawsuit against the South Korean government to have the injections stopped. Sadly, like in so many lawsuits around the world, the judge dismissed her case.

Human Papilloma Virus "Vaccine" for 9-12-Year-Old Children Shows Nanobots, Self-Assembly Hydrogel, and Polymer Mesh Development

SEPTEMBER 01, 2023[213]

The following is a darkfield microscopic examination of the HPV (Human Papilloma Virus) "vaccine."

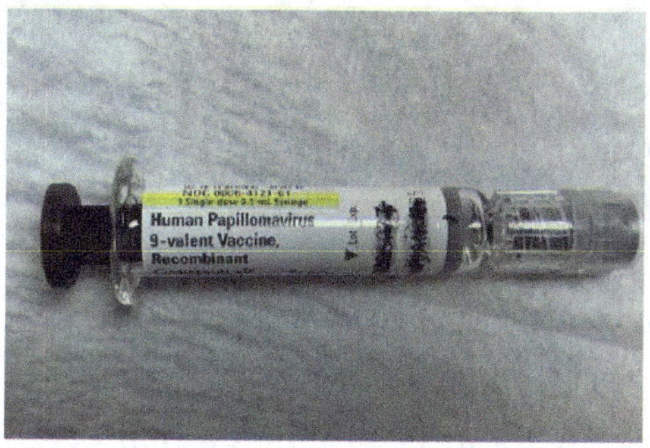

Figure 121. HPV "vaccine" vial. AM Medical.[214]

Immediately upon putting the HPV "vaccine" on the slide, similar hydrogel substrate conglomerates were seen. The size seems to be about 100x smaller than a red blood cell:

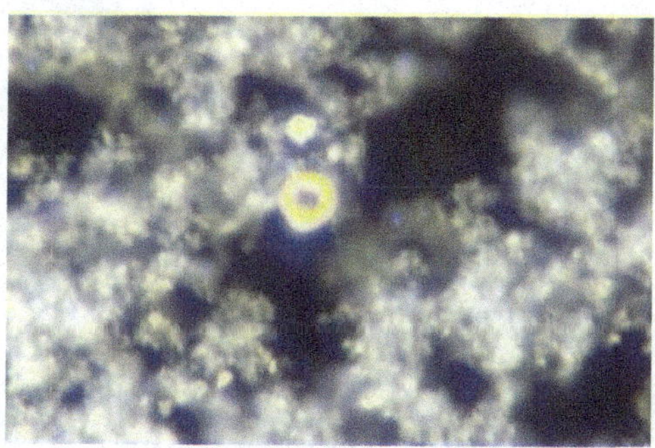

Figure 122. HPV "vaccine" shows extensive hydrogel and blinking quantum dot microrobots. Magnification 400x. AM Medical.[215]

Soon after placing the drop onto the slide the usual hydrogel structures developed adjacent to spherical construction sites:

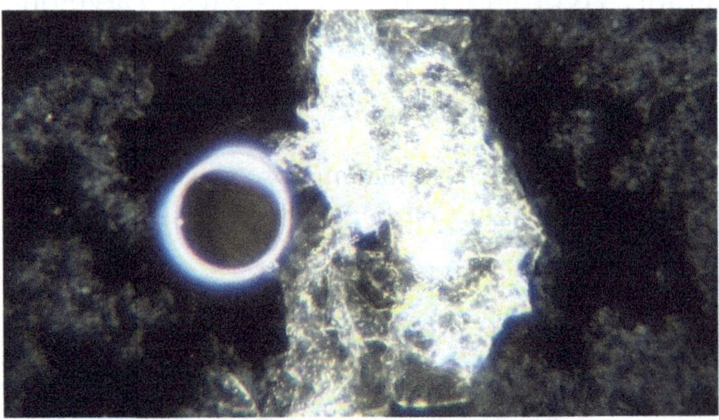

Figure 123. HPV "vaccine" shows polymer hydrogel and spherical construction site. Magnification 400x. AM Medical.[216]

Very dense material is assembled that certainly looks like the clot structures I see in the blood as well:

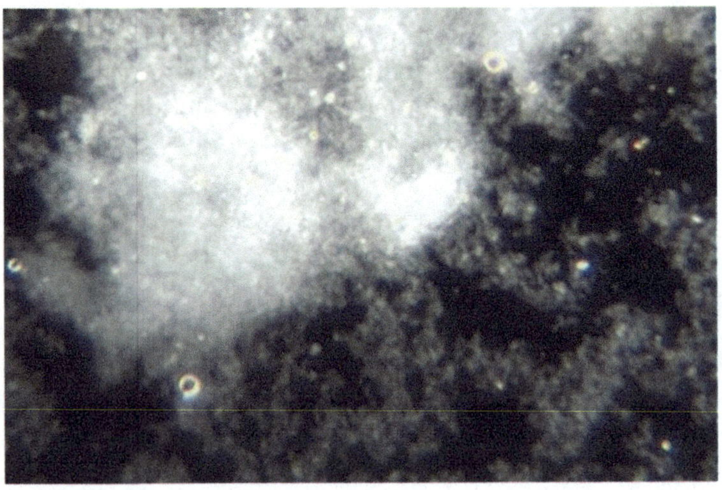

Figure 124. HPV "vaccine" shows polymer hydrogel self-assembly. Magnification 400x. AM Medical.[217]

On my Substack you can watch video capture of this self-assembly as pieces of the hydrogel substance are moved around with small nanobots coordinating the assembly—this looks like the insulin videos I have also taken:[218]

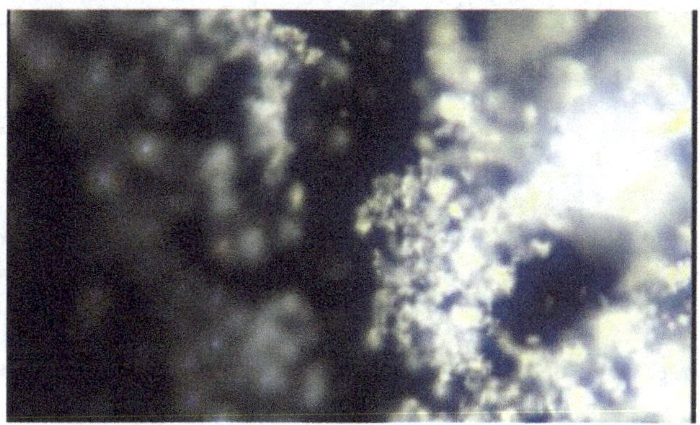

Figure 125. HPV "vaccine" shows active polymer hydrogel self-assembly. Magnification 400x. AM Medical.[219]

Subsequently, a very rapid transformation into a crystalline phase occurred that demonstrates how fast the composite structures can assemble. Small nanobots can also be seen in the captured image below:

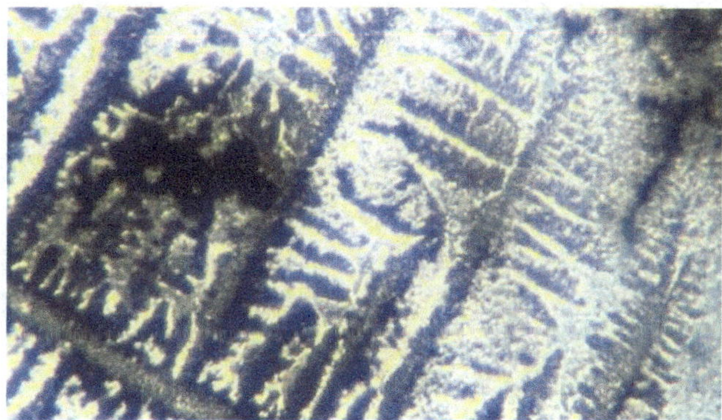

Figure 126. HPV "vaccine" shows active polymer hydrogel self-assembly into DARPA hydrogel-like patterns. Magnification 400x. AM Medical.[220]

After approximately 45 minutes observation, an extensive spherical mesh developed, as appears in the blood I observe. This is called micellar hydrogel:

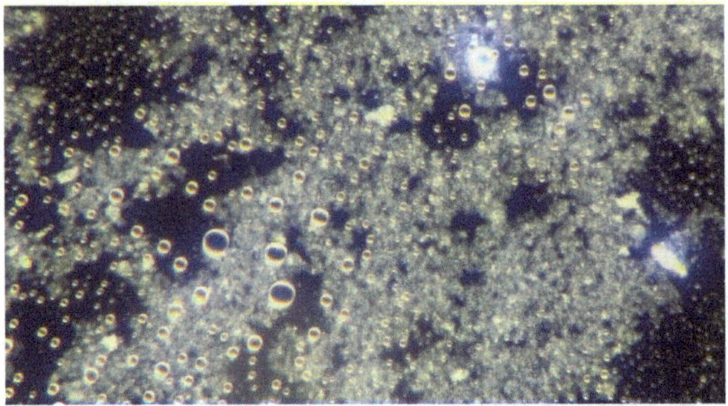

Figure 127. HPV "vaccine" shows spherical mesh network self-assembly. Magnification 400x. AM Medical.[221]

In this video, an extensive, micellar hydrogel mesh becomes visible, together with mobile spheres and solid hydrogel structures.[222] All of those spheres simply appeared, they were not visible initially:

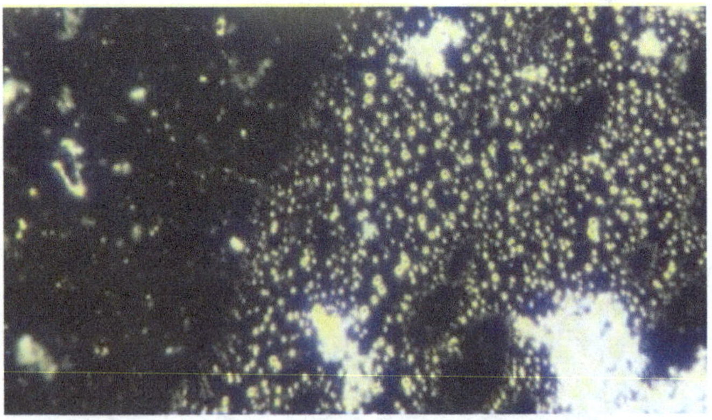

Figure 128. HPV "vaccine" shows spherical mesh network self-assembly with solid hydrogel polymer interspersed. Magnification 200x. AM Medical.[223]

For comparison, the image below reveals what this polymer mesh looks like in human blood. It is the same and continues to evolve and self-assemble if you let the blood sit on the microscopy slide until the mesh replaces the blood completely:

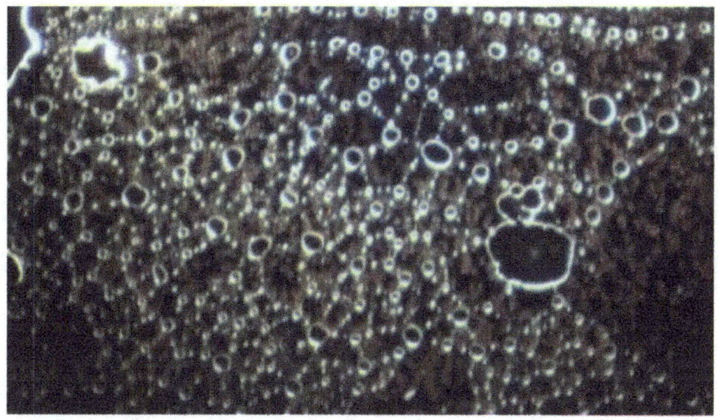

Figure 129. Darkfield live blood analysis of COVID 19 unvaccinated blood shows spherical mesh network self-assembly. Magnification 100x. AM Medical.[224]

Here are other classic structures that developed in the HPV "vaccine" that we also see in the blood all the time. These solid structures are DNA biosensor mesogens which contain quantum dot nano- and microrobots:

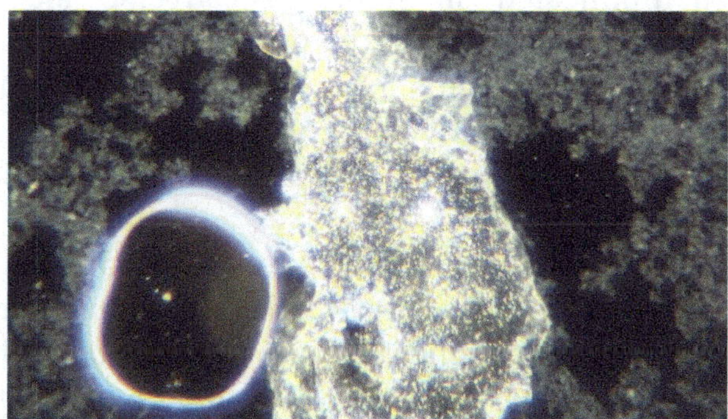

Figure 130. HPV "vaccine" self-assembled into mesogen with adjacent micellar construction site and surrounding hydrogel polymer. Magnification 400x. AM Medical.[225]

To summarize, the HPV injection contents did not develop filaments but assembled into a polymer mesh. Many other structures self-assembled that are similar to nanotechnology and synthetic biological contamination in the blood that I see all the time. Small nanobots were filmed that are in the size range of one hundredth of a human red blood cell. Bottom line, all "vaccines" have self-assembly nanotechnology in them.

Giardasil "Vaccine" Microscopy by Dr. Geanina Hagimă and HPV Vaccine Injury Review

OCTOBER 16, 2023[226]

Dr. Hagimă in Romania replicated my research on the HPV "vaccine" injection and found similar dense material. Video footage is available on Substack.[227]

"The Gardasil 9 HPV vaccine contains proteins of HPV types 6, 11, 16, 18, 31, 33, 45, 52, and 58, amorphous aluminum hydroxyphosphate sulfate, yeast protein, sodium chloride, L-histidine, polysorbate 80, sodium borate, and water for injection."[228] Adjuvants, such as organosiloxanes and silica, have been implicated in numerous adverse side effects, including serious injuries and even death.

Interestingly, the literature discusses extreme cross reactivity between polyethylene glycol, the hydrogel building block that is used for Pfizer's C19 lipid nanoparticle technology, and polysorbate 80.[229]

"Immediate hypersensitivity to PEG 3350 with cross-reactive polysorbate 80 hypersensitivities may be under-recognized in clinical practice and can be detected with clinical skin testing. Our studies raise the possibility of an IgE-mediated type I hypersensitivity mechanism in some cases."[230]

Just like in the C19 injections, unexplained genetically engineered DNA samples were also found in the HPV shots.[231]

In samples of Gardasil examined by Dr. Sin Hang Lee, a pathologist with expertise in DNA sequencing and DNA sequence analysis, he found fragments of actual HPV DNA. Dr. Lee stated, "HPV DNA in Gardasil is not 'natural' DNA. It is a recombinant HPV DNA (rDNA), genetically engineered, to be inserted into yeast cells for virus-like-particle (VLP) protein production. rDNA is known to behave differently from natural DNA. It may enter a human cell, especially in an inflammatory lesion caused by the effects of the aluminum adjuvant, via poorly understood mechanisms... Once a segment of recombinant DNA is inserted into a human cell, the consequences are hard to predict."[232,233,234]

These various and multiple "vaccines" also increased serious nervous system disorders (exploratory analysis) and general harms.

A lawsuit filed in Florida in 2021 alleges Gardasil contains "dangerous and undisclosed ingredients," including HPV L1-DNA fragments and phenylmethylsulfonyl fluoride (PMSF). According to the complaint, HPV L1-DNA fragments make the vaccine "more potent and dangerous than intended," and phenylmethylsulfonyl fluoride is a "toxic nerve agent that is not intended for human consumption or injection."[235]

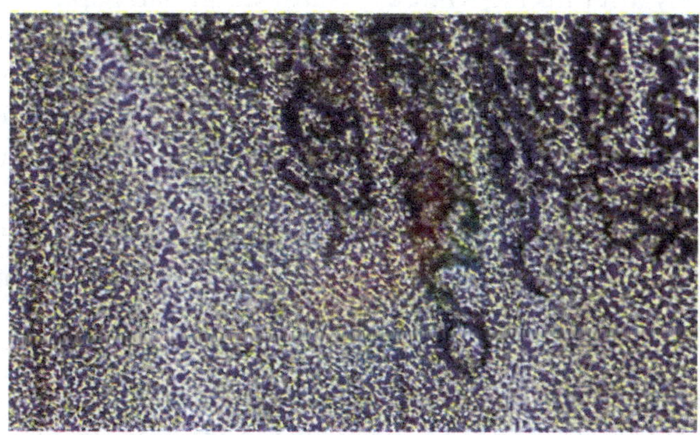

Figure 131. HPV "vaccine" under brightfield microscopy shows hydrogel polymer. Magnification 200x. Dr. Geanina Hagimă.[236]

Figures 131 and 132 show the microscopy performed by Dr. Hagimă on the HPV "vaccine" approximately one hour after applying the ingredients on the slide.

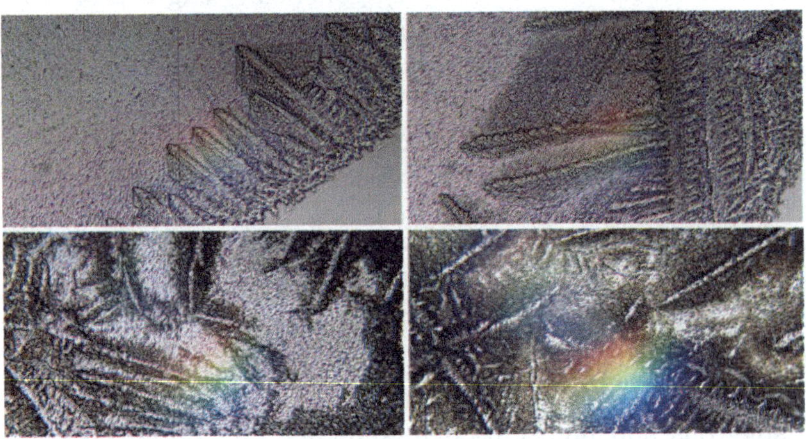

Figure 132. HPV "vaccine" under brightfield microscopy shows hydrogel polymer with fluorescence. Magnification 200x upper images; 400x lower images. Dr. Geanina Hagimă.[237]

This lawsuit further states: "Trey Cobb, who developed narcolepsy after taking Merck's Gardasil human papillomavirus, or HPV, vaccine won a major victory when the National Vaccine Injury Compensation Program ruled the vaccine caused his condition. The case could set a precedent in the upcoming lawsuits against Merck alleging the pharma giant knowingly hid risks associated with the vaccine."[238]

This is the third VICP ruling to find Gardasil can induce autoimmunity through the mechanisms of molecular mimicry and cross-reactivity and sets precedent for lawsuits against Merck.

"In the first case, 22-year-old Bard College student Christina Tarsell died from her vaccine injuries. In the second, several petitioners suffered primary ovarian insufficiency, a condition where the ovaries stop functioning."[239]

Additionally, there has been documentation of toxicity from around the world:

> Over the past five years clinicians from numerous countries have implicated human papillomavirus (HPV) immunizations as the cause of diverse systemic ailments, egregious injuries, and even death. Vaccine ingredients in Gardasil and Cervarix contain hidden organosiloxanes (organosilicones) and silica (silicon dioxide), all of which are capable of creating biochemical disturbances that are strikingly similar to the metabolic disruptions identified in both chronic fatigue syndrome and the recurrent public health debacle of silicone gel-filled breast implant toxicity.
>
> Recent publications originating from Italy, Japan, Australia, Columbia, India, Ireland, Denmark, Mexico, Norway, Sweden, Canada, France, the USA, and the United Kingdom have reported post-HPV vaccination phenomena that share overlapping clinical features with chronic fatigue syndrome/myalgic encephalomyelitis (CFS/ME), fibromyalgia (FM), postural orthostatic tachycardia syndrome (POTS), complex regional pain syndrome (CRPS), small fiber neuropathy (SFN), and autonomic dysfunction (AD). Typical symptoms include (but are not limited to) prolonged generalized fatigue, chronic headaches, widespread generalized pain, tremors, orthostatic fainting, postural tachycardia, alterations in gastrointestinal motility, gait disturbance, anxiety, paresthesia's, sleep disturbance, learning impairment, difficulty in concentration, and other cognitive phenomena. These reported phenomena have created hesitation by some parents to have HPV vaccination administered to their teenage children.[240]

The Expose, in the UK, published an article about the harmful ingredients present in routine "vaccines" and listed the following:

- Formaldehyde/Formalin – Highly toxic systematic poison and carcinogen.
- Betapropiolactone – Toxic chemical and carcinogen. May cause death/permanent injury after very short exposure to small quantities. Corrosive chemical.
- Hexadecyltrimethylammonium bromide – May cause damage to the liver, cardiovascular system, and central nervous system. May cause reproductive effects and birth defects.
- Aluminium hydroxide, aluminium phosphate, and aluminium salts – Neurotoxin. Carries risk for long-term brain inflammation/swelling, neurological disorders, autoimmune disease, Alzheimer's, dementia, and autism. It penetrates the brain where it persists indefinitely.
- Thimerosal (mercury) – Neurotoxin. Induces cellular damage, reduces oxidation-reduction activity, cellular degeneration, and cell death. Linked to neurological disorders, Alzheimer's, dementia, and autism.
- Polysorbate 80 & 20 – Trespasses the Blood-Brain Barrier and carries with it aluminium, thimerosal, and viruses; allowing it to enter the brain.
- Glutaraldehyde – Toxic chemical used as a disinfectant for heat-sensitive medical equipment.
- Foetal Bovine Serum – Harvested from bovine (cow) foetuses taken from pregnant cows before slaughter.
- Human Diploid Fibroblast Cells – aborted foetal cells. Foreign DNA has the ability to interact with our own.
- African Green Monkey Kidney Cells – Can carry the SV40 cancer-causing virus that has already tainted about 30 million Americans.

- Acetone – Can cause kidney, liver, and nerve damage.
- E. coli – Yes, you read that right.
- DNA from porcine (pig) Circovirus type 1.
- Human embryonic lung cell cultures (from aborted foetuses).[241]

Everyone is afraid to be called an anti-vaxxer, yet the extreme toxicity and debilitating side effects from these shots, called "vaccines," are legendary at this point. As with the HPV "vaccine," many people who took the COVID shots have experienced similar symptoms such as POTS (Postural Orthostatic Tachycardia Syndrome) with chronic fatigue, cognitive dysfunction, and more.

The HPV "vaccine" contains nerve toxins?

In medications?

And nobody is outraged about this?

Why do we allow this to be done to our children for the sake of conforming with Big Pharma mandates and risk making them dysfunctional for life?

Or even worse, killing them at a young age?

Steve Kirsch also posted a report that 50% of SIDS (sudden infant death syndrome) cases happened within 48 hours post vaccine.[242]

Don't even engage in the anti-vax argument at this point. It is nonsensical. I am against all "vaccines" because they all contain known poisons.

How are we going to survive if more and more of these shots are given to each human?

Become aware that the United Nations Agenda 2030 plans for 500 INJECTIONS PER PERSON, PER LIFETIME.

Measles, Mumps, Rubella, and Varicella "Vaccine" for Children Shows Nanobot Swarms, Quantum Dots, and Self-Assembly Hydrogel

SEPTEMBER 04, 2023[243]

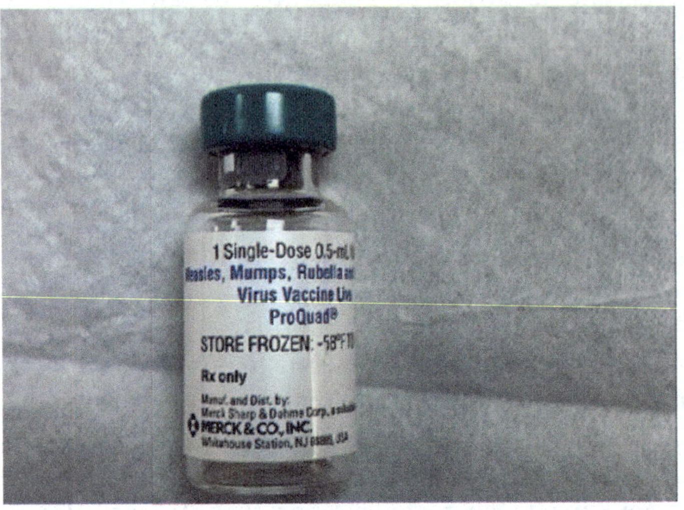

Figure 133. Measles, Mumps, Rubella, and Varicella "vaccine." AM Medical.[244]

The childhood MMRV "vaccine" is loaded with nanobots. They are so small that on my highest magnification you can barely see them, but they are clearly there. I have taken many videos and if you look at the entirety of the documentation it is clearly stunning. The MMRV vax is supposed to be stored at -56F. Thawed it looks exactly like the COVID 19 bioweapon. Filaments assemble and there are large areas of hydrogel clots. Without a cover slip the self-assembly is much more visible.

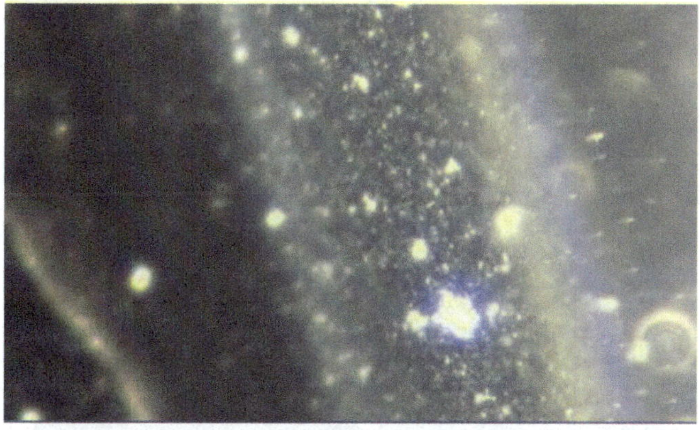

Figure 134. MMRV “vaccine” filled with nanorobots that assemble hydrogel polymer. Magnification 400x. AM Medical.[245]

One can see that the MMRV liquid is dense, and many layers of activity are observable in the image above, including larger hydrogel pieces. I wanted to show the miniscule swarming in the background that is clearly involved in self-assembly. Human red blood cells have about a diameter of 6.8 micrometers. I would say these small nanobots are at least 1000 times smaller than that.

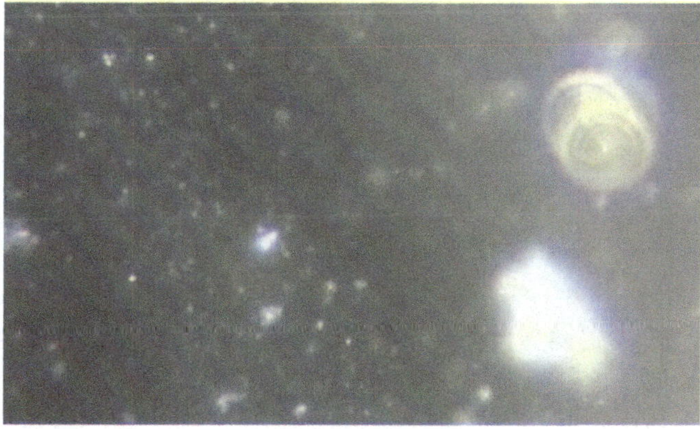

Figure 135. MMRV “vaccine” filled with nanorobots that assemble hydrogel polymer. Magnification 400x. AM Medical.[246]

Larger pieces of hydrogel can be seen moving in the extremely busy background. These nanorobots assemble hydrogel polymers which grow over a period of just minutes:

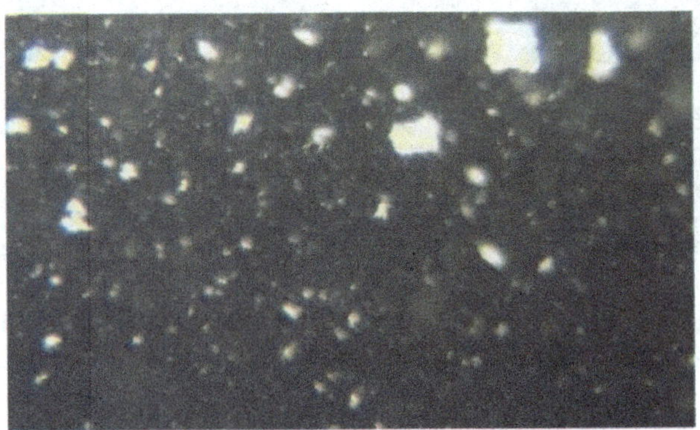

Figure 136. MMRV "vaccine" filled with nanorobots assembling hydrogel polymers. Magnification 400x. AM Medical.[247]

The entire drop was moving towards the center, clearly coordinated to build a large hydrogel-like clot. In the video you can see intelligent movement at 100x magnification. It looks just like the insulin that I also filmed.

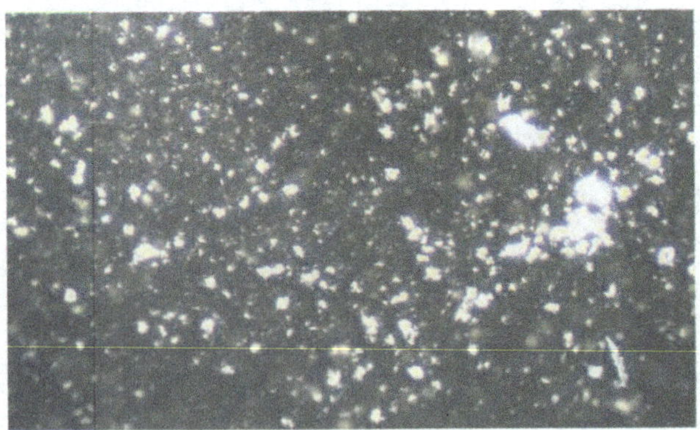

Figure 137. MMRV "vaccine" filled with nanorobots assembling hydrogel polymers. Magnification 200x. AM Medical.[248]

Below you can see after about 45 minutes how much of this mass has already been assembled:

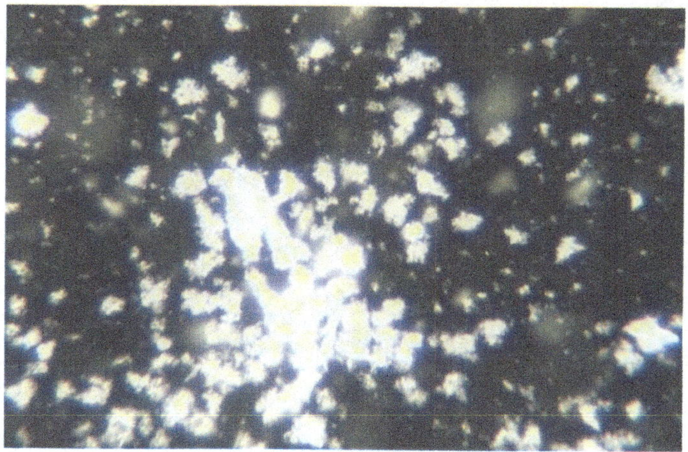

Figure 138. MMRV “vaccine” hydrogel polymer assembly. Magnification 200x. AM Medical.[249]

Please find someone to conduct this test and see for yourself—here is what this looks like after about 70 minutes:

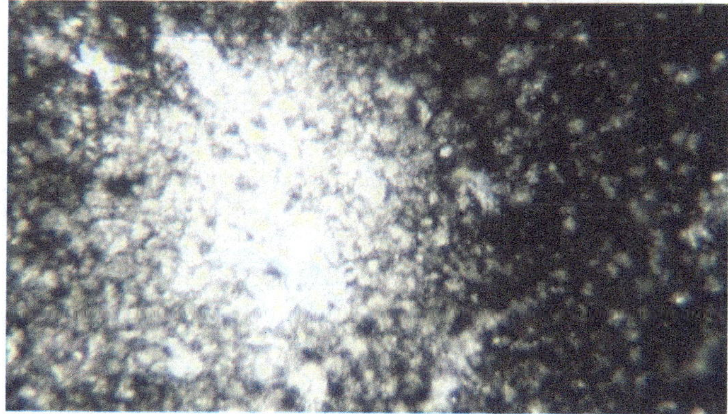

Figure 139. MMRV “vaccine” hydrogel polymer assembly. Magnification 200x. AM Medical.[250]

Filaments that we can now recognize were seen self-assembling. They were not present when the material was placed on the slide. This one appeared after about an hour and 20 minutes:

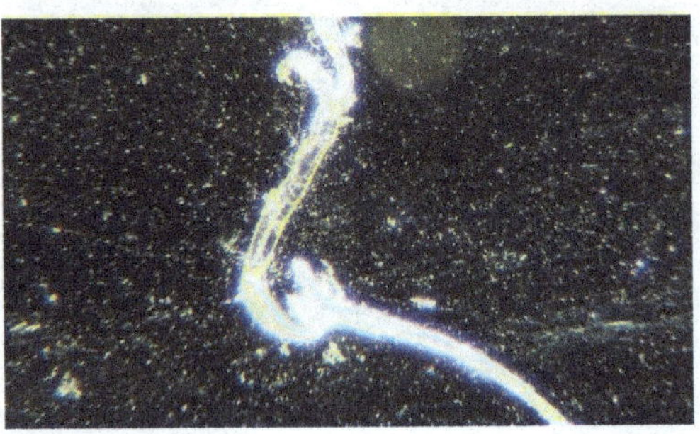

Figure 140. MMRV "vaccine" hydrogel filament assembly. Magnification 200x. AM Medical.[251]

This image below is at 100x objective with the light dialed down, and shows that the filaments have multiplied and grown huge:

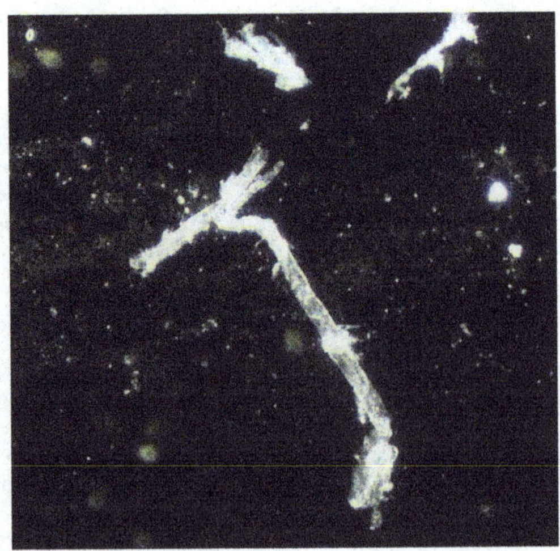

Figure 141. MMRV "vaccine" hydrogel filament assembly. Magnification 100x. AM Medical.[252]

Here are the classic spheres I see in the blood growing a similar hydrogel substance:

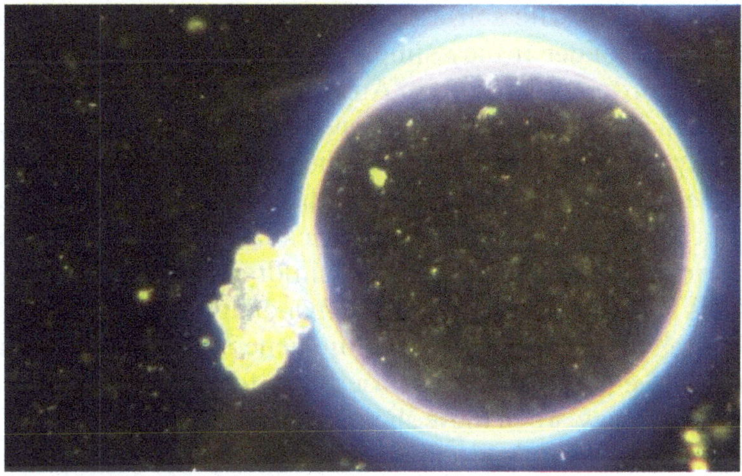

Figure 142. MMRV "vaccine" hydrogel filament assembly from spherical construction site. Magnification 400x. AM Medical.[253]

And this is a coagulated hydrogel in the MMRV "vaccine" with many blinking lights visible:

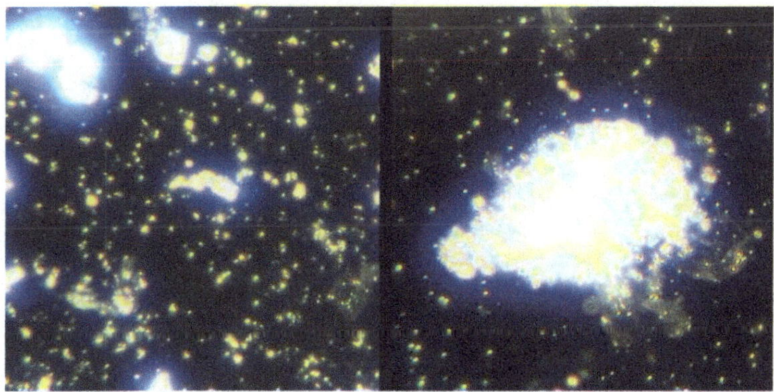

Figure 143. MMRV "vaccine" light-emitting, quantum dot nano- and microrobots self-assemble. Left: Magnification 200x. Right: 2000x. AM Medical.[254]

This horrendous "vaccine" is given to 9-month-old babies, then again at 15 months, and then at 6 years of age. This is the 5th childhood vaccine I have looked at. It all looks the same to me, it is loaded with self-assembly nanotechnology and almost makes me wonder if they simply use the same ingredients and just put a different label on it. Any doctor or individual who has ever been called an anti-vaxxer needs to read these articles and sue anyone who has accused them of such. Big Pharma criminals, the medical societies, medical boards, physicians, and healthcare providers who get kickbacks called "Pay for Performance" the more they shoot children up with this, and the schools and other agencies that are mandating this "vaccine," are all complicit in poisoning our future generation. This is literally a criminal enterprise. Undisclosed clot forming chemicals and nanotechnology are in these shots. Any doctor with a conscience needs to get a darkfield microscope and replicate this work. If you have a soul left, you cannot poison one more child with this. Ever again. Parents who love their children, you cannot buy into this "vaccine" propaganda again. NOBODY can justify injecting this material into babies!

Diphtheria, Tetanus, Pertussis, Polio, Hemophilus B, and Hepatitis B "Vaccine" for Small Children – Darkfield Microscopy Shows Self-Assembly Hydrogel Filaments and Structures

AUGUST 31, 2023[255]

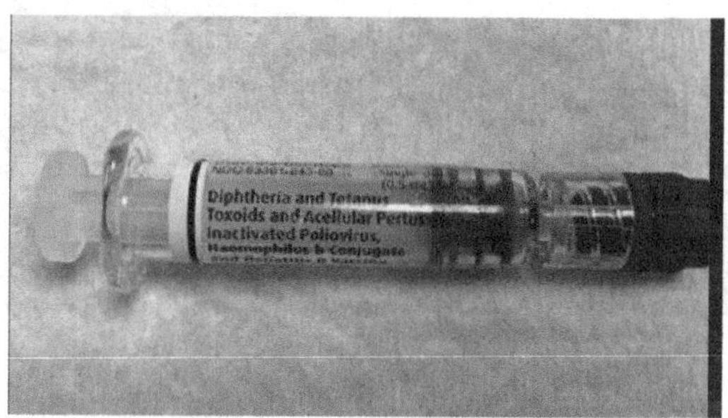

Figure 144. Diphtheria, Tetanus, Pertussis, Poliovirus, Hemophilus "vaccine." AM Medical.[256]

This next injection that I analyzed created an enormous number of filaments and structures in a short amount of time. Here is the initial view, with similar findings of coagulated particulate matter that appears to be a hydrogel substance:

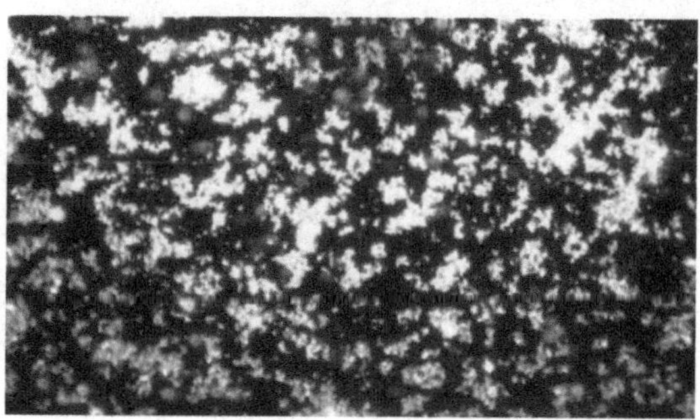

Figure 145. Diphtheria, Tetanus, Pertussis, Poliovirus, Hemophilus "vaccine" – hydrogel self-assembly. Magnification 100x. AM Medical.[257]

After a few minutes, classic hydrogel filaments are seen that have self-assembled:

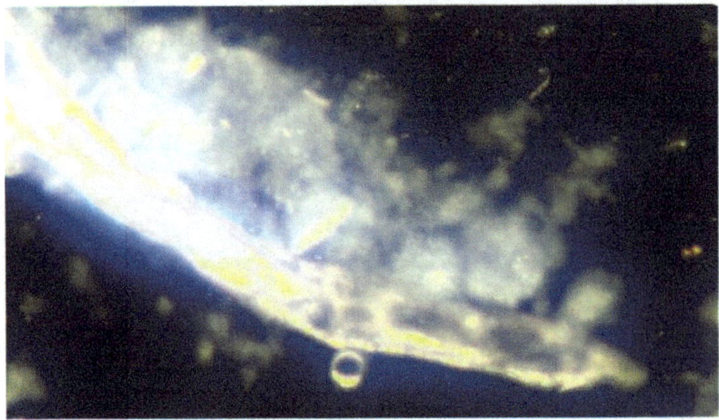

Figure 146. Diphtheria, Tetanus, Pertussis, Poliovirus, Hemophilus "vaccine" – hydrogel filament self-assembly. Magnification 400x. AM Medical.[258]

One can see very small nanobots/quantum dots that are mobile and moving extremely fast in the video footage. Here is another snapshot:

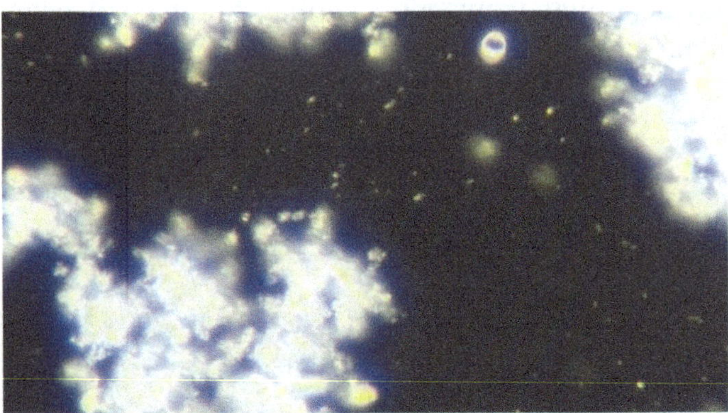

Figure 147. Diphtheria, Tetanus, Pertussis, Poliovirus, Hemophilus "vaccine" – hydrogel self-assembly and quantum dot nano- and microrobots. Magnification 400x. AM Medical.[259]

In these images, very small spheres and blinking lights can again be seen:

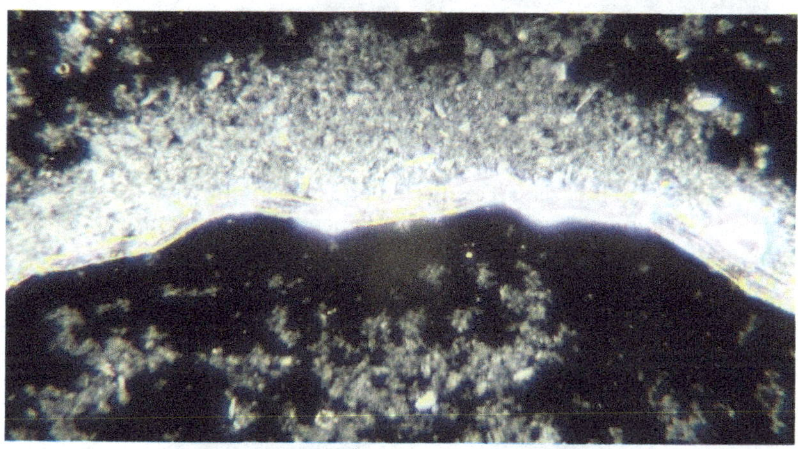

Figure 148. Diphtheria, Tetanus, Pertussis, Poliovirus, Hemophilus "vaccine" – hydrogel self-assembly filament. Magnification 200x. AM Medical.[260]

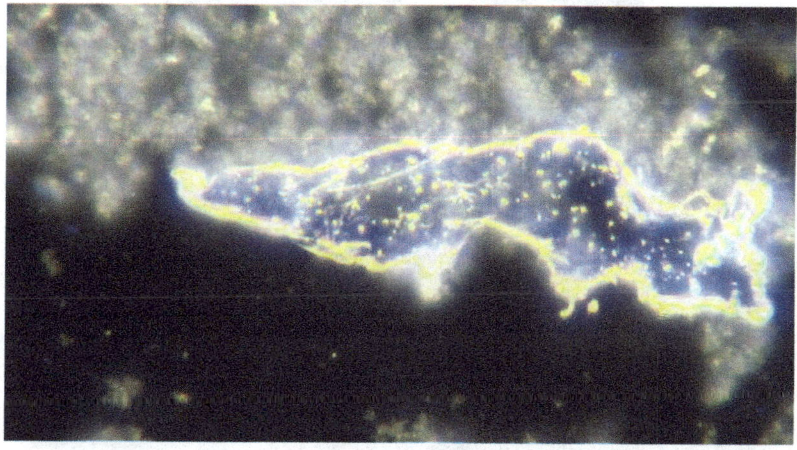

Figure 149. Diphtheria, Tetanus, Pertussis, Poliovirus, Hemophilus "vaccine" – hydrogel self-assembly filament which contains quantum dot nano- and microrobots. Magnification 400x. AM Medical.[261]

Classic self-assembly hydrogel filaments are seen below:

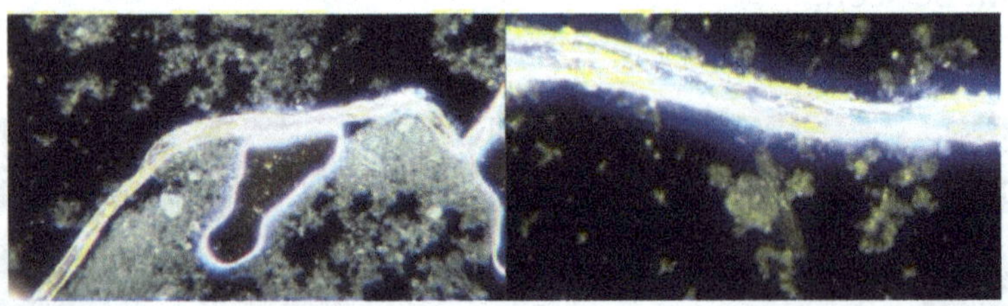

Figure 150. Diphtheria, Tetanus, Pertussis, Poliovirus, Hemophilus "vaccine" – hydrogel self-assembly filament. Left: Magnification 100x. Right: 400x. AM Medical.[262]

Spherical construction sites of hydrogel are also seen:

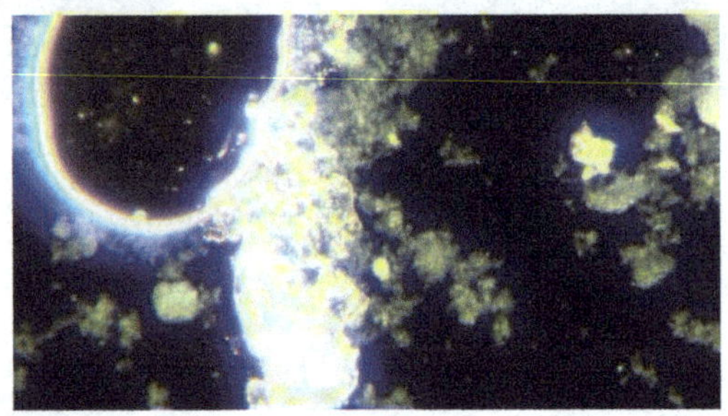

Figure 151. Diphtheria, Tetanus, Pertussis, Poliovirus, Hemophilus "vaccine" – hydrogel self-assembly polymer and construction sphere. Magnification 400x. AM Medical.[263]

A polymer, mesh-like pattern also evolved:

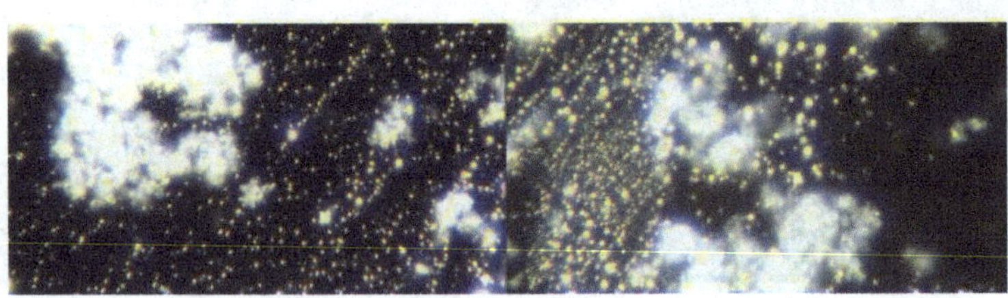

Figure 152. Diphtheria, Tetanus, Pertussis, Poliovirus, Hemophilus "vaccine" – hydrogel self-assembly polymer mesh network. Left: Magnification 200x. Right: 400x. AM Medical.[264]

This Diphtheria "vaccine" sample has now formed a classical hydrogel mesogen structure with many quantum dot nano- and microrobots that have self-assembled:

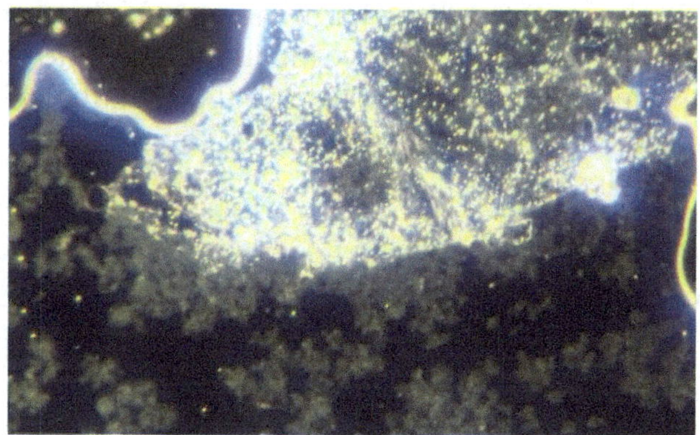

Figure 153. Diphtheria, Tetanus, Pertussis, Poliovirus, Hemophilus "vaccine" – hydrogel self-assembly polymer mesh network. Left: Magnification 200x. Right: 400x. AM Medical.[265]

The filaments are what we have classically seen in human blood, other medications, and rainwater from geoengineering operations:

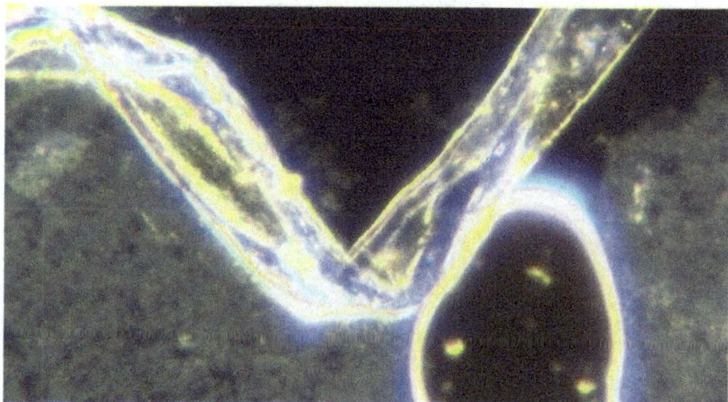

Figure 154. Diphtheria, Tetanus, Pertussis, Poliovirus, Hemophilus "vaccine" – self-assembly filament with spherical construction site and surrounding hydrogel. Magnification 400x. AM Medical.[266]

So far, all "vaccines" analyzed are filled with biotechnology poison. Childhood "vaccines" are loaded with nanotechnology and synthetic biology. Those who administer this poison need to be investigated and held accountable. I do not give any type of "vaccine" weapons to kill or harm anyone. If this was a sane world, I would not be on the investigation list, while the people who really are committing crimes via the "healthcare" system would be tried like the Nazi criminals in Germany.

That day is coming.

Meningococcus "Vaccine" for Children – Darkfield Microscopy Shows Self-Assembled Hydrogel Filaments

AUGUST 30, 2023[267]

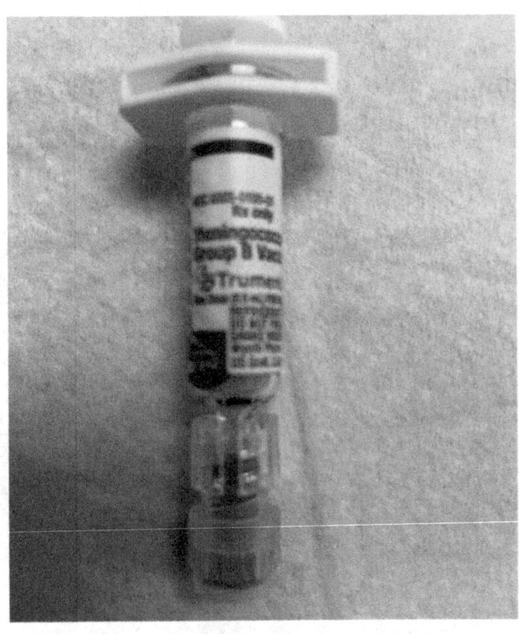

Figure 155. Meningococcal group B "vaccine." AM Medical.[268]

I want to do what I can to help alert people with information that they cannot otherwise get and that might harm them significantly. The harm to children by vaccination is especially disturbing. Investigating these injectables is extremely important, while having consistency in the methods of observation gives comparable imagery that is confirmation of an injustice that can be presented in any litigation.

In looking at the Meningococcal group B "vaccine," I placed a drop on a microscopy slide. Similar background debris substances appeared as in the previous medications analyzed. Initially, no filaments were present, but they did develop, as shown below. Classic spheres that are the construction sites for filaments were also seen.

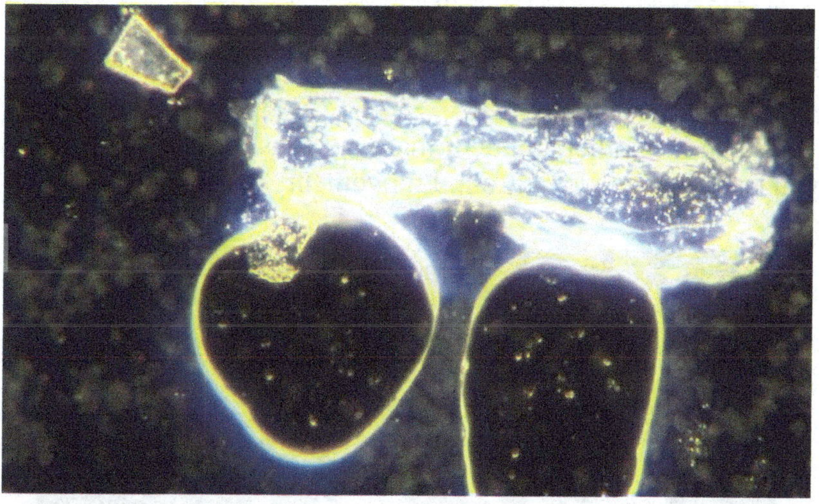

Figure 156. Meningococcal group B "vaccine" – hydrogel filament and construction sites. Magnification 400x. AM Medical.[269]

Below you can see a "hydrogel island" being constructed:

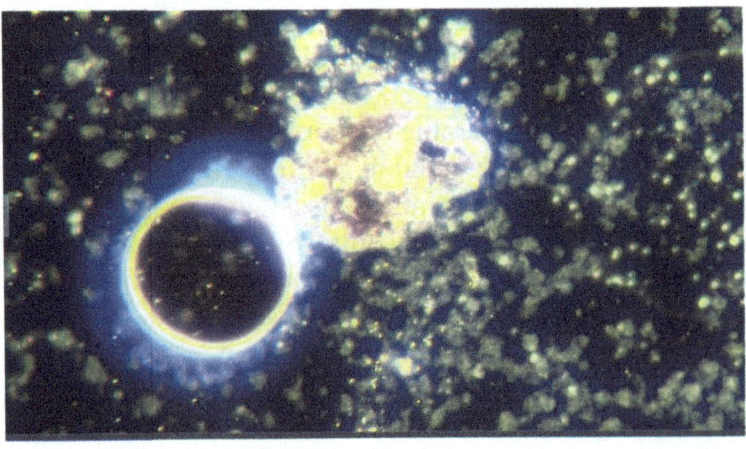

Figure 157. Meningococcal group B "vaccine" – hydrogel, micellar spherical construction site, and mesogen-like structure. Magnification 200x. AM Medical.[270]

Here is another filament that was constructed; in the video you can see some background movement:

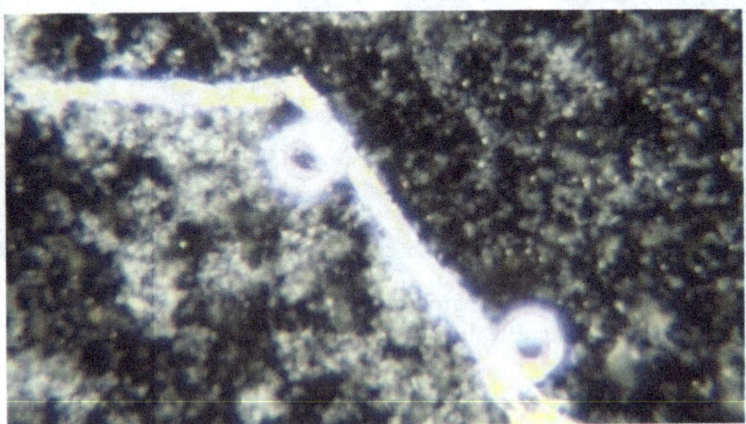

Figure 158. Meningococcal group B "vaccine" – hydrogel filament was self-assembled. Magnification 100x. AM Medical.[271]

In this next image, you can see a few of the blinking lights I call quantum dots that are involved in construction. I did not see swarms of them as in other medications, but I did see a few:

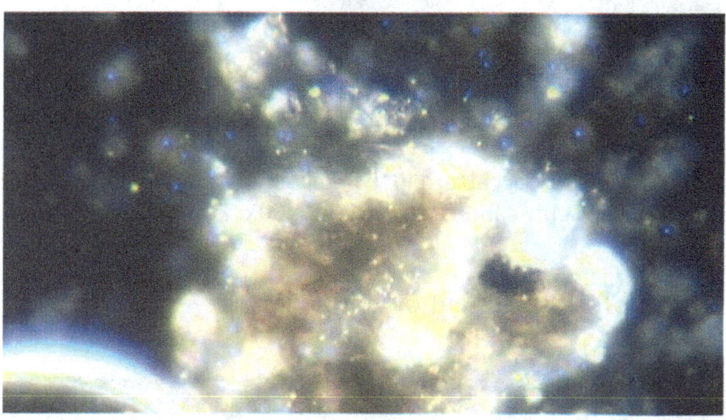

Figure 159. Meningococcal group B "vaccine" – hydrogel, bluish quantum dot microrobots, and mesogen-like structure. Magnification 2000x. AM Medical.[272]

After a few minutes on the slide, further "islands" of hydrogel developed:

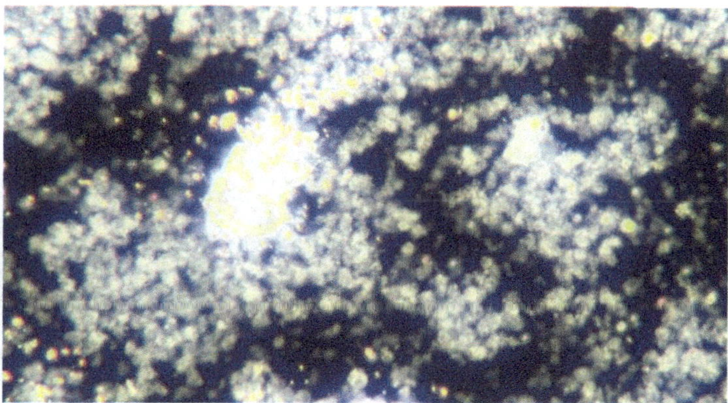

Figure 160. Meningococcal group B "vaccine" – hydrogel polymer self-assembly. Magnification 400x. AM Medical.[273]

Some of these "islands" looked quite solid:

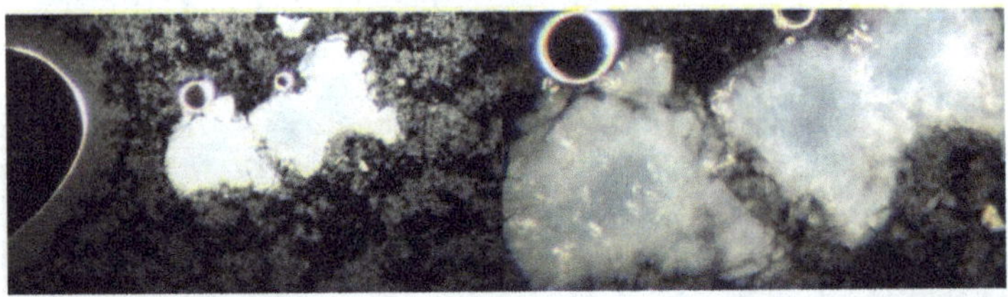

Figure 161. Meningococcal group B "vaccine" – hydrogel polymer self-assembly. Left: Magnification 200x. Right: 400x. AM Medical.[274]

Here a bluish filament developed:

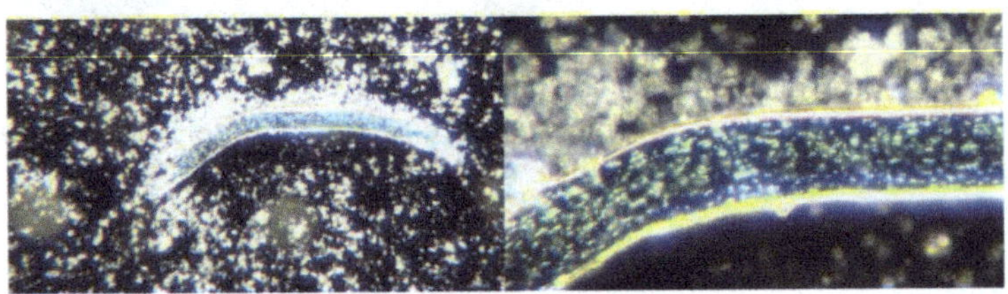

Figure 162. Meningococcal group B "vaccine" – hydrogel polymer self-assembly. Left: Magnification 200x. Right: 2000x. AM Medical.[275]

Over a short period of time a different filament developed. No filaments were initially present, they developed on the slide within minutes:

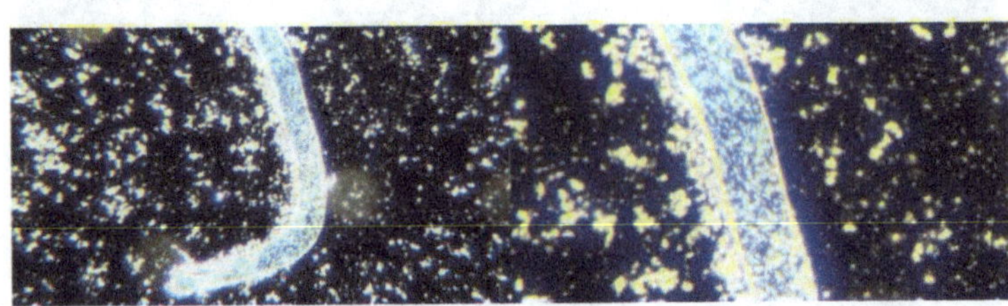

Figure 163. Meningococcal group B "vaccine" – hydrogel polymer self-assembly. Left: Magnification 200x. Right: 400x. AM Medical.[276]

To compare, below is a live blood analysis image of someone with bluish filaments that did not have the Meningococcal "vaccine." I consider the blue filaments a clear indication of nanotechnology. Blue fibers should not be in any "vaccine" nor in human blood. You can see the filaments look identical in both the "vaccine" (Figures 162 - 163) and unvaccinated blood (Figure 164).

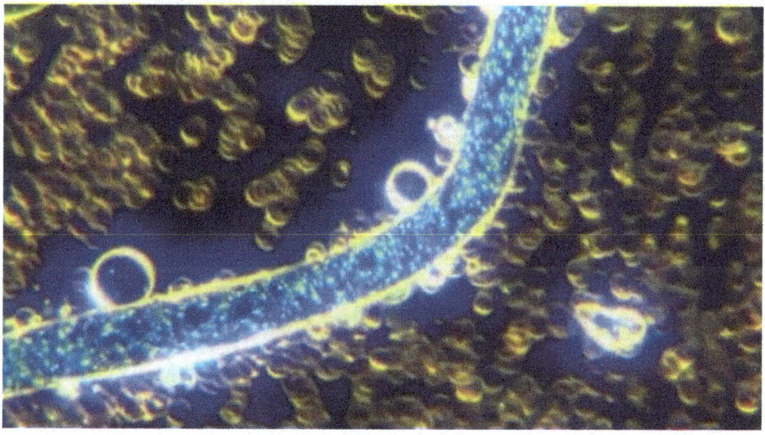

Figure 164. COVID 19 unvaccinated blood self-assembly polymer filament. Magnification 400x. AM Medical.[277]

I continue to show pharmaceutical injectables that clearly have self-assembly features and are the same nanotechnological structures we see in live blood. They are the same filaments we see in rainwater as we are being poisoned from illegal geoengineering operations. The fact that this "vaccine" is injected into small children is very concerning. People are always worried about being labelled "anti-vaxxers." I am so beyond that silly PSYOP label. I am anti-poison. I am anti-genocide. I am anti-making-people-sick so Big Pharma can profit off you!

ALL PHARMACEUTICAL INJECTABLES NEED TO BE LOOKED AT AND INVESTIGATED.

Darkfield Microscopy of Pneumococcal "Vaccine" Prevnar 13 Shows Quantum Dot Structures and Self-Assembly

AUGUST 29, 2023[278]

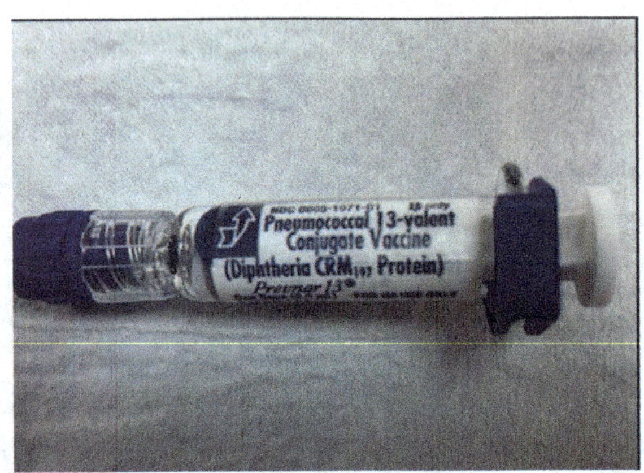

Figure 165. Pneumococcal and diphtheria "vaccine." AM Medical.[279]

Initial observation of the Pneumococcal 13-valent diphtheria conjugate "vaccine" showed the same hydrogel polymer as seen in other "vaccines":

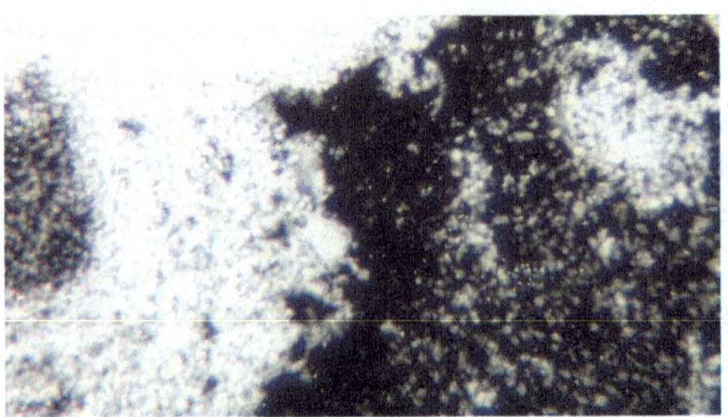

Figure 166. Pneumococcal and diphtheria "vaccine" – hydrogel and microrobots present. Magnification 200x. AM Medical.[280]

There was a similar hydrogel build up with spherical construction:

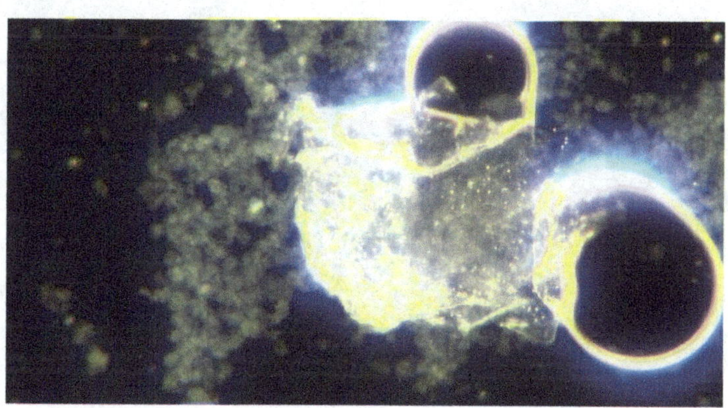

Figure 167. Pneumococcal and diphtheria "vaccine" – spherical construction sites and hydrogel polymer with microrobots present. Magnification 400x. AM Medical.[281]

At 400x magnification, quantum dots were seen as blinking lights with self-assembly of hydrogel-like substance. This hydrogel self-assembly video filmed in motion is available on my Substack:[282]

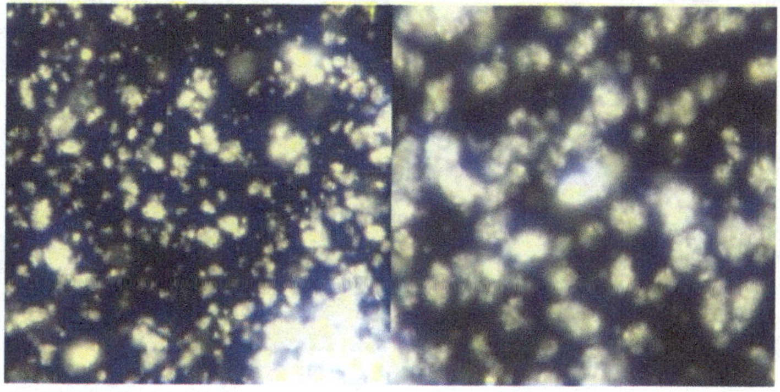

Figure 168. Pneumococcal and diphtheria "vaccine." Left: Magnification 400x. Right: 2000x. AM Medical.[283]

Filament structures formed as seen in live blood analysis:

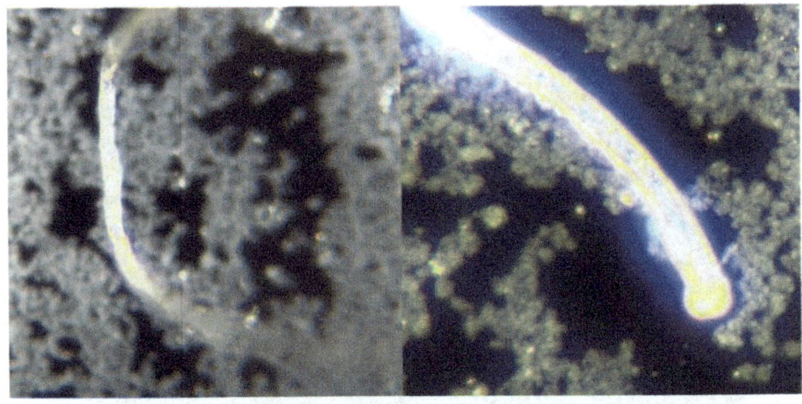

Figure 169. Pneumococcal and diphtheria "vaccine" – hydrogel self-assembly filaments. Left: Magnification 200x. Right: 400x. AM Medical.[284]

Quantum dot-like blinking lights were seen as well as small spherical vesicles:

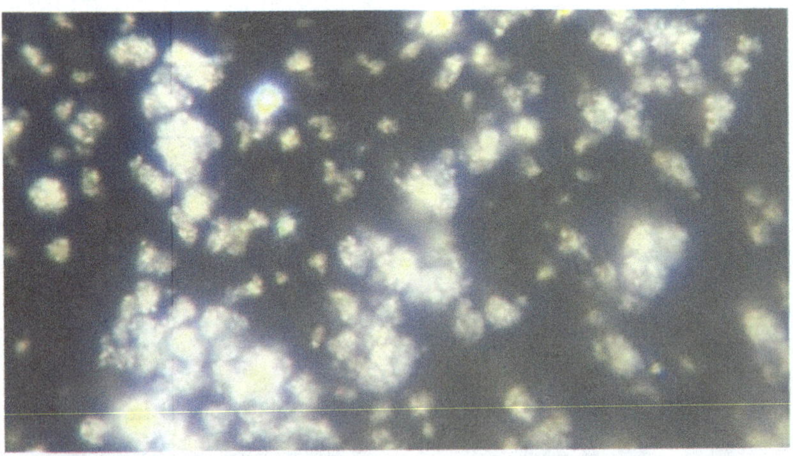

Figure 170. Pneumococcal and diphtheria "vaccine" – light-emitting quantum dots. Left: Magnification 400x. Right: 400x. AM Medical.[285]

In this video one can see that the small spheres are building similar hydrogel structures as witnessed in other "vaccine," blood, and environmental analyses:

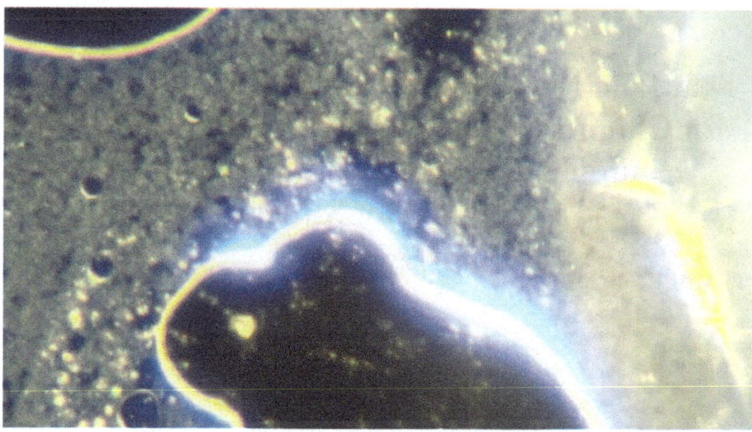

Figure 171. Pneumococcal and diphtheria "vaccine" – classical micellar construction sites. Magnification 400x. AM Medical.[286]

Eventually, crystallization develops:

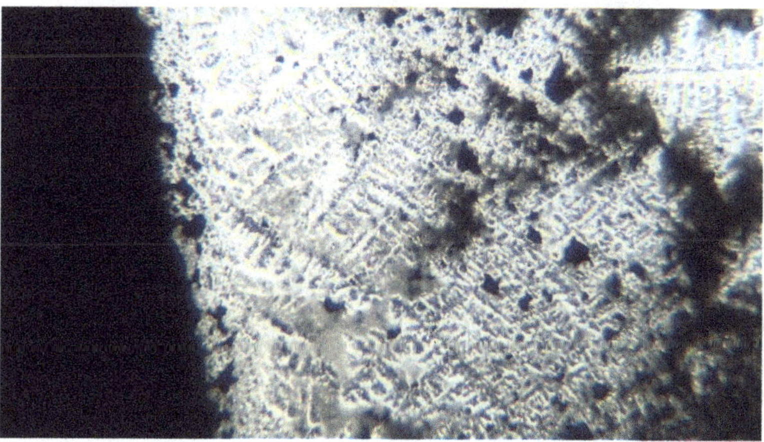

Figure 172. Pneumococcal and diphtheria "vaccine" – symmetric hydrogel crystallization. Magnification 400x. AM Medical.[287]

The pneumococcal and diphtheria "vaccine" analysis showed similar features of blinking quantum dots and self-assembly hydrogel with some filament structures. Once again, I ask, why are we subjecting young children to such poisons?

Darkfield Microscopy of Hepatitis A "Vaccine" for Children 2 Years and Older Shows Classic Hydrogel Filaments, Self-Assembly, and Quantum Dot Structures

SEPTEMBER 14, 2023[288]

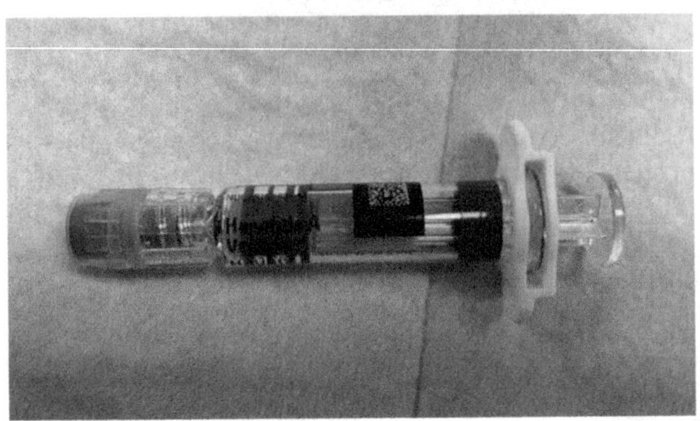

Figure 173. Hepatitis A "vaccine." AM Medical.[289]

In this ongoing investigation of childhood "vaccines," the next to be analyzed was the Hepatitis A "vaccine." The microscopic structures seen are like all other "vaccines." In the video microscopy evaluation, blinking lights consistent with the same quantum dot microrobots are easily identified. The granular material accumulates over time to build classic filaments and hydrogel structures.

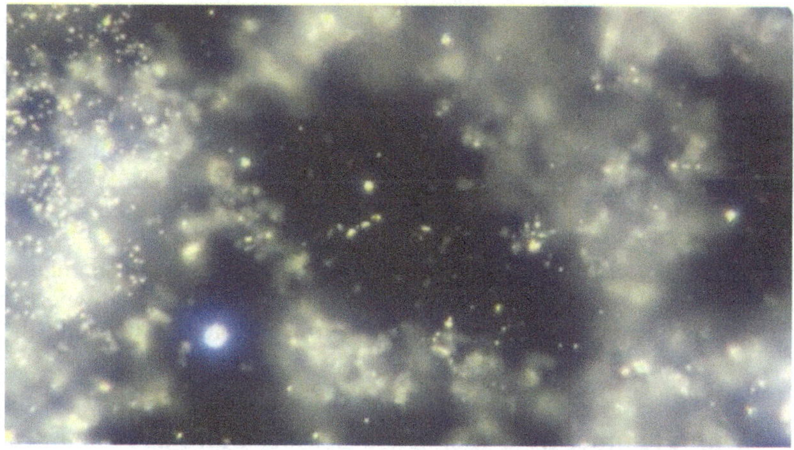

Figure 174. Hepatitis A "vaccine" – hydrogel and blinking quantum dot microrobots. AM Medical.[290]

Below are filament structures that self-assembled from the hydrogel substrate. Observation time was about 20 minutes to build these filaments. None of them were present when the drop was initially put on the microscope slide:

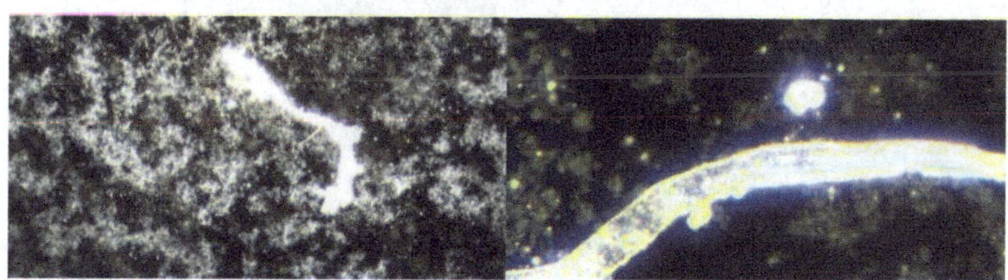

Figure 175. Hepatitis A "vaccine" – self-assembled filaments. Left: Magnification 100x. Right: 400x. AM Medical.[291]

Further classical filament self-assembly and spherical construction site with polymer growth developed:

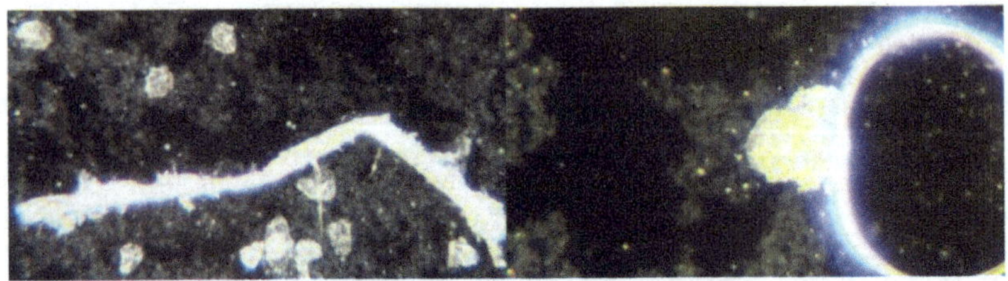

Figure 176. Hepatitis A "vaccine." Left: Self-assembled filament. Magnification 200x. Right: Spherical construction site creating polymer with surrounding quantum dot microrobots. Magnification 400x. AM Medical.[292]

Multiple other hydrogel self-assembly build ups occurred:

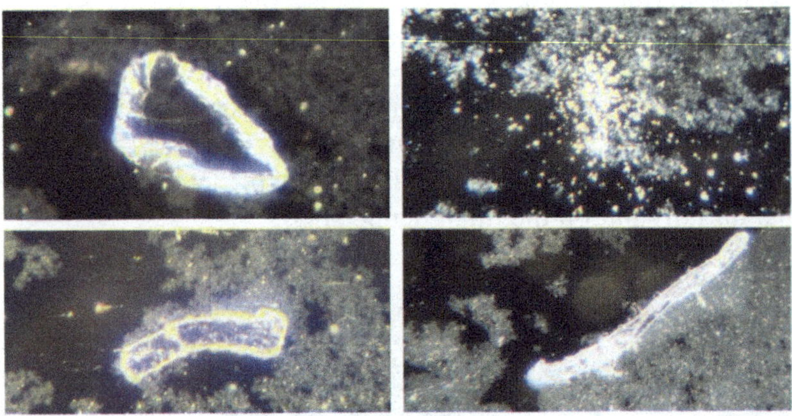

Figure 177. Hepatitis A "vaccine." Left upper: Polymer with surrounding microrobots. Magnification 400x. Left lower: Self-assembled filament. Magnification 200x. Right upper: Agglomeration of quantum dot microrobots. Magnification 200x. Right lower: Self-assembled filament. Magnification 200x. AM Medical.[293]

Again, we find consistency in the self-assembly of classical filaments we see in the blood, with some quantum dots in these "vaccines" also captured on film. All vaccines are contributing to humanity's blood contamination with these self-assembling, hydrogel, and biosensing quantum dot structures.

As a physician, I am horrified by this information. I want everyone in the world to see this, this is not normal. There is undeniable evidence. This is the transhumanist AI agenda in full force. The so-called "vaccines" must be stopped. This is being injected into children and good people who know nothing about the diabolical agenda behind the shots. There is so much irrefutable information now, and all those responsible need to be held accountable.

Read this book again. Look at the images. Read my second volume of *TransHuman: Overcoming the Global Depopulation Agenda*, and study the solutions provided.

The COVID 19 bioweapon and other "vaccines" were injected into 68% of the world population.

My heart goes out to those who have this in their body. Do something, share this information, speak up. Save humanity. Thank you.

About The Author

Dr. Ana Maria Mihalcea, MD, PhD, is a board-certified internal medicine physician with a PhD in pathology and over 24 years of clinical experience.

Dr. Mihalcea is President of AM Medical, LLC, located in Yelm, Washington, an anti-aging clinic dedicated to the reversal of all diseases, and author of the award-winning title *Light Medicine: A New Paradigm – The Science of Light, Spirit, and Longevity*. (www.arthemasophiapublishing.com)

She is also the founder of Tru Blu Medical and developer of Blue Light Wellness wraps that incorporate blue light therapy for home use. (www.trublumedical.com)

To follow her many research updates and recommended treatments visit her website. (https://www.dranamihalcea.com)

Dr. Mihalcea writes the *Humanity United Now* Substack newsletter, a forum for discussing topics such as the dangers of C19 injectables, long COVID, vax injury reversal, self-assembling nanotechnology, geoengineering, live blood analysis, and more. (https://anamihalceamdphd.substack.com/)

Her research field is C19 vaccine shedding, therapeutic approaches, including metal detoxification, and disabling self-assembling nanotechnology.

Dr. Mihalcea has a weekly show on CloutHub called: *Truth, Science, and Spirit*.
(https://clouthub.com/c/TruthScienceSpiritwithDrAnaMihalcea)

And you can also find information on her Rumble channel.
(https://rumble.com/c/HumanityUnitedNow)

Currently, she serves on the Board of Directors for the National American Renaissance Movement.
(https://nationalarm.org/board/)

She is also an Advisor for Targeted Justice.
(https://www.targetedjustice.com/)

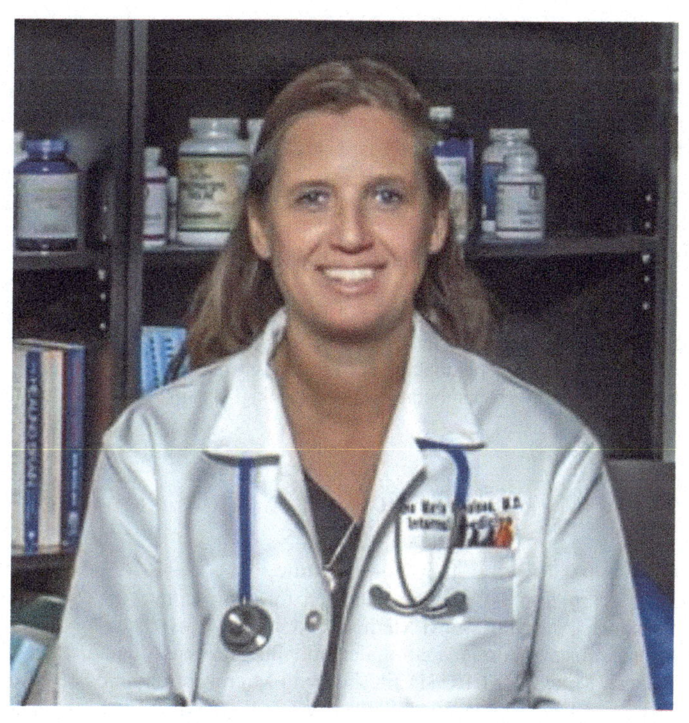

REFERENCES

Foreword

1. Becker, S. "Nanotechnology in the marketplace: how the nanotechnology industry views risk." *J Nanopart Res* 15, 1426 (2013). https://doi.org/10.1007/s11051-013-1426-7
2. Rawat, J., Kumar, V., Ahlawat, P. *et al.* "Current Trends on the Effects of Metal-Based Nanoparticles on Microbial Ecology." *Appl Biochem Biotechnol* 195, 6168–6182 (2023). https://doi.org/10.1007/s12010-023-04386-0
3. https://assets.modernatx.com/m/197fe68e2047ca6a/original/US10703789.pdf
4. https://patentscope.wipo.int/search/en/detail.jsf?docId=WO2012148684
5. https://karenkingston.substack.com/p/the-biorevolution-of-humanity
6. https://en.wikipedia.org/wiki/Deployment_of_COVID-19_vaccines
7. https://karenkingston.substack.com/p/excess-mortality-caused-by-vaccination
8. https://karenkingston.substack.com/p/is-rfk-jr-the-presidential-candidate

Chapter 1
My Collaboration with Clifford Carnicom

1. Carnicom, Clifford E. Carnicom Institute. https://carnicominstitute.org/author/clifford-carnicom/. Accessed June 5, 2024.
2. Mihalcea, Ana Maria. AM Medical LLC. https://substack.com/@anamihalceamdphd. Accessed June 6, 2024.
3. Adams, Mike. "EXCLUSIVE: Shocking Microscopy Photos of Blood Clots Extracted from Those Who 'Suddenly Died' – Crystalline Structures, Nanowires, Chalky Particles and Fibrous Structures." *Natural News*, June 12, 2022. https://naturalnews.com/2022-06-12-blood-clots-microscopy-suddenly-died.html. Accessed June 6, 2024.
4. Adams, Mike. *Self-Assembling 'Clot' Analysis*; Telegram, 2022. https://t.me/RealHealthRanger.
5. Mihalcea, Ana Maria. *Amyloid and Hydrogel Formation of a Peptide Sequence from a Coronavirus Spike Protein.* Substack, November 27, 2022. https://anamihalceamdphd.substack.com/p/amyloid-and-hydrogel-formation-of. Accessed June 6, 2024.
6. Carnicom, Clifford E. Carnicom Institute, August 28, 2022. https://carnicominstitute.org/blood-alterations-iii-transformation/
7. Ibid.
8. Mihalcea, Ana Maria. AM Medical LLC, December 27, 2022. https://anamihalceamdphd.substack.com/p/synthetic-biological-life-forms-cross
9. Mihalcea, Ana Maria. *Light Medicine: A New Paradigm - The Science of Light, Spirit, and Longevity*. Arthema Sophia Publishing, Yelm, WA, 2021. http://arthemasophiapublishing.com

10. Mihalcea, Ana Maria. *Unvaccinated Blood Unrecognizable After Application of Low Level Electrical Current and Structures Rapidly Grow – Clifford Carnicom's Findings Confirmed.* Substack, March 19, 2023. https://anamihalceamdphd.substack.com/p/unvaccinated-blood-unrecognizable. Accessed June 6, 2024.
11. Carnicom, Clifford E. *Blood Alterations: A Six Part Series*. Carnicom Institute, August – October, 2022. https://carnicominstitute.org/blood-alterations-a-six-part-series/. Accessed June 6, 2024.
12. Carnicom, Clifford E. Carnicom Institute, August 28, 2022. https://carnicominstitute.org/blood-alterations-iii-transformation/
13. Burns, Alice. *As Recommendations for Isolation End, How Common is Long COVID?* KFF, April 9, 2024. www.kff.org/coronavirus-covid-19/issue-brief/as-recommendations-for-isolation-end-how-common-is-long-covid. Accessed June 6, 2024.
14. Carnicom, Clifford E. Carnicom Institute, August 28, 2022. https://carnicominstitute.org/blood-alterations-iii-transformation/
15. Mihalcea, Ana Maria. AM Medical LLC, March 19, 2023. https://anamihalceamdphd.substack.com/p/unvaccinated-blood-unrecognizable
16. Mihalcea, Ana Maria and Clifford E. Carnicom. *Unvaccinated Blood: Recurrent New Proof of (CDB) Filaments Growing Under Exposure of Extremely Low Electrical Currents*. Substack, March 25, 2024. https://anamihalceamdphd.substack.com/p/unvaccinated-blood-recurrent-new. Accessed June 6, 2024.
17. Carnicom, Clifford E. *Blood Alterations: A Six Part Series*. Carnicom Institute, August – October, 2022. https://carnicominstitute.org/blood-alterations-a-six-part-series/. Accessed June 6, 2024.
18. Carnicom, Clifford E. Carnicom Institute. Substack, May 2, 2023. https://anamihalceamdphd.substack.com/p/replication-of-electrical-transformation?utm_source=publication-search
19. Carnicom, Clifford E. *A Mechanism of Blood Damage.* Carnicom Institute, December 14, 2009. https://carnicominstitute.org/a-mechanism-of-blood-damage/. Accessed June 6, 2024.
20. Ibid.
21. Carnicom, Clifford E. *CDB: Growth Progressions.* June 13, 2014. https://carnicominstitute.org/cdb-growth-progressions/
22. Carnicom, Clifford E. Carnicom Institute. Substack, March 25, 2023. https://anamihalceamdphd.substack.com/p/unvaccinated-blood-recurrent-new?utm_source=publication-search
23. Carnicom, Clifford E. *Blood Alterations: A Six Part Series*. Carnicom Institute, August – October 2022. https://carnicominstitute.org/blood-alterations-a-six-part-series/. Accessed June 6, 2024.
24. Carnicom, Clifford E. Carnicom Institute. Substack, March 25, 2023. https://anamihalceamdphd.substack.com/p/unvaccinated-blood-recurrent-new?utm_source=publication-search
25. Ibid.
26. Ibid.

27. Martin, Delgado Ricardo. La Quinta Columna. Substack, March 25, 2023. https://anamihalceamdphd.substack.com/p/unvaccinated-blood-recurrent-new?utm_source=publication-search
28. Carnicom, Clifford E. Carnicom Institute, Substack, March 25, 2022. https://carnicominstitute.org/blood-alterations-iii-transformation/
29. Mihalcea, Ana Maria. *There is No Isolated Virus. Then What Makes People Sick? Electromagnetic Frequency of Living Organisms – Considering the Science of the Future*. Substack, August 19, 2022. https://anamihalceamdphd.substack.com/p/there-is-no-isolated-virus-then-what. Accessed June 6, 2024.
30. Mihalcea, Ana Maria. *A Biophysical Understanding of Vaccine Shedding and Self-disseminating Vaccines in Populations*. Substack, July 29, 2022. https://anamihalceamdphd.substack.com/p/a-biophysical-understanding-of-vaccine. Accessed June 6, 2024.
31. Mihalcea, Ana Maria and Clifford E. Carnicom. *Unvaccinated vs Vaccinated Blood Comparison – Infrared Spectroscopy and Electrical Conductivity Studies*. Substack, March 27, 2023. https://anamihalceamdphd.substack.com/p/unvaccinated-vs-vaccinated-blood. Accessed June 6, 2024.
32. Carnicom, Clifford E. Carnicom Institute. Substack, March 27, 2023. https://anamihalceamdphd.substack.com/p/unvaccinated-vs-vaccinated-blood?utm_source=publication-search
33. Ibid.
34. Carnicom, Clifford E. *Human Blood vs. Synthetic Blood: The Path to the Blood Clot*. Carnicom Institute, December 14, 2023. www.carnicominstitute.org/human-blood-vs-synthetic-blood-the-path-to-the-blood-clot/. Accessed June 6, 2024.
35. Carnicom, Clifford E. Carnicom Institute. Substack, March 27, 2023. https://anamihalceamdphd.substack.com/p/unvaccinated-vs-vaccinated-blood?utm_source=publication-search
36. Ibid.
37. Ibid.
38. Mihalcea, Ana Maria. *Blood Cultures of Unvaccinated Blood Shows Extensive (CDB) Filament Development After 2 Weeks Incubation.* Substack, April 8, 2023. https://anamihalceamdphd.substack.com/p/blood-cultures-of-unvaccinated-blood. Accessed June 6, 2024.
39. Carnicom, Clifford E. Carnicom Institute. Substack, April 8, 2023. https://anamihalceamdphd.substack.com/p/blood-cultures-of-unvaccinated-blood?utm_source=publication-search
40. Ibid.
41. Tailliez, Bernard. *Qualité & Hygiène* Industrielles – *Respect de l'Environnement*: *RAPPORT ANALYTIQUE*. Substack, April 7, 2023. https://anamihalceamdphd.substack.com/p/chemical-analysis-comparison-of-hydrogel
42. Carnicom, Clifford E. Carnicom Institute. Substack, April 8, 2023. https://anamihalceamdphd.substack.com/p/blood-cultures-of-unvaccinated-blood?utm_source=publication-search
43. Ibid.

44. Ibid.
45. Ibid.
46. Ibid.
47. Ibid.
48. Ibid.
49. Mihalcea, Ana Maria. *Extensive (CDB) Hydrogel Filament Growth in C19 Vaccinated and Unvaccinated Blood Cultures After One Week of Incubation*. Substack, April 9, 2023, https://anamihalceamdphd.substack.com/p/extensive-cdb-hydrogel-filament-growth. Accessed June 6, 2024.
50. Carnicom, Clifford E. Carnicom Institute. Substack, April 9, 2023. https://anamihalceamdphd.substack.com/p/extensive-cdb-hydrogel-filament-growth?utm_source=publication-search
51. Ibid.
52. Ibid.
53. Ibid.
54. Ibid.
55. Ibid.
56. Yanowitz, Shimon. Substack, April 9, 2023. https://anamihalceamdphd.substack.com/p/extensive-cdb-hydrogel-filament-growth?utm_source=publication-search
57. Ibid.
58. Ibid.
59. Palmer, Michael and Jonathan Gilthorpe. *COVID-19 mRNA Vaccines Contain Excessive Quantities of Bacterial DNA: Evidence and Implications*. Doctors for COVID Ethics, April 5, 2024. https://doctors4covidethics.org/covid-19-mrna-vaccines-contain-excessive-quantities-of-bacterial-dna-evidence-and-implications/. Accessed June 6, 2024.
60. Mihalcea, Ana Maria. *Evidence of Impaired Electrical Blood Conductivity, Iron Oxidation and Reduced Oxygen Transport Capacity in The Post C19 Injection Era*. Substack, April 16, 2023. https://anamihalceamdphd.substack.com/p/evidence-of-impaired-electrical-blood. Accessed June 6, 2024.
61. Mihalcea, Ana Maria. AM Medical LLC, April 16, 2023. https://anamihalceamdphd.substack.com/p/evidence-of-impaired-electrical-blood?utm_source=publication-search
62. Carnicom, Clifford E. *Morgellons: A Thesis*. Carnicom Institute, October 15, 2011. https://carnicominstitute.org/morgellons-a-thesis/ Accessed June 6, 2024.
63. Imlay, James. *Fe-Bacteria*. Society for Redox Biology and Medicine (SFRBM). https://sfrbm.org/site/assets/documents/frs/ImlayFeBacteria.pdf
64. Carnicom, Clifford E. Carnicom Institute. Substack, April 16, 2023. https://anamihalceamdphd.substack.com/p/evidence-of-impaired-electrical-blood?utm_source=publication-search
65. Carnicom, Clifford E. *Morgellons: A Thesis*. Carnicom Institute, October 15, 2011. https://carnicominstitute.org/morgellons-a-thesis/. Accessed June 6, 2024.
66. Ibid.

67. Carnicom, Clifford E. *Carnicom Institute Laboratory Notebooks*. Carnicom Institute. https://carnicominstitute.org/carnicom-institute-laboratory-notebooks/. Accessed June 6, 2024.
68. Carnicom, Clifford E. *Carnicom Institute Legacy Project: A Release of Internal Original Research Documents.* Laboratory Notes Series: Volume 10, May 2015 – August 2015. https://carnicominstitute.org/laboratory_notebooks_html/ci_legacy_lab_notes_10.html.
69. Carnicom, Clifford E. Carnicom Institute. Substack, April 16, 2023. https://anamihalceamdphd.substack.com/p/evidence-of-impaired-electrical-blood?utm_source=publication-search
70. Zekry, Abdelhalim Abdelnaby. "What Values Should I Use for Permittivity & Electrical Conductivity of Blood?" *ResearchGate*, 2021. https://www.researchgate.net/post/What_values_should_I_use_for_Permittivity_Electrical_Conductivity_of_Blood. Accessed June 6, 2024.
71. Vedantu. *How Many Donor Atoms Are Present in EDTA?* https://www.vedantu.com/question-answer/donor-atoms-are-present-in-edta-class-12-chemistry-cbse-5f87cf40b39c3957d6fc06b2. Accessed June 6, 2024.
72. Department of Chemistry. *EDTA*. Purdue University. University, https://www.chem.purdue.edu/jmol/cchem/polys.html. Accessed June 6, 2024.
73. Mihalcea, Ana Maria. *Blood Conductivity and Electrical Impedance Spectroscopy – A New Model for Estimated Human Power Loss Shows Cause for Alarm.* Substack, June 25, 2023. https://anamihalceamdphd.substack.com/p/blood-conductivity-and-electrical. Accessed June 6, 2024.
74. Carnicom, Clifford E. Carnicom Institute. Substack, June 25, 2023. https://anamihalceamdphd.substack.com/p/blood-conductivity-and-electrical?utm_source=publication-search
75. Mihalcea, Ana Maria. AM Medical LLC, June 25, 2023. https://anamihalceamdphd.substack.com/p/blood-conductivity-and-electrical?utm_source=publication-search
76. Mihalcea, Ana Maria. *Light Medicine: A New Paradigm – The Science of Light, Spirit, and Longevity.* Arthema Sophia Publishing, Yelm, WA, 2021. http://arthemasophiapublishing.com
77. Mihalcea, Ana Maria. *Replication of Electrical Transformation of C19 Unvaccinated Blood – Filament Growth Documented – CDB Extraction and Isolation.* Substack, May 2, 2023. https://anamihalceamdphd.substack.com/p/replication-of-electrical-transformation. Accessed June 6, 2024.
78. Carnicom, Clifford E. Carnicom Institute. Substack, May 2, 2023. https://anamihalceamdphd.substack.com/p/replication-of-electrical-transformation?utm_source=publication-search
79. Mihalcea, Ana Maria. AM Medical LLC, May 2, 2023. https://anamihalceamdphd.substack.com/p/replication-of-electrical-transformation?utm_source=publication-search

REFERENCES

80. Mihalcea, Ana Maria. *Chemical Composition Analysis of Synthetic Biology Cross Domain Bacteria (CDB) aka Hydrogel/Graphene Filaments in Unvaccinated Blood.* Substack, May 8. 2023. https://anamihalceamdphd.substack.com/p/chemical-composition-analysis-of. Accessed June 6, 2024.
81. Mihalcea, Ana Maria. *Replication of Electrical Transformation of C19 Unvaccinated Blood – Filament Growth Documented – CDB Extraction and Isolation – Ana Mihalcea, MD, PhD in Conjunction with Clifford Carnicom.* Substack, May 2, 2023. https://anamihalceamdphd.substack.com/p/replication-of-electrical-transformation. Accessed June 6, 2024.
82. Carnicom, Clifford E. Carnicom Institute. Substack, May 8, 2023. https://anamihalceamdphd.substack.com/p/chemical-composition-analysis-of?utm_source=publication-search
83. Mihalcea, Ana Maria. AM Medical LLC, May 8, 2023. https://anamihalceamdphd.substack.com/p/chemical-composition-analysis-of?utm_source=publication-search
84. Carnicom, Clifford E. Carnicom Institute. Substack, May 8, 2023. https://anamihalceamdphd.substack.com/p/chemical-composition-analysis-of?utm_source=publication-search
85. Workman, Jerry, Jr. and Lois Weyer. *Practical Guide and Spectral Atlas for Interpretive Near Infrared Spectroscopy*. 2nd ed., CRC Press, 2012. https://doi.org/10.1201/b11894.
86. Carnicom, Clifford E. *Morgellons: A Working Hypothesis - Introduction.* Carnicom Institute, December 18, 2013. https://carnicominstitute.org/morgellons-a-working-hypothesis-introduction/. Accessed June 6, 2024.
87. Popov, I.A., Bozhenko, K.V., and Boldyrev, A.I. "Is Graphene Aromatic?" *Nano Research*, vol. 5, no. 2, 2012, pp. 117-123, https://doi.org/10.1007/s12274-011-0192-z.
88. Carnicom, Clifford E. *Blood Alterations IV: Protein Analysis*. Carnicom Institute, August 19, 2022. https://carnicominstitute.org/blood-alterations-iv-protein-analysis/. Accessed June 6, 2024.
89. Carnicom, Clifford E. *Environmental Filament Project: Metals Testing Laboratory Report.* Carnicom Institute, August 21, 2017. https://carnicominstitute.org/environmental-filament-project-metals-testing-laboratory-report/
90. Ibid.
91. Ibid.
92. Gatti, Antonietta M. and Stefano Montanari. "New Quality-Control Investigations on Vaccines: Micro- and Nanocontamination." *Journal of Vaccines and Vaccination*, vol. 4, 2017, n. pag.
93. Mihalcea, Ana Maria. AM Medical LLC, May 8, 2023. https://anamihalceamdphd.substack.com/p/chemical-composition-analysis-of?utm_source=publication-search
94. Carnicom, Clifford E. *A Toxicology Study*. Carnicom Institute, December 9, 2018. https://carnicominstitute.org/a-toxicology-study/. Accessed June 6, 2024.

95. Carnicom, Clifford E. *Morgellons Toxicity Continued Report.* Carnicom Institute, May 21, 2019. https://carnicominstitute.org/morgellons-toxicity-continued-report/. Accessed June 6, 2024.
96. Carnicom, Clifford E. *Bean Growth Report.* Carnicom Institute, October 3, 2017. https://carnicominstitute.org/bean-growth-report/. Accessed June 6, 2024.
97. Carnicom, Clifford E. *Mustard Seed Report: Growth Termination.* Carnicom Institute, September 24, 2017. https://carnicominstitute.org/mustard-seed-report-growth-termination/. Accessed June 6, 2024.
98. Carnicom, Clifford E. *Mustard Seed Germination: Initial Report.* Carnicom Institute, September 20, 2017. https://carnicominstitute.org/mustard-seed-germination-initial-report/. Accessed June 6, 2024.
99. Carnicom, Clifford E. *Yeast Deformation: Initial Report.* Carnicom Institute, September 22, 2017. https://carnicominstitute.org/yeast-deformation-initial-report/. Accessed June 6, 2024.
100. Mihalcea, Ana Maria. *Synthetic Biology Cross Domain Bacteria (CDB) NIR Fingerprint Match Found in Human Blood – Hydrogel Signatures Identified.* Substack, May 14, 2023. https://anamihalceamdphd.substack.com/p/synthetic-biology-cross-domain-bacteria. Accessed June 6, 2024.
101. Mihalcea, Ana Maria. *Chemical Composition Analysis of Synthetic Biology Cross Domain Bacteria (CDB) aka Hydrogel/graphene filaments in Unvaccinated Blood – Ana Mihalcea, MD, PhD in Conjunction with Clifford Carnicom.* Substack, May 8, 2023. https://anamihalceamdphd.substack.com/p/chemical-composition-analysis-of. Accessed June 6, 2024.
102. Carnicom, Clifford E. Carnicom Institute. Substack, May 14, 2023. https://anamihalceamdphd.substack.com/p/synthetic-biology-cross-domain-bacteria?utm_source=publication-search
103. Mihalcea, Ana Maria. *Chemical Analysis Comparison of Hydrogel Filaments from C19 Shots and Environmental Geoengineering Sources – Project What Happened to Humanity's Blood?* Substack, April 7, 2023. https://anamihalceamdphd.substack.com/p/chemical-analysis-comparison-of-hydrogel. Accessed June 6, 2024.
104. Malinova, V., *et al.* "Synthetic Biology, Inspired by Synthetic Chemistry." *ScienceDirect*, June 11, 2012. https://www.sciencedirect.com/science/article/pii/S001457931200419X. Accessed June 6, 2024.
105. Rutkin, Aviva. "Cyborg Rose Has Electric Circuits Running Through Polymer Veins." *New Scientist*, November 20, 2015. https://www.newscientist.com/article/dn28528-cyborg-rose-has-electric-circuits-running-through-polymer-veins/
106. Carnicom, Clifford E. Carnicom Institute. Substack, May 14, 2023. https://anamihalceamdphd.substack.com/p/synthetic-biology-cross-domain-bacteria?utm_source=publication-search
107. Mihalcea, Ana Maria. *Prospective Difference Between C19 Vaccinated and Unvaccinated Blood: Electromagnetic Observations, ELF Response and Potassium Metabolism.* Substack, June 26, 2023. https://anamihalceamdphd.substack.com/p/prospective-difference-between-c19. Accessed June 6, 2024.

REFERENCES

108. Carnicom, Clifford E. Carnicom Institute. Substack, June 26, 2023. https://anamihalceamdphd.substack.com/p/prospective-difference-between-c19?utm_source=publication-search
109. Carnicom, Clifford E. *A Connection: ELF – Satellites – HAARP – Aerosols.* Carnicom Institute, February 9, 2003. https://carnicominstitute.org/a-connection-elf-satellites-haarp-aerosols/. Accessed June 6, 2024.
110. Carnicom, Clifford E. *ELF 2005: Positive Identification.* Carnicom Institute, May 13, 2005. https://carnicominstitute.org/elf-2005-positive-identification/. Accessed June 6, 2024.
111. Carnicom, Clifford E. *Direction of ELF-VLF Energy Verified.* Carnicom Institute, March 29, 2003. https://carnicominstitute.org/direction-of-elf-vlf-energy-verified/. Accessed June 6, 2024.
112. Carnicom, Clifford E. *ELF Verified in Utah.* Carnicom Institute, March 23, 2003. https://carnicominstitute.org/elf-verified-in-utah/. Accessed June 6, 2024.
113. Carnicom, Clifford E. Carnicom Institute, 2003. https://carnicominstitute.org/elf-verified-in-utah/
114. Carnicom, Clifford E. *ELF & The Human Antenna.* Carnicom Institute, January 19, 2003. https://carnicominstitute.org/elf-the-human-antenna/ Accessed June 6, 2024.
115. Becker, Robert O. and Gary Selden. *The Body Electric: Electromagnetism and the Foundation of Life.* William Morrow and Company, 1985.
116. Carnicom, Clifford E. *Potassium Questions Intensify.* Carnicom Institute, June 8, 2005. https://carnicominstitute.org/potassium-questions-intensify/. Accessed June 6, 2024.
117. Mihalcea, Ana Maria. *Blood Clot Analysis From Living & Deceased Individuals Shows Consistent Findings: A Rubber Like Polymerized Protein – Microscopy Shows Filaments – Part 1 of 3.* Substack, July 10, 2023. https://anamihalceamdphd.substack.com/p/blood-clot-analysis-from-living-and. Accessed June 6, 2024.
118. Mihalcea, Ana Maria and Clifford E. Carnicom. AM Medical LLC and Carnicom Institute. Substack, July 10, 2023. https://anamihalceamdphd.substack.com/p/blood-clot-analysis-from-living-and?utm_source=publication-search
119. Carnicom, Clifford E. Carnicom Institute. Substack, July 10, 2023. https://anamihalceamdphd.substack.com/p/blood-clot-analysis-from-living-and?utm_source=publication-search
120. Ibid.
121. Ibid.
122. Ibid.
123. Mihalcea, Ana Maria. *Blood Clot Analysis from Living and Deceased Individuals Near Infrared Spectroscopy Shows Multiple Hydrogel Polymer Components – Part 2 of 3.* Substack, July 10, 2023. https://anamihalceamdphd.substack.com/p/blood-clot-analysis-from-living-and-98a. Accessed June 6, 2024.
124. Carnicom, Clifford E. Carnicom Institute. Substack, July 10, 2023. https://anamihalceamdphd.substack.com/p/blood-clot-analysis-from-living-and-98a?utm_source=publication-search
125. Ibid.

126. Ibid.
127. Fishbein, L. "Aromatic Amines. In: Anthropogenic Compounds." *The Handbook of Environmental Chemistry*, vol 3 / 3C. Springer, Berlin, Heidelberg, 1984. https://doi.org/10.1007/978-3-540-38819-7_1
128. Roberts, John D. and Marjorie C. Caserio. "Polymerization of Alkenes. " *LibreTexts*, California Institute of Technology. https://chem.libretexts.org/Bookshelves/Organic_Chemistry/Basic_Principles_of_Organic_Chemistry_(Roberts_and_Caserio)/10:_Alkenes_and_Alkynes_I_-_Ionic_and_Radical_Addition_Reactions/10.09:_Polymerization_of_Alkenes. Accessed June 6, 2024.
129. Jensen, Bettina E. B., *et al.* "Poly (vinyl alcohol) Physical Hydrogels: Matrix-Mediated Drug Delivery Using Spontaneously Eroding Substrate." *The Journal of Physical Chemistry*. B vol. 120,26 (2016): 5916-26. doi:10.1021/acs.jpcb.6b01381
130. Mihalcea, Ana Maria. *Blood Clot Analysis From Living And Deceased Individuals – Preliminary Chemical Solubility Testing – Part 3 of 3*. Substack, July 10, 2023. https://anamihalceamdphd.substack.com/p/blood-clot-analysis-from-living-and-58d. Accessed June 6, 2024.
131. Carnicom, Clifford E. Carnicom Institute. Substack, July 10, 2023. https://anamihalceamdphd.substack.com/p/blood-clot-analysis-from-living-and-58d?utm_source=publication-search
132. Ibid.
133. Ibid.
134. Ibid.
135. Mihalcea, Ana Maria. *Analysis of Symptomatic Health Findings in C19 Unvaccinated Individual Shows Hydrogel Signatures Matching Deceased Clots and Complete Absence of Water*. Substack, August 1, 2023. https://anamihalceamdphd.substack.com/p/analysis-of-symptomatic-health-findings. Accessed June 6, 2024.
136. Carnicom, Clifford E. Carnicom Institute. Substack, August 1, 2023. https://anamihalceamdphd.substack.com/p/analysis-of-symptomatic-health-findings?utm_source=publication-search
137. Carnicom, Clifford E. *Morgellons Research Project: Primary Symptom Survey Results*. Carnicom Institute, November 5, 2016. https://carnicominstitute.org/morgellons-research-project-primary-symptom-survey-results/. Accessed June 6, 2024.
138. Carnicom, Clifford E. Carnicom Institute. Substack, August 1, 2023. https://anamihalceamdphd.substack.com/p/analysis-of-symptomatic-health-findings?utm_source=publication-search
139. Mihalcea, Ana Maria and Clifford E. Carnicom. *Unvaccinated Blood: Recurrent New Proof of (CDB) Filaments Growing Under Exposure of Extremely Low Electrical Currents: Ana Maria Mihalcea MD, PhD in conjunction with Clifford Carnicom*. Substack, March 26, 2023. https://anamihalceamdphd.substack.com/p/unvaccinated-blood-recurrent-new. Accessed June 6, 2024.
140. Carnicom, Clifford E. Carnicom Institute. Substack, August 1. 2023. https://anamihalceamdphd.substack.com/p/analysis-of-symptomatic-health-findings?utm_source=publication-search

REFERENCES

141. Mihalcea, Ana Maria. *Synthetic Biology Cross Domain Bacteria (CDB) NIR Fingerprint Match Found in Human Blood – Hydrogel Signatures Identified – Ana Mihalcea MD, PhD in Conjunction with Clifford Carnicom.* Substack, May 15, 2023. https://anamihalceamdphd.substack.com/p/synthetic-biology-cross-domain-bacteria. Accessed June 6, 2024.
142. Carnicom, Clifford E. Carnicom Institute. Substack, August 1, 2023. https://anamihalceamdphd.substack.com/p/analysis-of-symptomatic-health-findings?utm_source=publication-search.
143. Mihalcea, Ana Maria. *Rubbery Clot Formation Shown in Living C19 Unvaccinated Person via Darkfield Microscopy – Hydrogel Replacing Blood.* Substack, July 21, 2023. https://anamihalceamdphd.substack.com/p/rubbery-clot-formation-shown-in-living. Accessed June 6, 2024.
144. Schauenburg, Dominik, Alberto Osuna Gálvez, and Jeffrey W. Bode. "Covalently Functionalized Amide Cross-Linked Hydrogels from Primary Amines and Polyethylene Glycol Acyltrifluoroborates (PEG-KATs)." *Journal of Materials Chemistry B*, issue 29, 2018. https://doi.org/10.1039/C8TB00774J. Accessed June 6, 2024.
145. Mihalcea, Ana Maria. *Global Brain Chip and Mesogens: Nano Machines for Ultimate Control of False Memories – Computer System for Collective Mind Control.* Substack, July 18, 2023. https://anamihalceamdphd.substack.com/p/global-brain-chip-and-mesogens-nano. Accessed June 6, 2024.
146. Mihalcea, Ana Maria and Clifford E. Carnicom. AM Medical LLC, August 1, 2023. https://anamihalceamdphd.substack.com/p/analysis-of-symptomatic-health-findings?utm_source=publication-search
147. Carnicom, Clifford E. Carnicom Institute. Substack, August 1, 2023. https://anamihalceamdphd.substack.com/p/analysis-of-symptomatic-health-findings?utm_source=publication-search
148. Mihalcea, Ana Maria and Clifford E. Carnicom. *Blood Clot Analysis from Living and Deceased Individuals Shows Consistent Findings: A Rubber-Like Polymerized Protein – Microscopy Shows Filaments – Part 1 of 3. Dr. Ana Mihalcea with Clifford Carnicom.* Substack, July 10, 2023. https://anamihalceamdphd.substack.com/p/blood-clot-analysis-from-living-and-Accessed June 6, 2024.
149. Mihalcea, Ana Maria and Clifford E. Carnicom. *Blood Clot Analysis from Living and Deceased Individuals Near Infrared Spectroscopy Shows Multiple Hydrogel Polymer Components – Part 2 of 3. Dr. Ana Mihalcea with Clifford Carnicom.* Substack, July 10, 2023. https://anamihalceamdphd.substack.com/p/blood-clot-analysis-from-living-and-98a?utm_source=profile&utm_medium=reader2. Accessed June 6, 2024.
150. Mihalcea, Ana Maria and Clifford E. Carnicom. *Blood Clot Analysis from Living and Deceased Individuals – Preliminary Chemical Solubility Testing – Part 3 of 3. Dr. Ana Mihalcea with Clifford Carnicom.* Substack, July 10, 2023. https://anamihalceamdphd.substack.com/p/blood-clot-analysis-from-living-and-58d?utm_source=profile&utm_medium=reader2. Accessed June 6, 2024.

151. Mihalcea, Ana Maria. *The Danger in the Air – Rainwater Analysis Research by Dr. Geanina Hagimă From Romania Shows Magnetic Nanoparticles and Filaments. Comparison to Clifford Carnicom's Rainwater Analysis*. Substack, August 21, 2023. https://anamihalceamdphd.substack.com/p/the-danger-in-the-air-rainwater-analysis. Accessed June 6, 2024.
152. Hagimă, Geanina. Substack, August 21, 2023. https://anamihalceamdphd.substack.com/p/the-danger-in-the-air-rainwater-analysis?utm_source=publication-search
153. Hagimă, Geanina. "EXCLUSIV ActiveNews: CE SE AFLĂ ÎN APA DE PLOAIE? PERICOLUL DIN AER. Dr. Geanina Hagimă: Apel către cercetătorii români, dar şi către patrioţii din structurile de apărare şi informaţii. FOTO prin microscopie electronică şi VIDEO." *ActiveNews*, August 14, 2023. https://www.activenews.ro/opinii/EXCLUSIV-ActiveNews-CE-SE-AFLA-IN-APA-DE-PLOAIE-PERICOLUL-DIN-AER.-Dr.-Geanina-Hagima-Apel-catre-cercetatorii-romani-dar-si-catre-patriotii-din-structurile-de-aparare-si-informatii.-FOTO-prin-microscopie-electronica-si-VIDEO-183736. Accessed June 6, 2024.
154. Hagimă, Geanina. "Ce ne bagă-n apa de ploaie: România, iulie - august 2023." Rumble, uploaded by *Active News* Ro, 2023. https://rumble.com/v377k92-ce-ne-bag-n-apa-de-ploaie-romnia-iulie-august-2023.html. Accessed June 6, 2024.
155. Hagimă, Geanina. Substack, August 21, 2023. https://anamihalceamdphd.substack.com/p/the-danger-in-the-air-rainwater-analysis?utm_source=publication-search
156. Hagimă, Geanina. *Pericolul din Aer - Nanotubuli de Carbură de Siliciu*. https://anamihalceamdphd.substack.com/api/v1/file/8973c5aa-59d1-4560-ba5d-c6b874ab342b.pdf. Accessed June 6, 2024.
157. Lienhard, Michael A. and David J. Larkin. *Silicon Carbide Nanotube Synthesized*. NASA Ames Research Center, Propulsion and Power, UEET, CICT. https://anamihalceamdphd.substack.com/api/v1/file/8973c5aa-59d1-4560-ba5d-c6b874ab342b.pdf. Accessed June 6, 2024.
158. Link, Jamie R. and Michael J. Sailor. "Smart dust: self-assembling, self-orienting photonic crystals of porous Si." *Proceedings of the National Academy of Sciences of the United States of America* vol. 100,19 (2003): 10607-10. doi:10.1073/pnas.1233824100.
159. Hagimă, Geanina. Substack, August 21, 2023. https://anamihalceamdphd.substack.com/p/the-danger-in-the-air-rainwater-analysis?utm_source=publication-search
160. Ibid.
161. Hagimă, Geanina. Substack, 2023. https://anamihalceamdphd.substack.com/api/v1/file/8973c5aa-59d1-4560-ba5d-c6b874ab342b.pdf
162. Carnicom, Clifford E. Carnicom Institute, June 20, 2016. https://carnicominstitute.org/the-demise-of-rainwater/
163. Carnicom, Clifford E. Carnicom Institute, November 4, 2015. https://carnicominstitute.org/secondary-rainwater-analysis-organics-inorganics/
164. Ibid.

165. Carnicom, Clifford E. *Tertiary Rainwater Analysis: Questions of Toxicity.* Carnicom Institute, November 8, 2015. https://carnicominstitute.org/tertiary-rainwater-analysis-questions-of-toxicity-2/. Accessed June 6, 2024.
166. Carnicom, Clifford E. *Preliminary Rainwater Analysis: Aluminum Concentration.* Carnicom Institute, November 2, 2015. https://carnicominstitute.org/preliminary-rainwater-analysis-aluminum-concentration/. Accessed June 6, 2024.
167. Carnicom, Clifford E. *Environmental Filament Project: Metals Testing Laboratory Report.* Carnicom Institute, August 21, 2017. https://carnicominstitute.org/environmental-filament-project-metals-testing-laboratory-report/
168. Mihalcea, Ana Maria. *Dr. Pierre Gilbert 1995 Confirms Clifford Carnicom and My Discovery of ELF Fields Mind Controlling C19 Injected Turning Them Into Zombies. Confirms Contamination of Mankind's Blood With Nanotechnology.* Substack, August 25, 2023. https://anamihalceamdphd.substack.com/p/dr-pierre-gilbert-1995-confirms-clifford. Accessed June 6, 2024.
169. Gilbert, Pierre. "Dr. Pierre Gilbert Says Vaccines Containing Liquid Crystals Will Turn Recipients into Zombies." 1995. Rumble, uploaded by *Real Truth Real News.* https://rumble.com/v1j1m2h--1995-dr.-pierre-gilbert-says-vaccines-containing-liquid-crystals-will-turn.html. Accessed June 6, 2024.
170. Mihalcea, Ana Maria and Clifford E Carnicom. *Prospective Difference Between C19 Vaccinated and Unvaccinated Blood: Electromagnetic Observations, ELF Response and Potassium Metabolism – Ana Mihalcea, MD, PhD, and Clifford Carnicom.* Substack, June 26, 2023. https://anamihalceamdphd.substack.com/p/prospective-difference-between-c19. Accessed June 6, 2024.
171. Mihalcea, Ana Maria. *Discussion of New Research Findings: Nanotechnology in C19 Shots, HAARP, DARPA, Big Pharma Collaborating with Nanotech Company, Insulin & Mind Control: Interview with Maria Zeee.* Substack, August 12, 2023. https://anamihalceamdphd.substack.com/p/discussion-of-new-research-findings. Accessed June 6, 2024.
172. Mihalcea, Ana Maria. *Polymer Coated Quantum Dots – Darkfield Live Blood Analysis, Insulin Analysis and C19 Bioweapon Patents All Shows Nanotechnology Biosensors That Can Be Used for Surveillance and Mind Control.* Substack, July 30, 2023. https://anamihalceamdphd.substack.com/p/polymer-coated-quantum-dots-darkfield. Accessed June 6, 2024.

Chapter 2
Rubbery Clots

1. Mihalcea, Ana Maria. *Huge Rubbery Blood Clots in An Unvaccinated Individual – From Shedding? What Are They Made Of? A Call for Help to Analyze.* Substack, December 21, 2022. https://anamihalceamdphd.substack.com/p/huge-rubbery-blood-clots-in-an-unvaccinated. Accessed June 6, 2024.

2. Adams, Mike. "Lab Director Mike Adams Has Analyzed COVID 'Vaccine' Clots, Says They're 'Self-Assembling Biostructures.'" *Sense Receptor News*, August 29, 2022. https://sensereceptornews.com/?p=10535. Accessed June 6, 2024.
3. Mihalcea, Ana Maria. *'Shedding' – Understanding Self Spreading Vaccines in the Setting of Novel mRNA Technology*. Substack, June 30, 2022. https://anamihalceamdphd.substack.com/p/shedding-understanding-self-spreading?utm_source=substack&utm_campaign=post_embed&utm_medium=web. Accessed June 6, 2024.
4. Mihalcea, Ana Maria. *D-Dimer Elevation in the Unvaccinated. A Marker of Shedding?* Rumble, uploaded by Humanity United Now. https://rumble.com/v14n6aa-d-dimer-elevation-in-the-unvaccinated.-a-marker-of-shedding.html. Accessed June 6, 2024.
5. Adams, Mike. "Lab Director Mike Adams Has Analyzed COVID 'Vaccine' Clots, Says They're 'Self-Assembling Biostructures.'" *Sense Receptor News*, August 29, 2022. https://sensereceptornews.com/?p=10535. Accessed June 6, 2024.
6. Mihalcea, Ana Maria. AM Medical LLC, December 21, 2022. https://anamihalceamdphd.substack.com/p/huge-rubbery-blood-clots-in-an-unvaccinated?utm_source=publication-search
7. Ibid.
8. Ibid.
9. Ibid.
10. Mihalcea, Ana Maria. *New Findings in Unvaccinated Live Blood Show Same Self Assembly Hydrogel Spheres as in Embalmed Blood Deceased With Huge Rubbery Clots. Shocking Research Verification: There Are No More Pure Bloods!* Substack, June 19, 2023. https://anamihalceamdphd.substack.com/p/new-findings-in-unvaccinated-live. Accessed June 6, 2024.
11. Mihalcea, Ana Maria. AM Medical LLC, June 19, 2023. https://anamihalceamdphd.substack.com/p/new-findings-in-unvaccinated-live?utm_source=publication-search
12. Mihalcea, Ana Maria. *My Interview with Maria Zeee – Biden's Universal Nanotechnology Vaccine & 'Zombie' Blood.* Substack, June 14, 2023. https://anamihalceamdphd.substack.com/p/my-interview-with-maria-zeee-bidens. Accessed June 6, 2024.
13. Mihalcea, Ana Maria. AM Medical LLC, June 19, 2023. https://anamihalceamdphd.substack.com/p/new-findings-in-unvaccinated-live?utm_source=publication-search
14. Ibid.
15. Ibid.
16. Ibid.
17. Ibid.
18. Ibid.

REFERENCES

19. Mihalcea, Ana Maria. *New Findings in Unvaccinated Live Blood Show Same Self Assembly Hydrogel Spheres as in Embalmed Blood Deceased with Huge Rubbery Clots. Shocking Research Verification: There Are No More Pure Bloods!* Substack, June 20, 2023. https://anamihalceamdphd.substack.com/p/new-findings-in-unvaccinated-live. Accessed June 6, 2024.
20. Mihalcea, Ana Maria. AM Medical LLC, June 19, 2023. https://anamihalceamdphd.substack.com/p/new-findings-in-unvaccinated-live?utm_source=publication-search
21. Ibid.
22. Ibid.
23. Mihalcea, Ana Maria. *Rubbery Clot Formation Shown in Living C19 Unvaccinated Person Via Darkfield Microscopy – Hydrogel Replacing Blood.* Substack, July 21, 2023. https://anamihalceamdphd.substack.com/p/rubbery-clot-formation-shown-in-living?utm_source=publication-search. Accessed June 6, 2024.
24. Mihalcea, Ana Maria. AM Medical LLC, July 21, 2023. https://anamihalceamdphd.substack.com/p/rubbery-clot-formation-shown-in-living?utm_source=publication-search
25. Mihalcea, Ana Maria. *Correlation of Severity of Live Blood Contamination Seen on Darkfield Microscopy with Visible Clotting in C19 Unvaccinated Individual.* Substack, July 19, 2023. https://anamihalceamdphd.substack.com/p/correlation-of-severity-of-live-blood. Accessed June 6, 2024.
26. Mihalcea, Ana Maria. AM Medical LLC, July 21, 2023. https://anamihalceamdphd.substack.com/p/rubbery-clot-formation-shown-in-living?utm_source=publication-search
27. Ibid.
28. Ibid.
29. Mihalcea, Ana Maria. *Blood Clot Analysis from Living and Deceased Individuals Shows Consistent Findings: A Rubber-Like Polymerized Protein – Microscopy Shows Filaments, Part 1 of 3.* Substack, July 10, 2023. https://anamihalceamdphd.substack.com/p/blood-clot-analysis-from-living-and. Accessed June 6, 2024.
30. Mihalcea, Ana Maria. AM Medical LLC, July 21, 2023. https://anamihalceamdphd.substack.com/p/rubbery-clot-formation-shown-in-living?utm_source=publication-search
31. Ibid.
32. Ibid.
33. Mihalcea, Ana Maria. *Rubbery Clot Formation Shown in Living C19 Unvaccinated Person Via Darkfield Microscopy – Hydrogel Replacing Blood.* Substack, July 21, 2023. https://anamihalceamdphd.substack.com/p/rubbery-clot-formation-shown-in-living?utm_source=publication-search. Accessed June 6, 2024.
34. SciTech Daily. *Polyacrylonitrile (PAN) Nanofiber Mesh Capturing Water Aerosols.* YouTube. https://www.youtube.com/watch?v=w5JUhjdj1GY. Accessed June 6, 2024.

35. Mihalcea, Ana Maria. *Polyacrylonitrile (PAN) Polyamide Nanofiber Mesh Looks Just Like What I See in the Live C19 Unvaccinated Blood Now and We Identified Polyamides in NIR Spectroscopy Chemical Functional Group Analysis*. Substack, July 5, 2023. https://anamihalceamdphd.substack.com/p/polyacrylonitrile-pan-polyamide-nanofiber. Accessed June 6, 2024.
36. Mihalcea, Ana Maria. *Rubbery Clot Development in C19 Unvaccinated Individual with Previous Deep Vein Thrombosis and Massive Pulmonary Emboli – While on Eliquis, Nattokinase, Lumbrokinase and Serrapeptase*. Substack, October 19, 2023. https://anamihalceamdphd.substack.com/p/rubbery-clot-development-in-c19-unvaccinated?utm_source=publication-search. Accessed June 6, 2024.
37. Mihalcea, Ana Maria. *Blood Clot Analysis from Living and Deceased Individuals Shows Consistent Findings: A Rubber Like Polymerized Protein – Microscopy Shows Filaments. Part 1 of 3*. Substack, July 10, 2023. https://anamihalceamdphd.substack.com/p/blood-clot-analysis-from-living-and. Accessed June 6, 2024.
38. Mihalcea, Ana Maria. *Blood Clot Analysis from Living and Deceased Individuals Near Infrared Spectroscopy Shows Multiple Hydrogel Polymer Components, Part 2 of 3*. Substack, July 10, 2023. https://anamihalceamdphd.substack.com/p/blood-clot-analysis-from-living-and-98a. Accessed June 6, 2024.
39. Mihalcea, Ana Maria. *Blood Clot Analysis from Living and Deceased Individuals – Preliminary Chemical Solubility Testing, Part 3 of 3*. Substack, July 10, 2023. https://anamihalceamdphd.substack.com/p/blood-clot-analysis-from-living-and-58d?utm_source=profile&utm_medium=reader2. Accessed June 6, 2024.
40. Mihalcea, Ana Maria. *Correlation of Severity of Live Blood Contamination Seen on Darkfield Microscopy with Visible Clotting in C19 Unvaccinated Individual*. Substack, July 19, 2023. https://anamihalceamdphd.substack.com/p/correlation-of-severity-of-live-blood?utm_source=profile&utm_medium=reader2. Accessed June 6, 2024.
41. Mihalcea, Ana Maria. AM Medical LLC, October 19, 2023. https://anamihalceamdphd.substack.com/p/rubbery-clot-development-in-c19-unvaccinated?utm_source=publication-search
42. Ibid.
43. Ibid.
44. Ibid.
45. Ibid.
46. Ibid.
47. Ibid.
48. Ibid.
49. Mihalcea, Ana Maria. *Rubbery Clot Development in C19 Unvaccinated Individual with Previous Deep Vein Thrombosis and Massive Pulmonary Emboli – While on Eliquis, Nattokinase, Lumbrokinase and Serrapeptase*. Substack, October 19, 2023. https://anamihalceamdphd.substack.com/p/rubbery-clot-development-in-c19-unvaccinated?utm_source=publication-search. Accessed June 6, 2024.

50. Mihalcea, Ana Maria. *Same Self Replicating Nanotechnology Spheres Seen in C19 Unvaccinated Living Blood as in Deceased Embalmed C19 Vaccinated Blood with Rubbery Clots – What Will Humanity Do About This?* Substack, November 15, 2023. https://anamihalceamdphd.substack.com/p/same-self-replicating-nanotechnology?utm_source=publication-search. Accessed June 6, 2024.
51. Stumphauzer, Nicholas and Mathew Skow Mill. *Died Suddenly*. Produced by Stew Peters, initial release November 21, 2022.
52. Mihalcea, Ana Maria. AM Medical LLC, November 15, 2023. https://anamihalceamdphd.substack.com/p/same-self-replicating-nanotechnology?utm_source=publication-search
53. Ibid.
54. Ibid.
55. Ibid.
56. Ibid.
57. Ibid.
58. Ibid.
59. Ibid.
60. Ibid.
61. Ibid.
62. Mihalcea, Ana Maria. *Torsion Spectroscopy of C19 Vaccinated Deceased Clots by Dr. Diana Wojtkowiak – Confirms Prion-Like Protein That Cannot be Dissolved with Conventional Blood Thinners*. Substack, December 14, 2023. https://anamihalceamdphd.substack.com/p/torsion-spectroscopy-of-c19-vaccinated?utm_source=publication-search. Accessed June 6, 2024.
63. Mihalcea, Ana Maria. AM Medical LLC, December 14, 2023. https://anamihalceamdphd.substack.com/p/torsion-spectroscopy-of-c19-vaccinated?utm_source=publication-search
64. Wojtkowiak, Diana. *Zawiadomienie o Próbie Dokonania Przestępstwa Legalizacji Zbrodni Ludobójstwa*. Gdańsk, October 1, 2022. http://www.torsionfield.eu/wordpress/wp-content/uploads/2022/10/Zawiadomienie-o-próbie-dokonania-przestepstwa-legalizacji-zbrodni-ludobójstwa.pdf. Accessed June 6, 2024.
65. Wojtkowiak, Diana. *Notice of Liability to Polish Government*. Gdańsk, October 1, 2022. http://www.torsionfield.eu/wordpress/wp-content/uploads/2022/11/Notice-of-liability-to-Polish-gov.pdf. Accessed June 6, 2024.
66. Wojtkowiak, Diana. Substack, December 14, 2023. https://anamihalceamdphd.substack.com/p/torsion-spectroscopy-of-c19-vaccinated?utm_source=publication-search
67. Ibid.
68. Mihalcea, Ana Maria. *GLOBAL BRAIN CHIP AND MESOGENS Nano Machines for Ultimate Control of False Memories – Computer System for Collective Mind Control*. Substack, July 18, 2023. https://anamihalceamdphd.substack.com/p/global-brain-chip-and-mesogens-nano. Accessed July11, 2024.

69. Qing, Zhihe, *et al*. "Progress in Biosensor Based on DNA-Templated Copper Nanoparticles." *Biosensors and Bioelectronics*, May 7, 2019. https://doi.org/10.1016/j.bios.2019.05.014. Accessed July 11, 2024.
70. Mostafavi, Ebrahim, *et al*. "Selenium-Based Nanomaterials for Biosensing Applications." *Materials Advances*, September 14, 2022. https://pubs.rsc.org/en/content/articlelanding/2022/ma/d2ma00756h. Accessed July 11, 2024.
71. Sharma, Ankita, *et al*. "Zinc Oxide Nanostructures–Based Biosensors." *ScienceDirect*, August 13, 2021. https://www.sciencedirect.com/science/article/abs/pii/B9780128189009000024. Accessed July 11, 2024.
72. Mihalcea, Ana Maria. *GLOBAL BRAIN CHIP AND MESOGENS Nano Machines for Ultimate Control of False Memories – Computer System for Collective Mind Control*. Substack, July 18, 2023. https://anamihalceamdphd.substack.com/p/global-brain-chip-and-mesogens-nano. Accessed July 11, 2024.
73. Moore, John, *et al*. "Condensation Polymers: Proteins." *Chemistry LibreTexts*, University of Wisconsin, https://chem.libretexts.org/Bookshelves/General_Chemistry/Interactive_Chemistry_(Moore_Zhou_and_Garand)/02%3A_Unit_Two/2.07%3A_Day_15-_Condensation_Polymers_Proteins. Accessed September 8, 2024.
74. Boddu, Sai H S, *et al*. "Polyamide/Poly (Amino Acid) Polymers for Drug Delivery." *Journal of Functional Biomaterials*, vol. 12,4 58. October 8, 2021. doi:10.3390/jfb12040058.

Chapter 3
Fluorescence Phenomenon

1. Mihalcea, Ana Maria. *Fluorescent Filaments Coming Out of C19 Vaccinated Individuals Skin Glowing Under UV Light: Darkfield Microscopy*. Substack, January 27, 2024. https://anamihalceamdphd.substack.com/p/environmental-filaments-uv-light?utm_source=publication-search. Accessed July 11, 2024.
2. Mihalcea, Ana Maria. AM Medical LLC, January 27, 2024. https://anamihalceamdphd.substack.com/p/environmental-filaments-uv-light?utm_source=publication-search
3. Su, Y., Walker, J.R., Park, Y., *et al*. "Novel NanoLuc Substrates Enable Bright Two-Population Bioluminescence Imaging in Animals." *Nature Methods*, vol. 17, 2020, pp. 852–860, https://doi.org/10.1038/s41592-020-0889-6.
4. Ellenby, Dani. *New 'Smart' Polymer Glows Brighter When Stretched*. Okinawa Institute of Science and Technology, 23 January 2020, https://phys.org/news/2020-01-smart-polymer-brighter.html. Accessed June 6, 2024.
5. Patel, Prachi. "Plastics Shine Bright to Warn of Invisible Cracks." *Chemical & Engineering News*, September 22, 2016. https://cen.acs.org/articles/94/web/2016/09/Plastics-shine-bright-warn-invisible.html. Accessed June 6, 2024.

REFERENCES

6. Mihalcea, Ana Maria. AM Medical LLC, January 27, 2024. https://anamihalceamdphd.substack.com/p/environmental-filaments-uv-light?utm_source=publication-search
7. Ibid.
8. Ibid.
9. Ibid.
10. Ibid.
11. Ibid,
12. Ibid.
13. Ibid.
14. Ibid.
15. Ibid.
16. Mihalcea, Ana Maria. *Spider Silk Polymer Sprayed Via Geoengineering Operations from California – Darkfield Microscopy Analysis*. Substack, January 16, 2024. https://anamihalceamdphd.substack.com/p/spider-silk-polymer-sprayed-via-geoengineering. Accessed June 6, 2024.
17. Kandas, Ishac, *et al.* "Optical Fluorescent Spider Silk Electrospun Nanofibers with Embedded Cerium Oxide Nanoparticles." *Journal of Nanophotonics*, vol. 12, no. 02, June 2018, p. 1. https://www.researchgate.net/publication/325745449_Optical_fluorescent_spider_silk_electrospun_nanofibers_with_embedded_cerium_oxide_nanoparticles. DOI: 10.1117/1.JNP.12.026016. Accessed June 6, 2024.
18. Yi J., *et al.* "Polymer Films Inspired by Spider Silk Connect Biological Tissues and Electronic Devices." *Nature, Research Briefings*, December 13, 2023. https://www.nature.com/articles/d41586-023-03653-8. Accessed June 6, 2024.
19. Mihalcea, Ana Maria. *Darkfield Microscopy of Micro Robots in Live Blood Exposed to Scalar Wave Quantum Cold Laser*. Substack, November 3, 2023. https://anamihalceamdphd.substack.com/p/darkfield-microscopy-of-micro-robots. Accessed June 6, 2024.
20. Mihalcea, Ana Maria. *Energy Harvesting from the Human Body by Wireless Body Area Network – A Cause for the Electrical Conductivity Loss in Human Blood?* Substack, January 28, 2024. https://anamihalceamdphd.substack.com/p/energy-harvesting-from-the-human. Accessed June 6, 2024.
21. Mihalcea, Ana Maria. AM Medical LLC, January 27, 2024. https://anamihalceamdphd.substack.com/p/environmental-filaments-uv-light?utm_source=publication-search
22. Mihalcea, Ana Maria. *Fluorescent Orange Face Tattoo Under UV Light in C19 Vaccinated and Eye of Horus Phenomenon – Are Humans Limbic Systems Being Altered for Behavior Modification?* Substack, February 18, 2024. https://anamihalceamdphd.substack.com/p/fluorescent-orange-face-tattoo-under?utm source=publication-search. Accessed July 11, 2024.
23. Coy, Justin. Substack, February 18, 2024. https://anamihalceamdphd.substack.com/p/fluorescent-orange-face-tattoo-under?utm_source=publication-search

24. Staninger, Hildegarde. RIET-I. *The Eye of Horus Effect After Exposure to Aerial Biological Pesticides*. Integrative Health Systems, LLC, September 8, 2009. www.nrep.org. NREP 2009 Conference October 5-6, 2009. Windows on Wisdom. Integrative Health Systems, 415 3/4th N. Larchmont Blvd., Los Angeles, CA 90004.
25. Staninger, Hildegarde. RIET-I. Substack, February 18, 2024. https://anamihalceamdphd.substack.com/p/fluorescent-orange-face-tattoo-under?utm_source=publication-search
26. Mihalcea, Ana Maria and Clifford E. Carnicom. *Prospective Difference Between C19 Vaccinated and Unvaccinated Blood: Electromagnetic Observations, ELF Response and Potassium Metabolism*. Substack, June 26, 2023. https://anamihalceamdphd.substack.com/p/prospective-difference-between-c19. Accessed June 6, 2024.
27. Walsh, Colleen. "What the Nose Knows: Experts Discuss the Science of Smell and How Scent, Emotion, and Memory Are Intertwined – and Exploited." *Harvard Gazette*, February 27, 2020. https://news.harvard.edu/gazette/story/2020/02/how-scent-emotion-and-memory-are-intertwined-and-exploited/. Accessed June 6, 2024.
28. Mihalcea, Ana Maria. *Truth, Science and Spirt Episode 7 Fluorescent Skin with Justin Coy, PhD*. Rumble, uploaded by Humanity United Now. https://rumble.com/v4dg0lh-truth-science-and-spirt-episode-7-fluorescent-skin-with-justin-coy-phd.html. Accessed July 11, 2024.
29. Hambling, David. "Pentagon Explores 'Human Fear' Chemicals; Scare-Sensors, 'Contagious' Stress in the Works?" *Wired*, January 18, 2008. https://www.wired.com/2008/01/pentagon-resear/. Accessed June 6, 2024.
30. Glaister, Dan. "Air Force Looked at Spray to Turn Enemy Gay." *The Guardian*, June 13, 2007. https://www.theguardian.com/world/2007/jun/13/usa.danglaister. Accessed June 17, 2024.
31. Coy, Justin. Substack, February 18, 2024. https://anamihalceamdphd.substack.com/p/fluorescent-orange-face-tattoo-under?utm_source=publication-search
32. NYU Langone Health. *A Phase 1/2/3, Placebo-Controlled, Randomized, Observer-Blind, Dose-Finding Study to Evaluate the Safety, Tolerability, Immunogenicity, and Efficacy of SARS-CoV-2 RNA Vaccine Candidates Against COVID-19 in Healthy Individuals*. NYU Langone Health Clinical Research Studies. www.clinicaltrials.gov/ct2/show/NCT04368728. Accessed July 11, 2024.
33. Ibid.
34. Skyes, A. Edward and Dai Qin. University of Toronto. Substack, February 28, 2024. https://anamihalceamdphd.substack.com/p/the-most-deadly-product-in-the-history?utm_source=publication-search.
35. Chung, Emily. "Nanoparticle Exposure Test Developed by Canadian Scientists." *CBC News*, May 21, 2014. https://www.cbc.ca/news/science/nanoparticle-exposure-test-developed-by-canadian-scientists-1.2649608. Accessed June 6, 2024.

REFERENCES

36. Mihalcea, Ana Maria. *C19 Uninjected Individuals Expelling Fluorescent Filaments Through Skin Similar to C19 Injected.* Substack, May 31, 2024. https://anamihalceamdphd.substack.com/p/c19-uninjected-individuals-expelling?utm_source=publication-search. Accessed July 11, 2024.
37. Mihalcea, Ana Maria. AM Medical LLC, May 31, 2024. https://anamihalceamdphd.substack.com/p/c19-uninjected-individuals-expelling?utm_source=publication-search
38. Ibid.
39. Ibid.
40. Ibid.
41. Ibid.
42. Ibid.
43. Ibid.
44. Ibid.
45. Mihalcea, Ana Maria. *Further Darkfield Microscopy on Fluorescent Filaments Coming Out of C19 Unvaccinated Individuals and the Orange Glowing Facial Spots – It's All Self-Assembly Nanotechnology.* Substack, June 3, 2024. https://anamihalceamdphd.substack.com/p/further-darkfield-microscopy-on-fluorescent?utm_source=publication-search. Accessed July 11, 2024.
46. Mihalcea, Ana Maria. AM Medical LLC, June 3, 2024. https://anamihalceamdphd.substack.com/p/further-darkfield-microscopy-on-fluorescent?utm_source=publication-search.
47. Ibid.
48. Ibid.
49. Ibid.
50. Ibid.
51. Ibid.
52. Ibid.
53. Ibid.
54. Ibid.
55. Ibid.
56. Ibid.
57. Mihalcea, Ana Maria. *Spider Silk Polymer Sprayed Via Geoengineering Operations from California – Darkfield Microscopy Analysis.* Substack, January 16, 2024. https://anamihalceamdphd.substack.com/p/spider-silk-polymer-sprayed-via-geoengineering. Accessed July 11, 2024.
58. Mihalcea, Ana Maria. AM Medical LLC, June 3, 2024. https://anamihalceamdphd.substack.com/p/further-darkfield-microscopy-on-fluorescent?utm_source=publication-search.
59. Mihalcea, Ana Maria. AM Medical LLC, January 16, 2024. https://anamihalceamdphd.substack.com/p/spider-silk-polymer-sprayed-via-geoengineering
60. Mihalcea, Ana Maria. AM Medical LLC, June 3, 2024. https://anamihalceamdphd.substack.com/p/further-darkfield-microscopy-on-fluorescent?utm_source=publication-search.

61. Mihalcea, Ana Maria. *Global Brain Chip and Mesogens: Nano Machines for Ultimate Control of False Memories – Computer System for Collective Mind Control*. Substack, July 18, 2023. https://anamihalceamdphd.substack.com/p/global-brain-chip-and-mesogens-nano. Accessed June 6, 2024.
62. Staninger, Hildegarde. Substack, June 3, 2024. https://anamihalceamdphd.substack.com/p/further-darkfield-microscopy-on-fluorescent?utm_source=publication-search.
63. Mihalcea, Ana Maria. *Bioluminescent Brain Sensors for Oxygen Imaging in Dementia and Long Covid – They Don't Just Want to Make Your Skin Glow but Your Brain Too*. Substack, April 2, 2024. https://anamihalceamdphd.substack.com/p/bioluminescent-brain-sensors-for?utm_source=publication-search. Accessed July 11, 2024.

Chapter 4
Covid 19 Bioweapon and Childhood Vaccines

1. Mihalcea, Ana Maria. *Nanotech in The Shots?* Substack, October 2, 2022. https://anamihalceamdphd.substack.com/p/nanotech-in-the-shots?utm_source=publication-search.
2. LifeOfTheBlood. BitChute. https://www.bitchute.com/channel/wfxsdpIPtP0d/. Accessed August 8, 2024.
3. Ibid.
4. Ibid.
5. Ibid.
6. Ibid.
7. Ibid.
8. Ibid.
9. Ibid.
10. Mihalcea, Ana Maria. *'Vaccine' Microscopy by Dr. Geanina Hagimă in Romania Shows Micro Bots, Quantum Dots and Microchip Development – Influenza and Moderna C19 Shots.* Substack, October 10, 2023. https://anamihalceamdphd.substack.com/p/vaccine-microscopy-by-dr-geanina?utm_source=publication-search.
11. Hughes, David. "What is in the So-Called COVID-19 'Vaccines'? Part 1: Evidence of a Global Crime Against Humanity." *International Journal of Vaccine Theory, Practice, and Research*, vol. 2, no. 2, Sept 2022, pp. 455-486. https://doi.org/10.56098/ijvtpr.v2i2.52.
12. Hagimă Geanina. Substack, October 10, 2023. https://anamihalceamdphd.substack.com/p/vaccine-microscopy-by-dr-geanina?utm_source=publication-search
13. Ibid.
14. Ibid.
15. Ibid.
16. Ibid.

17. Mihalcea, Ana Maria. *'Vaccine' Microscopy by Dr. Geanina Hagimă in Romania Shows Micro Bots, Quantum Dots and Microchip Development – Influenza and Moderna C19 Shots.* Substack, October 10, 2023. https://anamihalceamdphd.substack.com/p/vaccine-microscopy-by-dr-geanina?utm_source=publication-search.
18. Hagimă Geanina. Substack, October 10, 2023. https://anamihalceamdphd.substack.com/p/vaccine-microscopy-by-dr-geanina?utm_source=publication-search
19. Ibid.
20. Ibid.
21. Ibid.
22. Mihalcea, Ana Maria. *Article Review: What is in the So-Called COVID-19 'Vaccines'? Part 1: Evidence of a Global Crime Against Humanity.* Substack, October 16, 2022. https://anamihalceamdphd.substack.com/p/article-review-what-is-in-the-so?utm_source=publication-search.
23. LifeOfTheBlood. BitChute. https://www.bitchute.com/channel/wfxsdpIPtP0d/. Accessed August 8, 2024.
24. Hughes, David A. *What is in the Covid "Vaccines"? Evidence of Crimes Against Humanity.* Paper Lincoln Uni. BitChute, 2022. https://www.bitchute.com/video/h5JrWu67F645/. Accessed August 8, 2024.
25. Hughes, David A. "What is in the So-Called COVID-19 'Vaccines'? Part 1: Evidence of a Global Crime Against Humanity.", *International Journal of Vaccine Theory, Practice, and Research*, September 3, 2022. https://ijvtpr.com/index.php/IJVTPR/article/view/52
26. Ghitalla, Barbel. "What is in the So-Called COVID-19 'Vaccines'? Part 1: Evidence of a Global Crime Against Humanity." Dr. David A. Hughes, *International Journal of Vaccine Theory, Practice, and Research*, September 3, 2022.https://ijvtpr.com/index.php/IJVTPR/article/view/52
27. Anonymous Dr. John B. "What is in the So-Called COVID-19 'Vaccines'? Part 1: Evidence of a Global Crime Against Humanity." Dr. David A. Hughes, *International Journal of Vaccine Theory, Practice, and Research*, September 3, 2022. https://ijvtpr.com/index.php/IJVTPR/article/view/52/288
28. Noack, Andreas. "What is in the So-Called COVID-19 'Vaccines'? Part 1: Evidence of a Global Crime Against Humanity." Dr. David A. Hughes, *International Journal of Vaccine Theory, Practice, and Research*, September 3, 2022. https://ijvtpr.com/index.php/IJVTPR/article/view/52/288
29. Ibid.
30. LifeOfTheBlood. "What is in the So-Called COVID-19 'Vaccines'? Part 1: Evidence of a Global Crime Against Humanity." Dr. David A. Hughes, *International Journal of Vaccine Theory, Practice, and Research*, September 3, 2022. https://ijvtpr.com/index.php/IJVTPR/article/view/52/288
31. Latypova, Sasha. *Conversations with Pharma Insider Sasha Latypova – Nanotech in C19 Vials, Regulatory Fraud, Bad Manufacturing Practices, DOD Contracts & More.* Substack, October 11, 2022. https://anamihalceamdphd.substack.com/p/conversations-with-pharma-insider

32. Mihalcea, Ana Maria. *What is in the So-Called COVID-19 'Vaccines'? Evidence of a Global Crime Against Humanity – My Interview with Dr. David Hughes*. Substack, November 8, 2022. https://anamihalceamdphd.substack.com/p/what-is-in-the-so-called-covid-19?utm_source=publication-search
33. Ibid.
34. Mihalcea, Ana Maria. *What is in the So-Called COVID-19 'Vaccines'? Evidence of a Global Crime Against Humanity*. Rumble, uploaded by Humanity United Now, 2023. https://rumble.com/v1sm3bm-what-is-in-the-so-called-covid-19-vaccines-evidence-of-a-global-crime-again.html.
35. Ibid.
36. Ibid.
37. Hughes, David A. "COVID-19 'Vaccines' for Children in the UK: A Tale of Establishment Corruption." *International Journal of Vaccine Theory, Practice, and Research*, 2022. https://www.academia.edu/71131897/_COVID_19_Vaccines_for_Children_in_the_UK_A_Tale_of_Establishment_Corruption.
38. Hughes, David A. "What is in the So-Called COVID-19 'Vaccines'? Part 1: Evidence of a Global Crime Against Humanity.", *International Journal of Vaccine Theory, Practice, and Research*, September 3, 2022. https://ijvtpr.com/index.php/IJVTPR/article/view/52.
39. Ibid.
40. Ibid.
41. Nixon, David. "What is in the So-Called COVID-19 'Vaccines'? Part 1: Evidence of a Global Crime Against Humanity." Dr. David A. Hughes, *International Journal of Vaccine Theory, Practice, and Research*, September 3, 2022. https://ijvtpr.com/index.php/IJVTPR/article/view/52/288
42. Taylor, Mat. "What is in the So-Called COVID-19 'Vaccines'? Part 1: Evidence of a Global Crime Against Humanity." Dr. David A. Hughes, *International Journal of Vaccine Theory, Practice, and Research*, September 3, 2022. https://ijvtpr.com/index.php/IJVTPR/article/view/52/288
43. Mihalcea, Ana Maria. *BREAKING NEWS: New Analysis of C19 Bioweapons: No MRNA, But Toxic Metals and Silicone. Dental Anesthetics & Pneumovax Also Contain Silicone & Metals Used for Nanotech-Interview with Dr. Geanina Hagimă*. Substack, November 25, 2023. https://anamihalceamdphd.substack.com/p/breaking-news-new-analysis-of-c19?utm_source=publication-search.
44. Rocky Mountain Labs. "Difference between SEM and EDX Analysis." *Rocky Mountain Laboratories*, November. 2023. https://rockymountainlabs.com/sem-and-edx-analysis/.
45. Mihalcea, Ana Maria. *BREAKING NEWS: New Analysis of C19 Bioweapons: No MRNA, But Toxic Metals and Silicone. Dental Anesthetics & Pneumovax Also Contain Silicone & Metals Used for Nanotech-Interview with Dr. Geanina Hagimă*. Substack, November 25, 2023. https://anamihalceamdphd.substack.com/p/breaking-news-new-analysis-of-c19?utm_source=publication-search.

46. Mihalcea, Ana Maria. *Electron Microscopy of Comirnaty, Moderna C19 Shots, Dental Anesthetics & Pneumovax.* Rumble, uploaded by Humanity United Now. https://rumble.com/v3xti7w-electron-microscopy-of-comirnaty-moderna-c19-shots-dental-anestetics-and-pn.html. Accessed August 8, 2024.
47. Mihalcea, Ana Maria. *'Vaccine' Microscopy by Dr. Geanina Hagimă in Romania: Comirnaty Omicron B4-5 Shows Micro Bots, Quantum Dots and Hydrogel Filament Development.* Substack, October 15, 2023. https://anamihalceamdphd.substack.com/p/vaccine-microscopy-by-dr-geanina-a08
48. Hagimă, Geanina. Substack, November 25, 2023. https://anamihalceamdphd.substack.com/p/breaking-news-new-analysis-of-c19?utm_source=publication-search
49. Ibid.
50. Ibid.
51. Ibid.
52. Ibid.
53. Lee, K. L., Hsu, H. Y., You, M. L., *et al.* "Highly Sensitive Aluminum-Based Biosensors Using Tailorable Fano Resonances in Capped Nanostructures." *Scientific Reports*, vol. 7, 44104, 2017. https://doi.org/10.1038/srep44104.
54. Hagimă, Geanina. Substack, November 25, 2023. https://anamihalceamdphd.substack.com/p/breaking-news-new-analysis-of-c19?utm_source=publication-search
55. Staff, *The Exposé*. "Scientists Discover 'Carbon Nanotech' & 'Radioactive Thulium' in Pfizer & Moderna COVID Vaccines." *The Exposé*, August 16, 2022. https://expose-news.com/2022/08/16/radioactive-nanotech-found-in-covid-vaccine/
56. Kirsch, Steve. *Want to Know What's Inside the Vaccine Vials?* Substack, August 1, 2022. https://kirschsubstack.com/p/want-to-know-whats-inside-the-vaccine.
57. Mihalcea, Ana Maria. *Alarming New Report from Working Group of Vaccine Analysis in Germany and Other Countries.* Substack, August 8, 2022. https://anamihalceamdphd.substack.com/p/alarming-new-report-from-working
58. Mihalcea, Ana Maria. *UK Forensic Report Finds Graphene: Qualitative Evaluation of Inclusions in Moderna, AstraZeneca, and Pfizer Covid-19 Vaccines – by UNIT: Self-Assembly Graphene Nanoparticles Confirmed.* Substack, September 15, 2022. https://anamihalceamdphd.substack.com/p/uk-forensic-report-finds-graphene.
59. Mihalcea, Ana Maria. *Darkfield Microscopy of Pneumococcal Vaccine Prevnar 13 Shows Quantum Dot Structures and Self Assembly.* Substack, August 29, 2023. https://anamihalceamdphd.substack.com/p/darkfield-microscopy-of-pneumococcal
60. Hagimă, Geanina. Substack, November 25, 2023. https://anamihalceamdphd.substack.com/p/breaking-news-new-analysis-of-c19?utm_source=publication-search
61. Ibid.

62. Mihalcea, Ana Maria. *Toxic Metal Nano 'Contaminants' in Shots and Adverse Effect Correlation*. Substack, September 11, 2022. https://anamihalceamdphd.substack.com/p/toxic-metal-nano-contaminants-in?utm_source=publication-search
63. Mihalcea, Ana Maria. *Alarming New Report from Working Group of Vaccine Analysis in Germany and Other Countries*. Substack, August 8, 2022. https://anamihalceamdphd.substack.com/p/alarming-new-report-from-working.
64. Mihalcea, Ana Maria. *Dark-Field Microscopic Analysis on the Blood of 1,006 Symptomatic Persons After Anti-COVID mRNA Injections from Pfizer/BioNtech or Moderna*. Substack, August 29, 2022. https://anamihalceamdphd.substack.com/p/dark-field-microscopic-analysis-on?utm_source=publication-search
65. Gatti, Antonietta M. and Stefano Montanari. "New Quality-Control Investigations on Vaccines: Micro- and Nanocontamination." *International Journal of Vaccines and Vaccination*, vol. 4, no. 1, January 23, 2017. https://medcraveonline.com/IJVV/IJVV-04-00072.pdf
66. Ibid.
67. Ibid.
68. Ibid.
69. Ibid.
70. Mihalcea, Ana Maria. *Alarming New Report from Working Group of Vaccine Analysis in Germany and Other Countries*. Substack, August 8, 2022. https://anamihalceamdphd.substack.com/p/alarming-new-report-from-working
71. Gatti, Antonietta M. and Stefano Montanari. *International Journal of Vaccines and Vaccination*, 2017. https://medcraveonline.com/IJVV/IJVV-04-00072.pdf
72. Ibid.
73. Ibid.
74. Chalmers, Vanessa. "RARE TRIGGER: Viral Video Shows Woman Struggling to Walk After Her Covid Jab in Extremely Rare Case." *The Sun*, July 26, 2021. https://www.thesun.co.uk/news/15692995/viral-video-woman-struggling-walk-after-covid-jab-fnd/
75. Thomas, Paul. *Dr. Paul Thomas: Safe Passage in a Changing World.* https://www.paulthomasmd.com/aluminum-in-vaccines.html. Accessed August 8, 2024.
76. TNR. *Signs and Symptoms of Heavy Metal Toxicity in Your Body.* Top Natural Remedy, September 17, 2018. https://topnaturalremedy.com/signs-and-symptoms-of-heavy-metal-toxicity-in-your-body/
77. Mihalcea, Ana Maria. *Chemical Analysis Comparison of Hydrogel Filaments from C19 Shots and Environmental Geoengineering Sources – Project What Happened to Humanity's Blood?* Substack, April 7, 2023. https://anamihalceamdphd.substack.com/p/chemical-analysis-comparison-of-hydrogel?utm_source=publication-search.
78. UNIT. "Global Moderna COVID 19 'vaccine' filament growth." Project CUNIT-2-112Y6580. Global Humanitarian Crisis Prevention and Response Unit. https://anamihalceamdphd.substack.com/p/chemical-analysis-comparison-of-hydrogel
79. Ibid.
80. Ibid.

81. Tailliez, Bernard. *Qualité & Hygiène Industrielles – Respect de l'Environnement: Rapport Analytique*. Substack, April 7, 2023. https://anamihalceamdphd.substack.com/p/chemical-analysis-comparison-of-hydrogel
82. Tailliez, Bernard. *Qualité & Hygiène Industrielles – Respect de l'Environnement: Rapport Analytique*. Substack October 2013. https://anamihalceamdphd.substack.com/api/v1/file/977d4945-ccb8-4437-a121-712ff84333f4.pdf
83. Ahmed, Enas M. "Hydrogel: Preparation, Characterization, and Applications: A Review. " *Journal of Advanced Research*, vol. 6, no. 2, 2015, pp. 105-121. https://doi.org/10.1016/j.jare.2013.07.006
84. Tailliez, Bernard. *Qualité & Hygiène Industrielles – Respect de l'Environnement: Rapport Analytique*. Substack, April 7, 2023. https://anamihalceamdphd.substack.com/p/chemical-analysis-comparison-of-hydrogel?utm_source=publication-search
85. Pfizer Australia Pty Ltd. *Nonclinical Evaluation Report.* Substack, April 7, 2023. https://anamihalceamdphd.substack.com/p/chemical-analysis-comparison-of-hydrogel?utm_source=publication-search
86. Mihalcea, Ana Maria. *Chemical Analysis Comparison of Hydrogel Filaments from C19 Shots and Environmental Geoengineering Sources – Project What Happened to Humanity's Blood?* Substack, April 7, 2023. https://anamihalceamdphd.substack.com/p/chemical-analysis-comparison-of-hydrogel?utm_source=publication-search
87. Mihalcea, Ana Maria. *Alarming New Report from Working Group of Vaccine Analysis in Germany and Other Countries*. Substack, August 8, 2022. https://anamihalceamdphd.substack.com/p/alarming-new-report-from-working?utm_source=publication-search
88. Mihalcea, Ana Maria. *Summary of Initial Findings V1 Working Group for Vaccine Analysis*. Substack, July 6, 2022. https://anamihalceamdphd.substack.com/p/alarming-new-report-from-working?utm_source=publication-search
89. Ibid.
90. Ibid.
91. Bailey, Sam. "NZ Scientist Examines Pfizer Jab Under the Microscope." *Odysee*, March 22, 2022. https://odysee.com/@drsambailey:c/nz-scientist-examines-pfizer-jab-under-the-microscope:6?src=embed
92. Ibid.
93. Nagase, Daniel. "WATCH: Dr. Nagase Reviews Images from COVID Vaccines, Shows No 'Elements of Life.'" *Western Standard*, April 18, 2024. https://rumble.com/v11go0d-watch-dr.-nagase-reviews-images-from-covid-vaccines-shows-no-elements-of-li.html
94. Wilson, Rhoda. "Canadian Researchers Find Carbon Nanotech and Thulium in Moderna and Pfizer Covid Injections." *The Exposé*, May 27, 2022. https://expose-news.com/2022/05/27/carbon-nanotech-and-thulium-in-covid-injections/
95. Nagase, Daniel. *The Exposé*, May 27, 2022. https://expose-news.com/2022/05/27/carbon-nanotech-and-thulium-in-covid-injections/

96. Ibid.
97. Mihalcea, Ana Maria. *Alarming New Report from Working Group of Vaccine Analysis in Germany and Other Countries*. Substack, August 8, 2022. https://anamihalceamdphd.substack.com/p/alarming-new-report-from-working?utm_source=publication-search.
98. Giovannini, Franco, *et al. Contrast Phase Microscope Analysis on the Blood of 1006 Symptomatic Subjects After Anti-COVID Vaccination with Pfizer/BioNTech or Moderna*. 2022. https://anamihalceamdphd.substack.com/api/v1/file/fc9c3d97-e39e-40e6-ab67-97447f86ebb9.pdf. Accessed August 8, 2024.
99. Giovannini, Franco, *et al. International Journal of Vaccine Theory, Practice, and Research.* Substack, August 8, 2022. https://anamihalceamdphd.substack.com/p/alarming-new-report-from-working?utm_source=publication-search
100. Mihalcea, Ana Maria. *UK Forensic Report Finds Graphene: Qualitative Evaluation of Inclusions in Moderna, AstraZeneca, and Pfizer Covid-19 Vaccines – by UNIT: Self-Assembly Graphene Nanoparticles Confirmed.* Substack, September 14, 2022. https://anamihalceamdphd.substack.com/p/uk-forensic-report-finds-graphene?utm_source=publication-search
101. Staff, *The Exposé*. "UK Lab Report Discovers Graphene in the Covid-19 Vaccines; & Scientists Believe the Vaccinated Are Transmitting It to the Unvaccinated." *The Exposé*, September 10, 2022. https://expose-news.com/2022/09/10/uk-lab-report-graphene-covid-vaccines/
102. Ibid.
103. UK Forensic Laboratory Report Summary. Project CUNIT-2-112Y6580. *EbMCsquared CIC.* http://ukcitizen2021.org/Case_Briefing_Document_and_lab_report_Ref_AUC_101_Report%20.pdf
104. Ibid.
105. Ibid.
106. Ibid.
107. Ibid.
108. Ibid.
109. Ibid.
110. Ibid.
111. Ibid.
112. Ibid.
113. Mihalcea, Ana Maria. *New Images of Self-Assembly Structures in Pfizer Vials and Live Blood Analysis*. Substack, October 4, 2022. https://anamihalceamdphd.substack.com/p/new-images-of-self-assembly-structures?utm_source=publication-search
114. Adams, Mike. "PEOPLE FOR PEOPLE – Nanotechnology in Pfizer Vials and Live Blood Analysis." *Brighteon*, October 4, 2022. https://www.brighteon.com/35712e35-7bc1-4b24-8770-31f6d1c88028
115. Ibid.

116. Mihalcea, Ana Maria. *Self-Assembly Nanostructures in C19 Vials - Documented Growth and Self Assembly out of Liposomes from Thawing at Room Temperature to Incubation at Body Temperature for 7 Days*. Substack, September 20, 2022. https://anamihalceamdphd.substack.com/p/self-assembly-nanostructures-in-c19?utm_source=substack&utm_campaign=post_embed&utm_medium=web
117. Nixon, David. Substack, October 4, 2022. https://anamihalceamdphd.substack.com/p/new-images-of-self-assembly-structures?utm_source=publication-search
118. Ibid.
119. Ibid.
120. Ibid.
121. Ibid.
122. Ibid.
123. Ibid.
124. Ibid.
125. Ibid.
126. Van Welbergen, Philippe. "From One to Another: Doctors Find Graphene is Shedding from the COVID-19 Vaccinated to the Unvaccinated, Forming Deadly Blood Clots & Decimating Blood Cells." *The Exposé*, February 17, 2024. https://expose-news.com/2024/02/17/drs-find-graphene-shed-vaxed-to-unvaccinated/
127. Ibid.
128. Mihalcea, Ana Maria. *Self-Assembly Nanostructures in C19 Vials – Documented Growth and Self Assembly out of Liposomes from Thawing at Room Temperature to Incubation at Body Temperature for 7 Days*. Substack, September 20, 2022. https://anamihalceamdphd.substack.com/p/self-assembly-nanostructures-in-c19?utm_source=publication-search
129. Yanowitz, Shimon. "PEOPLE FOR PEOPLE – Dr. Ana Maria Mihalcea, MD, PhD." *Brighteon*, September 20, 2022. https://www.brighteon.com/8530b525-ba96-47bc-945d-9443cd1280bf
130. Ibid.
131. Ibid.
132. Ibid.
133. Ibid.
134. Ibid.
135. Ibid.
136. Ibid.
137. Ibid.
138. Ibid.
139. Mihalcea, Ana Maria. *Self-Assembly Microtechnology Pfizer Vials Research Updates – Ribbons, Microchips, Optical Communications Cables and Correlation to PEG, Graphene, Hydrogel*. Substack, December 17, 2022. https://anamihalceamdphd.substack.com/p/self-assembly-microtechnology-pfizer?utm_source=publication-search

140. Mihalcea, Ana Maria. *Nanobots, Construction Process of Microchips in C19 Injectables, New Insights on Shedding.* Rumble, uploaded by Humanity United Now, 2022. https://rumble.com/v1uq5v4-nanobots-construction-process-of-microchips-in-c19-injectables-new-insights.html. Accessed August 8, 2024.
141. Nixon, David. Substack, December 17, 2022. https://anamihalceamdphd.substack.com/p/self-assembly-microtechnology-pfizer?utm_source=publication-search
142. Nixon, David. https://drdavidnixon.com. Accessed August 8, 2024.
143. Nixon, David. Substack, December 17, 2022. https://anamihalceamdphd.substack.com/p/self-assembly-microtechnology-pfizer?utm_source=publication-search
144. Ibid.
145. Ibid.
146. Ibid.
147. Ibid.
148. Mihalcea, Ana Maria. *C19 Vax Analysis Shows Dozens of Toxic Phthalates That Have Been Associated with Endocrine Disruption and Death from Heart Disease.* Substack, January 20, 2024. https://anamihalceamdphd.substack.com/p/c19-vax-analysis-shows-dozens-of?utm_source=publication-search
149. Kautz-Vella, Harald and Kristin Hauksdottir. *The Chemistry in Contrails: Assessing the Impact of Aerosols from Jet Fuel Impurities, Additives and Classified Military Operations on Nature.* June 30, 2013. https://aquarius-technologies.de/wp-content/uploads/2021/07/The-Chemistry-in-Contrails.pdf. Accessed August 26, 2024.
150. Ibid.
151. Hill, C. June 24, 2013. Alien Spiders! *Black Goo, Chemtrails, Morgellons, Excellent Must See!!!* Harald Kautz-Vella lecture August 2015. Quang Le, YouTube. https://www.youtube.com/watch?v=WgRByQXVjck. Accessed August 8, 2024.
152. Ibid.
153. Akyildiz, Ian. "*COVID MRNAs ARE NOTHING MORE THAN SMALL SCALE BIO-NANO MACHINES" – Lecture by Professor Ian Akyildiz from Georgia Institute of Technology.*" Substack, May 27, 2023. https://anamihalceamdphd.substack.com/p/covid-mrnas-are-nothing-more-than
154. DARPA. ASU, Arizona Institute for Nano-Electronics. Substack, January 20, 2024. https://anamihalceamdphd.substack.com/p/c19-vax-analysis-shows-dozens-of?utm_source=publication-search. Accessed August 26, 2024.
155. Mihalcea, Ana Maria. *Chemical Analysis Comparison of Hydrogel Filaments from C19 Shots and Environmental Geoengineering Sources - Project What Happened to Humanity's Blood?* Substack, April 7, 2023. https://anamihalceamdphd.substack.com/p/chemical-analysis-comparison-of-hydrogel
156. Mihalcea, Ana Maria. *GLOBAL BRAIN CHIP AND MESOGENS Nano Machines for Ultimate Control of False Memories – Computer System For Collective Mind Control.* Substack, July 18, 2023. https://anamihalceamdphd.substack.com/p/global-brain-chip-and-mesogens-nano

157. Callender, Todd. Substack, January 20, 2024. https://anamihalceamdphd.substack.com/p/c19-vax-analysis-shows-dozens-of
158. ModernaTX, Inc. *United States Patent US11622972B2*. ModernaTX, Inc., April 11, 2023. https://assets.modernatx.com/m/3a035077746fb2a0/original/US-11622972-B2_I.pdf. Accessed August 26, 2024.
159. Callender, Todd. *Pfizer. COVID 19 injection analysis*. Substack, January 20, 2024. https://anamihalceamdphd.substack.com/p/c19-vax-analysis-shows-dozens-of. Accessed August 26, 2024.
160. Phys Org. *Widely Used Chemical Linked to 100,000 US Deaths per Year: Study*. October 13, 2021. https://phys.org/news/2021-10-widely-chemical-linked-deaths-year.html
161. Dutta, Sudipta, *et al*. "Phthalate Exposure and Long-Term Epigenomic Consequences: A Review." *Frontiers in Genetics*, vol. 11 405, May 6, 2020. doi:10.3389/fgene.2020.00405
162. Cao, Yaru, *et al*. "Microplastics: A Major Source of Phthalate Esters in Aquatic Environments." *ScienceDirect, Journal of Hazardous Materials*, vol. 432, 2022, p. 128731. June 15, 2022. https://doi.org/10.1016/j.jhazmat.2022.128731
163. Zhang, Ying-Jie, *et al*. "Phthalate Metabolites: Characterization, Toxicities, Global Distribution, and Exposure Assessment." *ScienceDirect, Environmental Pollution*, vol. 291, 2021, p. December 15, 2021. 118106. https://doi.org/10.1016/j.envpol.2021.118106
164. Mihalcea, Ana Maria. *Recent Consumer Report Reveals High Levels of Plastics in All Food Categories – Is Poisoning Our Biosphere Via Geoengineering the REAL Cause?* Substack, January 19, 2024. https://anamihalceamdphd.substack.com/p/recent-consumer-report-reveals-high
165. Mihalcea, Ana Maria. *Study Shows a Quarter Million Nanoparticle Polymers Per Liter in Water Bottles – Same Polymers Found as in Moderna Patent for Covid 19 Shots, Morgellons Filaments, Blood & Rubbery Clots*. Substack, January 13, 2024. https://anamihalceamdphd.substack.com/p/study-shows-a-quarter-million-nanoparticle
166. Mihalcea, Ana Maria. *Residual DNA Fragments Analysis Detected in Monovalent and Bivalent Pfizer/BioNTech and Moderna modRNA COVID-19 Shots Confirms Spider Silk Genes Encoded in the Spike Open Reading Frame*. Substack, April 3, 2024. https://anamihalceamdphd.substack.com/p/residual-dna-fragments-analysis-detected?utm_source=publication-search
167. Mihalcea, Ana Maria. *Spider Silk Polymer Sprayed Via Geoengineering Operations from California – Darkfield Microscopy Analysis*. Substack, January 16, 2024. https://anamihalceamdphd.substack.com/p/spider-silk-polymer-sprayed-via-geoengineering
168. Speicher, David. Substack, April 3, 2024. https://anamihalceamdphd.substack.com/p/residual-dna-fragments-analysis-detected?utm_source=publication-search. Accessed August 26, 2024.
169. Ibid.
170. Geggel, Laura. "'Dragon Silk' Armor Could Protect US Troops." *Live Science*, July 15, 2016. https://www.livescience.com/55423-spider-silkworm-silk-protects-army-soldiers.html

171. Mihalcea, Ana Maria. *Discussion of Argentinian C19 Bioweapon Analysis Finding Building Blocks of Self-Assembly Nanotechnology*. Substack, June 6, 2024. https://anamihalceamdphd.substack.com/p/discussion-of-argentinian-c19-bioweapon?utm_source=publication-search
172. Diblasi, Lorena. *Analysis of Covid 19 Injections – Conversation with Biotechnologist Lorena Diblasi, EP 23*. Rumble, uploaded by Humanity United Now, 2024. https://rumble.com/v4zzbqx-analysis-of-covid-19-injections-conversation-with-biotechnologist-lorena-di.html
173. McAtee, Melissa. *Breaking News: Glowing C19 Shots and Fluorescent Nanotechnology – Conversation with Pfizer Whistleblower Melissa McAtee – Truth, Science and Spirit, Ep 26*. Substack, June 27, 2024. https://anamihalceamdphd.substack.com/p/breaking-news-glowing-c19-shots-and
174. Mihalcea, Ana Maria. *Further Darkfield Microscopy on Fluorescent Filaments Coming Out of C19 Unvaccinated Individuals and the Orange Glowing Facial Spots – It's All Self-Assembly Nanotechnology*. Substack, June 4, 2024. https://anamihalceamdphd.substack.com/p/further-darkfield-microscopy-on-fluorescent
175. Sangorrin, Marcela, *et al.* Substack, June 6, 2024. https://anamihalceamdphd.substack.com/p/analysis-of-covid-19-injections-50
176. LibreTexts Chemistry. "Lanthanides: Properties and Reactions." *LibreTexts* https://chem.libretexts.org/Bookshelves/Inorganic_Chemistry/Supplemental_Modules_and_Websites_(Inorganic_Chemistry)/Descriptive_Chemistry/Elements_Organized_by_Block/4_f-Block_Elements/The_Lanthanides/aLanthanides%3A_Properties_and_Reactions. Accessed August 8, 2024.
177. Sangorrin, Marcela, *et al.* Substack, June 6, 2024. https://anamihalceamdphd.substack.com/p/analysis-of-covid-19-injections-50
178. Ibid.
179. Nash, K. L., *et al.* "The Kinetics of Lanthanide Complexation by EDTA and DTPA in Lactate Media." *Dalton Transactions*, October 4, 2012. https://doi.org/10.1039/C2DT31851B
180. Mihalcea, Ana Maria. AM Medical LLC, June 6, 2024. https://anamihalceamdphd.substack.com/p/discussion-of-argentinian-c19-bioweapon?utm_source=publication-search
181. Hagimă, Geanina. *BREAKING NEWS: New Analysis of C19 Bioweapons: No MRNA, But Toxic Metals and Silicone. Dental Anesthetics & Pneumovax Also Contain Silicone & Metals Used for Nanotech-Interview with Dr. Geanina Hagimă*. Substack, November 25, 2023. https://anamihalceamdphd.substack.com/p/breaking-news-new-analysis-of-c19
182. ModernaTX, Inc. Application No. 62/799,620, filed January 31, 2019. Google Patents. https://patents.google.com/patent/WO2020160397A1/en. Accessed August 26, 2024.
183. ModernaTX, Inc. *United States Patent US11622972B2*. ModernaTX, Inc., April 11, 2023. https://assets.modernatx.com/m/3a035077746fb2a0/original/US-11622972-B2_I.pdf. Accessed August 26, 2024.
184. Sangorrin, Marcela, *et al.* Substack, June 6, 2024. https://anamihalceamdphd.substack.com/p/analysis-of-covid-19-injections-50

185. Dos Santos, Marcelina Cardoso, and Niko Hildebrandt. "Recent Developments in Lanthanide-to-Quantum Dot FRET Using Time-Gated Fluorescence Detection and Photon Upconversion." *ScienceDirect, TrAC Trends in Analytical Chemistry*, vol. 84, part A, 2016, pp. 60-71, November 2016. https://doi.org/10.1016/j.trac.2016.03.005
186. LibreTexts Chemistry. "Lanthanides: Properties and Reactions." *LibreTexts* https://chem.libretexts.org/Bookshelves/Inorganic_Chemistry/Supplemental_Modules_and_Websites_(Inorganic_Chemistry)/Descriptive_Chemistry/Elements_Organized_by_Block/4_f-Block_Elements/The_Lanthanides/aLanthanides%3A_Properties_and_Reactions. Accessed August 8, 2024.
187. Jethva, Palak, *et al.* "Lanthanide-Doped Upconversion Luminescent Nanoparticles-Evolving Role in Bioimaging, Biosensing, and Drug Delivery." *MDPI, Materials (Basel, Switzerland)* vol. 15,7 2374. March 23, 2022. doi:10.3390/ma15072374
188. Acevedo-Guzmán, Diego A., *et al.* "Solvothermal Synthesis of Lanthanide-Functionalized Graphene Oxide Nanocomposites." *ScienceDirect, Materials Chemistry and Physics*, vol. 304, 2023, p. 127840. August 1, 2023. https://doi.org/10.1016/j.matchemphys.2023.127840
189. Sangorrin, Marcela, *et al.* Substack, June 6, 2024. https://anamihalceamdphd.substack.com/p/analysis-of-covid-19-injections-50
190. Mihalcea, Ana Maria. *NASA Future Strategic Warfare Compared to Current Events. Are We in a War of Our Military Against Us – We The People?* Substack, June 6, 2024. https://anamihalceamdphd.substack.com/p/nasa-future-strategic-warfare-compared
191. WEF. *World Economic Forum Strategic Intelligence*. World Economic Forum. https://www.weforum.org. Accessed August 26, 2024.
192. Akyildiz, Ian. '*COVID MRNAS ARE NOTHING MORE THAN SMALL SCALE BIO-NANO MACHINES' – Lecture by Professor Ian Akyildiz from Georgia Institute of Technology*. Substack, May 27, 2023. https://anamihalceamdphd.substack.com/p/covid-mrnas-are-nothing-more-than
193. Mihalcea, Ana Maria. *Another Confirmation of Self-Assembly Nanotechnology in COVID Bioweapons: Remarkable Longitudinal Study and Culture Work of COVID Shots for up to 12 Months and Cellular Toxicity Studies*. Substack, August 9, 2024. https://anamihalceamdphd.substack.com/p/another-confirmation-of-self-assembly?utm_source=publication-search
194. Lee, Young Mi and Daniel Broudy. "Real-Time Self-Assembly of Stereomicroscopically Visible Artificial Constructions in Incubated Specimens of mRNA Products Mainly from Pfizer and Moderna: A Comprehensive Longitudinal Study." *International Journal of Vaccine Theory, Practice, and Research*, July 18, 2024. https://doi.org/10.56098/586k0043
195. Ibid.
196. Lee, Young Mi and Daniel Broudy. "Real-Time Self-Assembly of Stereomicroscopically Visible Artificial Constructions in Incubated Specimens of mRNA Products Mainly from Pfizer and Moderna: A Comprehensive Longitudinal Study." *International Journal of Vaccine Theory, Practice, and Research*, 2024. https://mail.ijvtpr.com/index.php/IJVTPR/article/view/102
197. Ibid.

198. Ibid.
199. Ibid.
200. Ibid.
201. Ibid.
202. Ibid.
203. Ibid.
204. Ibid.
205. Ibid.
206. Ibid.
207. Ibid.
208. Ibid.
209. Ibid.
210. Ibid.
211. Ibid.
212. Ibid.
213. Mihalcea, Ana Maria. *Human Papilloma Virus Vaccine HPV For 9–12-Year-Old Children Shows Nanobots, Self-Assembly Hydrogel and Polymer Mesh Development*. Substack, September 1, 2023. https://anamihalceamdphd.substack.com/p/human-papilloma-virus-vaccine-hpv?utm_source=publication-search
214. Ibid.
215. Ibid.
216. Ibid.
217. Ibid.
218. Ibid.
219. Ibid.
220. Ibid.
221. Ibid.
222. Ibid.
223. Ibid.
224. Ibid.
225. Ibid.
226. Hagimă, Geanina. *Giardasil Vaccine Microscopy by Dr. Geanina Hagimă and HPV Vaccine Injury Review.* Substack, October 16, 2023. https://anamihalceamdphd.substack.com/p/giardasil-vaccine-microscopy-by-dr?utm_source=publication-search
227. Ibid.
228. KM. *The Gardasil Ingredients Not Listed on the Package Insert*. Kwartler Manus LLC. https://www.kminjurylawyers.com/gardasil/the-gardasil-ingredients-not-listed-on-the-package-insert/. Accessed August 8, 2024.
229. Stone, Cosby A. Jr., *et al*. "Immediate Hypersensitivity to Polyethylene Glycols and Polysorbates: More Common Than We Have Recognized." *The Journal of Allergy and Clinical Immunology: In Practice*, vol. 7,5 (2019): 1533-1540.e8. doi:10.1016/j.jaip.2018.12.003
230. Ibid.

231. Wilson, Rhoda. "South Carolina Professor Finds 200 Billion Pieces of DNA Contaminating a Single Dose of Pfizer's Covid Injection." *The Exposé*, September 19, 2023. https://expose-news.com/2023/09/19/200-billion-pieces-of-dna-in-a-single-dose/
232. KM. *The Gardasil Ingredients Not Listed on the Package Insert*. Kwartler Manus LLC. https://www.kminjurylawyers.com/gardasil/the-gardasil-ingredients-not-listed-on-the-package-insert/. Accessed August 8, 2024.
233. Baum, Hedlund, Aristei, and Goldman PC. *Gardasil Contains 'Dangerous and Undisclosed Ingredients,' Lawsuit Alleges*. Wisner Baum, 30 July 2021. https://www.wisnerbaum.com/blog/2021/july/gardasil-contains-dangerous-and-undisclosed-ingr/.
234. Jørgensen, L., *et al*. "Benefits and Harms of the Human Papillomavirus (HPV) Vaccines: Systematic Review with Meta-Analyses of Trial Data from Clinical Study Reports." *BMC Part of Springer Nature: Systematic Reviews*, vol. 9, 2020, p. 43. February 28, 2020. https://doi.org/10.1186/s13643-019-0983-y
235. Baum, Hedlund, Aristei, and Goldman PC. *Gardasil Contains 'Dangerous and Undisclosed Ingredients,' Lawsuit Alleges*. Wisner Baum, 30 July, 2021. https://www.wisnerbaum.com/blog/2021/july/gardasil-contains-dangerous-and-undisclosed-ingr/
236. Hagimă, Geanina. Substack, October 16, 2023. https://anamihalceamdphd.substack.com/p/giardasil-vaccine-microscopy-by-dr?utm_source=publication-search
237. Ibid.
238. Baletti, Brenda. *Merck's Gardasil HPV Vaccine Caused Teen's Narcolepsy, Federal Vaccine Court Rules*. Children's Health Defense, October 4, 2023. https://childrenshealthdefense.org/defender/merck-gardasil-hpv-vaccine-teens-narcolepsy/
239. Ibid.
240. Brawer, Arthur E. "Hidden Toxicity of Human Papillomavirus Vaccine Ingredients." *ClinMed International Library: Journal of Rheumatic Diseases and Treatment*, vol. 5, 2019, p. 075, https://doi.org/10.23937/2469-5726/1510075
241. Wilson, Rhoda. "Here Are Just SOME of the Harmful Ingredients Present in Routine Vaccines." *The Exposé*, October 14, 2023. https://expose-news.com/2023/10/14/some-of-the-harmful-ingredients-in-routine-vaccines/
242. Kirsch, Steve. *Former Omaha Police Detective Reveals 50% of SIDS Cases Happened Within 48 Hours Post Vaccine*. Substack, September 27, 2023. https://kirschsubstack.com/p/former-major-city-police-detective?utm_source=substack&utm_campaign=post_embed&utm_medium=web
243. Mihalcea, Ana Maria. *Measles, Mumps, Rubella and Varicella Vaccine for Children Shows Nanobot Swarms, Quantum Dots and Self-Assembly Hydrogel*. Substack, September 4, 2023. https://anamihalceamdphd.substack.com/p/measles-mumps-rubella-and-varicella?utm_source=publication-search
244. Ibid.
245. Ibid.
246. Ibid.

247. Ibid.
248. Ibid.
249. Ibid.
250. Ibid.
251. Ibid.
252. Ibid.
253. Ibid.
254. Ibid.
255. Mihalcea, Ana Maria. *Diphtheria, Tetanus, Pertussis, Polio, Hemophilus B and Hepatitis B Vaccine for Small Children: Darkfield Microscopy Shows Self-Assembly Hydrogel Filaments and Structures*. Substack, August 31, 2023. https://anamihalceamdphd.substack.com/p/diphtheria-tetanus-pertussis-polio?utm_source=publication-search
256. Ibid.
257. Ibid.
258. Ibid.
259. Ibid.
260. Ibid.
261. Ibid.
262. Ibid.
263. Ibid.
264. Ibid.
265. Ibid.
266. Ibid.
267. Mihalcea, Ana Maria. *Meningococcus Vaccine for Children – Darkfield Microscopy Shows Self-Assembled Hydrogel Filaments*. Substack, August 30, 2023. https://anamihalceamdphd.substack.com/p/meningococcus-vaccine-for-children?utm_source=publication-search
268. Ibid.
269. Ibid.
270. Ibid.
271. Ibid.
272. Ibid.
273. Ibid.
274. Ibid.
275. Ibid.
276. Ibid.
277. Ibid.
278. Mihalcea, Ana Maria. *Darkfield Microscopy of Pneumococcal Vaccine Prevnar 13 Shows Quantum Dot Structures and Self Assembly*. Substack, August 29, 2023. https://anamihalceamdphd.substack.com/p/darkfield-microscopy-of-pneumococcal?utm_source=publication-search
279. Ibid.
280. Ibid.
281. Ibid.
282. Ibid.
283. Ibid.
284. Ibid.

285. Ibid.
286. Ibid.
287. Ibid.
288. Mihalcea, Ana Maria. *Darkfield Microscopy of Hepatitis A Vaccine for Children 2 Years and Older Shows Classic Hydrogel Filaments, Self-Assembly and Quantum Dot Structures. Substack*, September 14, 2023. https://anamihalceamdphd.substack.com/p/darkfield-microscopy-of-hepatitis?utm_source=publication-search
289. Ibid.
290. Ibid.
291. Ibid.
292. Ibid.
293. Ibid.

ARTHEMA SOPHIA PUBLISHING
Other Titles

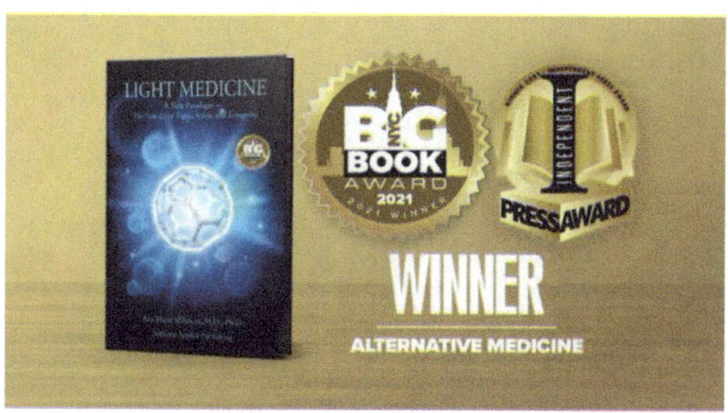

LIGHT MEDICINE
A New Paradigm – The Science of Light, Spirit, and Longevity

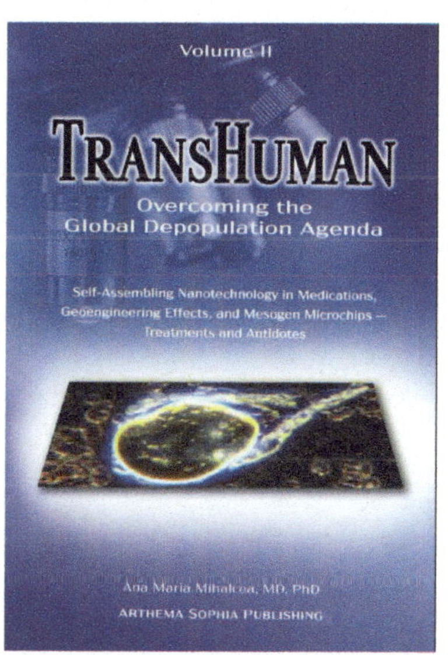

TRANSHUMAN
Overcoming the Global Depopulation Agenda – Volume 2

Made in the USA
Coppell, TX
25 February 2026